FUNDAMENTAL LABORATORY MATHEMATICS

REQUIRED CALCULATIONS *for the*
MEDICAL LABORATORY PROFESSIONAL

FUNDAMENTAL LABORATORY MATHEMATICS

REQUIRED CALCULATIONS *for the*
MEDICAL LABORATORY PROFESSIONAL

Lela Buckingham, PhD, MB (ASCP), DLM (ASCP)
Unit Director, Molecular Oncology
Department of Pathology
Rush Medical Laboratories
Rush University Medical Center
Chicago, Illinois

 F.A. Davis Company • Philadelphia

F.A. Davis Company
1915 Arch Street
Philadelphia, PA 19103
www.fadavis.com

Printed in the United States of America

Last digit indicates print number: 10 9 8 7 6 5 4 3 2 1

Senior Acquisitions Editor: Christa A. Fratantoro
Manager of Content Development: George W. Lang
Developmental Editor: Richard Morel
Design and Illustration Manager: Carolyn O'Brien

As new scientific information becomes available through basic and clinical research, recommended treatments and drug therapies undergo changes. The author(s) and publisher have done everything possible to make this book accurate, up to date, and in accord with accepted standards at the time of publication. The author(s), editors, and publisher are not responsible for errors or omissions or for consequences from application of the book, and make no warranty, expressed or implied, in regard to the contents of the book. Any practice described in this book should be applied by the reader in accordance with professional standards of care used in regard to the unique circumstances that may apply in each situation. The reader is advised always to check product information (package inserts) for changes and new information regarding dose and contraindications before administering any drug. Caution is especially urged when using new or infrequently ordered drugs.

Library of Congress Cataloging-in-Publication Data

Buckingham, Lela, author.
  Fundamental laboratory mathematics : required calculations for the medical laboratory professional /
Lela Buckingham.
      p. ; cm.
  Includes index.
  ISBN 978-0-8036-2949-3
  I. Title.
  [DNLM: 1. Clinical Laboratory Techniques—methods—Problems and Exercises. 2. Mathematics—
methods—Problems and Exercises. QY 18.2]
  R853.M3
  610.1'5195—dc 3
                    2014010269

PREFACE

Mathematical calculations are important even in the increasingly automated medical laboratory. Instrument software, computers and calculators facilitate accurate and efficient computations, however, a strong basic knowledge of math is still required for the medical laboratory professional. For this reason, laboratory mathematics is taught in our program and in many other MLS and MLT programs. Students come to these programs with varied levels of math proficiency. Even for those students with good math ability, review is beneficial.

This work is intended as a basic treatment of laboratory math skills directed toward the current practice in the medical laboratory. This book was written to fulfill the requirement for a basic math book for students studying medical technology. As professionals, these students will be required to perform laboratory procedures that include a variety of mathematical skills. For this reason, the problems in the book are designed to encourage students to apply math concepts in the context of medical laboratory practice. Electronic case studies available on the F.A. Davis "DavisPlus" website provide additional practice in applying math concepts to students.

To support faculty in developing courses in laboratory mathematics, Power Point presentations, an Electronic Bank of Test Questions, and an Instructor's Guide accompany this textbook. A searchable Digital Version of the text is also available to instructors.

Lela Buckingham, PhD, MB^{CM}(ASCP), DLM^{CM}(ASCP)

REVIEWERS

Brenda C. Barnes, MSEd, MT(ASCP^CM^SBB^CM^)

Director, Medical Laboratory Science Program
& Assistant Professor
Medical Laboratory Science
Allen College
Waterloo, Iowa

Philip Campbell, MSEd, MT(ASCP)

Program Director and Associate Professor
Department of Medical Laboratory Science
Eastern Kentucky University
Richmond, Kentucky

Mary Coleman, MS

Assistant Professor
Pathology
University of North Dakota
Grand Forks, North Dakota

Muneeza Esani, MHA, MT(ASCP)

Assistant Professor
Clinical Laboratory Science
University of Texas Medical Branch at Galveston,
School of Health Professions
Galveston, Texas

Jennifer B. Jones, BS, MT(ASCP)

Clinical Instructor
Clinical Laboratory Sciences
University of Kansas Medical Center
Kansas City, Kansas

Mary Anne Lefevre, MT (ASCP)

General Laboratory
Banner Good Samaritan Medical Center
Phoenix, Arizona

Tina McDaniel, MA, MT (ASCP)

Program Director
Medical Laboratory Technology
Davidson County Community College
Thomasville, North Carolina

Susan M. Orton, PhD, D(ABMLI), MT(ASCP)

Associate Professor
Division of Clinical Laboratory Science
The University of North Carolina, School of Medicine
Chapel Hill, North Carolina

Kathleen T. Paff, MA, CLS(NCA); MT(ASCP)

Director (retired)
Medical Laboratory Technology Program
Kellogg Community College
Battle Creek, Michigan

Deborah M. Parks, BSMT (ASCP)

Medical Laboratory Technician Program
Wytheville Community College
Wytheville, Virginia

Cathreen D. Pawlik, BA, MA

Editor
Bonsall, CA

Clair S. Wylie, MT (ASCP)

Faculty
Health Technology
Davidson County Community College
Thomasville, North Carolina

ACKNOWLEDGMENTS

Thanks and gratitude are extended to all who helped in the completion of this work. The useful input provided by the reviewers who gave their valuable time is greatly appreciated. I owe thanks to my colleagues at Rush University Medical Center, Dr. Brett Mahon and Dr. Robert DeCresce in the Department of Pathology.

Thanks to Dr. Herbert Miller, who first suggested the writing of this book, and the Medical Laboratory Science faculty in the Rush University College of Health Sciences for the opportunity to participate in medical science education. I greatly appreciate the guidance and support of the staff at F.A. Davis, and my knowledgeable and well-organized developmental editor, Richard Morel.

Finally, I would like to thank the graduate and undergraduate students, colleagues and friends who provided intellectual and moral support through the preparation of this manuscript.

Lela Buckingham

Contents

CHAPTER 1

BASIC MATHEMATICS

The practice of Medical Laboratory Science requires a firm understanding of mathematics. Even with increased automation in the laboratory, the technologist is required to use mathematics to interpret, analyze, and report instrument output. Raw data and final laboratory results are expressed in numerical values. Some quantitative (numerical) data require translation to qualitative results, such as positive or negative. A viral infection measured in viral particles per unit volume of blood may be reported as positive when the virus is detectable or above a predetermined level or negative when the virus is undetectable or detectable below a predetermined level.

NUMBERS AND NUMBERING SYSTEMS

Numerical information is central to laboratory science. Test methods and final reports use numerical data. Test methods or standard operating procedures (SOPs) direct the use of specified concentrations, incubation times, and data units. The medical laboratory professional must understand basic mathematic processes that are used to evaluate and analyze these data (Box 1-1).

LEARNING OUTCOMES

- Describe the base-10 numbering system.
- Review basic mathematical operations: addition, subtraction, multiplication, and division.
- Use and manipulate fractions.
- Describe reciprocals.
- Describe decimal fractions and percent expressions.
- Present the rules for orders of calculations.
- Round off numbers to express confidence.
- Relate uncertainty to significant figures.
- Explain basic concepts in laboratory practice.

Box 1-1 **Numbering Systems**

Place-value systems for numbering were used as far back as 4,000 years ago. Numbers were designated as marks or other symbols whose value depended on the location or placement with respect to other symbols. Because these systems were used for counting and keeping track, they used whole numbers or integers. With the emergence of primitive algebra and other calculations, more defined numerical systems evolved.

Numbers are also used to describe other numbers. Performance of quantitative tests is tracked by the reproducibility of control values from day to day or from run to run. This reproducibility (precision) is expressed as a number describing the group of individual control values for each batch of tests performed. Differences from standard reference values measure uncertainty (expected error) and define the degree of confidence in a test result. Uncertainty, error, and precision are as important as the absolute values they describe. The laboratory professional should be familiar with the concepts of uncertainty, error, and precision, to appreciate and recognize the limitations and potential pitfalls of testing processes.

Arabic Numbers

Laboratory practice uses primarily a **base-10** system; that is, there are 10 numerals: 0, 1, 2, 3, 4, 5, 6, 7, 8, and 9 (Box 1-2). The value of numbers is determined by their position with regard to a **decimal point**. In 10.0, the "1" has a value of 10, whereas the "1" in 0.1 has a value of one-tenth. Numerals increase 10-fold in value with each position moving leftward from the decimal point, so 0.1 is 10 times less than 1. Base-10 numbers are expressed in order of decreasing value:

...Thousands, hundreds, tens, units (**decimal point**) tenths, hundredths, thousandths...

Consider the number 3,915.807. The relationship of values and the decimal point is illustrated as follows:

Thousands	3
Hundreds	9
Tens	1
Units	5
Decimal	.
Tenths	8
Hundredths	0
Thousandths	7

Values expressing very large or very small values (such as millions or billionths) may have many numerals. The English numbering system uses a period for the decimal point and a comma to separate very large numbers into groups

---

Box 1-2 **Arabic Numerals**

The Babylonians, Egyptians, and Hindus devised a place-value system using 10 different symbols, which were later replaced by the Hindu-Arabic numbers. The use of a base of 10 may have arisen from the use of 10 fingers in counting. There is historical evidence of base-20 systems that may have been based on fingers and toes. Arabic numerals express values or numbers of units.

of three digits. The commas are not used to the right of the decimal point. Numbers in this system would be written as follows:

0.279088
0.32
1,900
25,000.83
15,879,000.983433

Laboratory work now uses computing instruments and analyzers running on number systems other than the base-10 system, such as the 2-digit binary system. The technologist should have to understand only the final output of these systems (Box 1-3), which will be expressed in the base-10 digits 0 to 9. Bar codes (Fig. 1-1) are read by instruments to track specimens through laboratory processing. These patterns are based on a binary number system that uses bar width and position to represent base-10 digits 0 to 9. The technologist uses a bar code reader or scanner to interpret the codes and transfer the information to base-10 or textual output.

Roman Numerals

An alternate numbering system, Roman numerals (Box 1-4) have several applications in the laboratory. Names of some proteins or enzymes such as polymerase I, or pol I, include Roman numerals. Gene names may also contain Roman numerals. Blood clotting regulators such as factor V and factor II are identified by Roman numerals. Biological agents and diseases are sometimes grouped and numbered with Roman numerals as type I or type II.

In addition Roman numerals are commonly used in written documents to organize information in outline form. Procedures in the laboratory may be written using such outline form.

THE NUMBER LINE

Decimal numbers allow expression of values very close to zero in practical terms. A "mirror" set of numbers is represented as less than zero, as well. Values greater than zero are called **positive** numbers. Values less than zero

---

Box 1-3	The Binary System

The base-10 system developed in the 13th century may have arisen from the use of 10 fingers (and 10 toes) to enumerate objects, that is, starting over after every 10th number. It still is the most common system used for practical applications. Computers make use of the base-2 system because all numbers can be expressed as either of two numerals: 0 or 1. Although this two-option on/off system is well-suited for digital instruments, it is unwieldy in that the expressions can be very long. The number 379 in the base-10 system would be 101111011 in the binary system. Computing also uses the octal (base-8) and hexadecimal (base-16) systems.

Figure 1-1 Bar codes are numbers in binary language using line (bar) width and position to represent ordinal values.

Box 1-4 Roman Numerals

Letters, I, V, X, L, D, M, are used for numbers in the Roman numbering system.

---

are called **negative** numbers. Negative numbers are designated by a minus sign (–), to the left of the number. Positive numbers may be similarly designated by a plus sign (+), but they usually carry no sign. A number with no sign designation is considered positive. Numbers are arranged from left to right according to their numerical value, and they form a **number line**. Negative and positive numbers are centered around zero in the number line:

...–10 –9 –8 –7 –6 –5 –4 –3 –2 –1 0 1 2 3 4 5 6 7 8 9 10...

The value of a number without consideration of sign is the **absolute value** of that number, designated by vertical lines to either side of the number ($|n|$), where n is any number. For example, the absolute value of -9 and 9 is the same: $|9|$.

> On an electronic calculator, the "(–)" key symbol denotes a negative number. It should be distinguished from the "–" key symbol for subtraction of one number from another. To enter a negative number in some calculators, press the sign key (–) first and then the number (direct entry). In other calculators, press the number first and then the sign key. The sign key may also be designated "+/–" on some keypads. The placement of these keys will depend on the make and manufacturer of the calculator.

BASIC MATHEMATICAL OPERATIONS

Numbers are manipulated through mathematical operations of addition, subtraction, multiplication, and division. These manipulations produce numerical results that describe the relationships between values such as numerical results from instrument output.

Addition

Addition, designated by the plus sign (+), is the increase in a value by the amount of another value. Each value counted is an **addend**. The total of all addend values is the **sum**.

$$
\begin{array}{r}
5 \text{ (addend)} \\
+ \quad 3 \text{ (addend)} \\
\hline
8 \text{ (sum)}
\end{array}
$$

Or, written in linear format: $5 + 3 = 8$. Most laboratory procedures involve mixtures of reagents. The amount of the mixture is the sum of its components.

When adding negative numbers, the sum is decreased by the negative value.

$$
\begin{array}{r}
5 \text{ (addend)} \\
+ \quad (-3) \text{ (addend)} \\
\hline
2 \text{ (sum)}
\end{array}
$$

If one or more negative addends has a negative value in excess of the others, the sum will be a negative number.

$$
\begin{array}{r}
(-5) \text{ (addend)} \\
+ \quad 3 \text{ (addend)} \\
\hline
-2 \text{ (sum)}
\end{array}
$$

Subtraction

Subtraction, designated by the minus sign (–), is the decrease in a value by the amount of another value. The value from which another value is subtracted is the **minuend**. The value that is subtracted from the minuend is the **subtrahend**. The resulting diminished value of the minuend is the **difference**.

$$
\begin{array}{r}
5 \ (\text{minuend}) \\
-\ \underline{3\ (\text{subtrahend})} \\
2\ (\text{difference})
\end{array}
$$

Or, written in linear format: $5 - 3 = 2$.
With a negative subtrahend, the difference is increased by the absolute value of the subtrahend.

$$
\begin{array}{r}
5 \ (\text{minuend}) \\
-\ \underline{(-3)\ (\text{subtrahend})} \\
8\ (\text{difference})
\end{array}
$$

When the minuend and the subtrahend are both negative, the value of the minuend (–5) is subtracted from the absolute value of the subtrahend ($|3|$).

$$
\begin{array}{r}
(-5) \ (\text{minuend}) \\
-\ \underline{(-3)\ (\text{subtrahend})} \\
-\ 2\ (\text{difference})
\end{array}
$$

Multiplication

Multiplication, designated by the multiplication sign ($\times$, $\cdot$, or *), is the addition of a value to itself a designated number of times. The value of 12 added to itself 3 times is $12 + 12 + 12$, expressed as 12×3. The value being increased, 12, is the **multiplicand**. The **multiplier**, 3, is the number of times the multiplicand is added to itself. The resulting value is the **product**, 36.

$$
\begin{array}{r}
12 \ (\text{multiplicand}) \\
\times\ \underline{3\ (\text{multiplier})} \\
36\ (\text{product})
\end{array}
$$

Multiplications may also be written in linear format: $12 \times 3 = 36$ or $12 \cdot 3 = 36$ or $12*3 = 36$. The last expression is found in software spreadsheet programs sometimes used in preparing laboratory results.

If the multiplicand and the multiplier are of different signs, the product will be a negative number.

$$
\begin{array}{r}
(-12) \ (\text{multiplicand}) \\
\times\ \underline{3\ (\text{multiplier})} \\
-36\ (\text{product})
\end{array}
$$

If the multiplicand and the multiplier are both negative numbers, the product will be a positive number.

```
    (-12) (multiplicand)
x    (-3) (multiplier)
        36 (product)
```

Division

Division is designated by the division sign (÷ or /), such as 36/3 or 36 ÷ 3. Division is the number of times the value of one number (the **divisor**), 3 in this case, can be subtracted from another number, 36 (the **dividend**). The resulting number of times is the **quotient**, 12.

```
36 (dividend) ÷ 3 (divisor) = 12 (quotient)
```

or

```
36 (dividend) / 3 (divisor) = 12 (quotient)
```

or

```
           quotient
divisor)dividend
```

When the divisor and the dividend are of opposite signs, the quotient will be negative.

```
36 (dividend) / (-3) (divisor) = -12 (quotient)
```

When the divisor and the dividend are both negative, the quotient will be positive.

```
(-36) (dividend) / (-3) (divisor) = 12 (quotient)
```

Numbers are not always exactly divisible by other numbers; that is, a residual amount less than the divisor may remain after the maximum subtractions of the divisor have been made. This residual number may be expressed as a decimal or fraction of the divisor.

Addition, subtraction, multiplication, and division are performed on the calculator using the appropriate function keys (+, −, ×, and ÷). Care should be taken when using calculators to perform simple operations because errors in entering data will produce an incorrect result from the calculator. For this reason, it is useful to estimate an approximate answer mentally, both with regard to sign and value.

ZERO NUMBER PROPERTIES

Zero (Box 1-5) has certain properties in mathematical functions. The sum of a number and zero is the same number:

$$5 + 0 = 5$$

The difference of a number and zero is the same number:

$$5 - 0 = 5$$

The difference of a zero and a number is the negative number:

$$0 - 5 = -5$$

The product of a number and zero is zero:

$$5 \times 0 = 0$$

Zero divided by any number is zero:

$$0 \div 5 = 0$$

Numbers cannot be divided by zero.

FRACTIONS

Fractions are used to express parts of whole numbers. Fractions are indications of one number divided by another (Fig. 1-2). Fractions can be used to express probability. In terms of probability, ½ means one chance in two. When a coin is tossed, the probability of getting heads is ½. In the fraction ½, the top number 1 is the **numerator**, and the number 2 is the **denominator**. In a fraction, the numerator (dividend) is divided by the denominator (divisor).

$$\frac{7}{14} \text{ (numerator)} \atop \text{ (denominator)}$$

A whole number is a fraction with a denominator of 1. Twelve (12) expressed as a fraction is ¹²⁄₁.

Box 1-5　The Absence of Quantity

Zero, the central point in the number line, represents the absence of quantity. Although zero is included as the 10th symbol in the decimal number set, this concept was not always appreciated as a value. The early numbering systems were intended to express the quantity of things. If there were no things to count, no expression was required. Some numbering systems, such as Roman numerals, had no symbol to represent nothing.

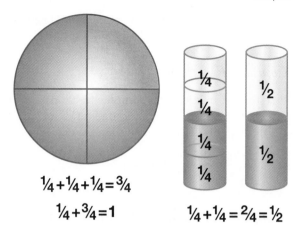

Figure 1-2 Fractions are parts of whole numbers. The denominators express the number of parts (four in this case) into which the whole is divided. The numerators express the number of fourths. Equivalent fractions represent the same value; for example, ¾ is equivalent to ½.

Common Fractions

There are several types of fractions. In **common fractions**, the numerator and denominator are whole numbers. Common fractions are either **proper**, in which the numerator is smaller than the denominator, or **improper**, in which the denominator is smaller than the numerator. A fraction in which the numerator and denominator are the same, also termed as **unity**, is equivalent to 1.

$$\text{Proper: } \frac{3}{7} \qquad \text{Improper: } \frac{89}{3} \qquad \text{Unity: } \frac{3}{3}$$

An improper fraction may also be expressed as a **mixed number**, consisting of a combination of a whole number and a proper fraction. To convert an improper fraction to a mixed number, divide the numerator by the denominator and leave the residual amount as a fraction. The improper fraction, ⁸⁹⁄₅, may be expressed as:

$$\frac{89}{5} = 5\overline{)89} \quad \begin{array}{r} 17 \\ \underline{5} \\ 39 \\ \underline{35} \\ 4 \end{array} = 17\tfrac{4}{5}$$

An improper fraction and its mixed number are said to be **equivalent**; that is, they express the same value. Both proper and improper fractions are sometimes expressed as **equivalent fractions** to facilitate calculations. Any fraction can be expressed in infinite ways without changing the value. To do this, multiply the numerator and denominator by the same number, which is the same as multiplying the fraction by 1. The following fractions are all equivalent to ½:

$$\frac{5}{10} \qquad \frac{100}{200} \qquad \frac{357}{714} \qquad \frac{12,500}{25,000}$$

In the foregoing fractions, the numerator (1) and denominator (2) were multiplied by 5, 100, 357, and 12,500, respectively.

Complex Fractions

Fractions of fractions are **complex fractions**. To simplify complex fractions, invert the fraction in the denominator, ¼ to ⁴⁄₁ in this example, and multiply the numerators, 1 and 4, and then the denominators, 2 and 1.

$$\frac{\frac{1}{2}}{\frac{1}{4}} = \frac{1}{2} \times \frac{4}{1} = \frac{4}{2} = 2$$

Comparative Values of Common Fractions

In all fractions, as the size of the denominator increases for a given numerator, the value of the fraction decreases. Conversely, as the size of the denominator decreases, the value of the fraction increases.

$$\frac{5}{2} \text{ is greater than } \frac{5}{10}$$

$$\frac{1}{\frac{1}{2}} \text{ is less than } \frac{1}{\frac{1}{8}}$$

Decimal Fractions

A **decimal fraction** is written as a whole number with a decimal point. Decimal fractions always have denominators of 10 or multiples of 10 (100, 1,000, 10,000, and so forth). Common fractions can be converted to decimal fractions by dividing the numerator by the denominator. The fraction ½ can be converted to a decimal fraction by dividing 2 into 1 or by finding a fraction equivalent to ½ with a denominator of 10. (In this case, multiply the numerator and denominator by 5.) The numerator is then written to the right of the decimal point and is expressed as the number of tenths:

$$\frac{1}{2} \times \frac{5}{5} = \frac{5}{10} = 0.5 = \text{"zero point five" or "five-tenths"}$$

A decimal fraction may have any power of 10 as a denominator:

$$\frac{1}{10} = 0.1 = \text{"zero point one" or "one-tenth"}$$

$$\frac{1}{100} = 0.01 = \text{"zero point zero one" or "one-hundredth"}$$

$$\frac{1}{1,000} = 0.001 = \text{"one-thousandth"}$$

$$\frac{1}{10,000} = 0.0001 = \text{"one-ten thousandth"}$$

$$\frac{1}{100,000} = 0.00001 = \text{"one-hundred thousandth"}$$

$$\frac{1}{1,00,000} = 0.000001 = \text{"one-millionth"}$$

A fraction of $\frac{5}{100}$ would be equivalent to a decimal fraction of 0.05, indicating the division by 100, whereas $\frac{5}{1,000}$ would be 0.005, indicating division by 1,000. Thus, the decimal point keeps track of the **order of magnitude**, or the power of 10 that the fraction represents:

If n is any whole number:

Tenths: first decimal place $(0.\mathbf{n})$
Hundredths: second decimal place $(0.\mathbf{0n})$
Thousandths: third decimal place $(0.\mathbf{00n})$
Ten thousandths: fourth decimal place $(0.\mathbf{000n})$
Hundred thousandths: fifth decimal place $(0.\mathbf{0000n})$
Millionths: sixth decimal place $(0.\mathbf{00000n})$

When the numerator of an improper fraction is divided by the denominator, the quotient will be more than one. Consider the following fractions:

$$\frac{11}{2} \times \frac{5}{5} = \frac{55}{10} = 5.5 = \text{"five point five"} = \text{"five and five-tenths"}$$

$$\frac{111}{5} \times \frac{2}{2} = \frac{222}{10} = 22.2 = \text{"22 point two"} = \text{"22 and two-tenths"}$$

Not all numerators are evenly divisible by their denominators. The fraction $\frac{1}{3}$ represents a decimal with 3 in an infinite number of places, 0.3333333333333.... When this occurs, the decimal fraction can be rounded off, as discussed later, or it can be written as $0.3\overline{3}$.

$$\frac{1}{3} = 0.3333333333333.... = 0.33 \sim 0.3$$

Percentages

Percent, or "per 100," indicates a decimal fraction with a denominator of 100. The symbol % is used to express per 100. A decimal fraction is converted to percent by moving the decimal point two places to the right (multiplying by 100). Be careful when numbers are expressed this way, because the value represented by the decimal point is still $\frac{1}{100}$th of the expressed percent.

$$\frac{45}{100} = 0.45 = 45\%$$

$$\frac{8}{100} = 8\%$$

$$\frac{150}{100} = 150\%$$

$$\frac{1,055}{100} = 1,055\%$$

$$\frac{0.07}{100} = 0.0007 = 0.07\%$$

Common fractions are converted to percent as described earlier for conversion to decimal fractions, using a denominator of 100. The fraction ¼ expressed as a percentage would be:

$$\frac{1}{4} \times \frac{25}{25} = \frac{25}{100} = 25\%$$

or, more simply,

$$\frac{1}{4} = \frac{25}{100} = 0.25$$

$$0.25 \times 100 = 25\%$$

Note that a value of 1 is equal to 100% (1.00 × 100). Values more than 1 are equal to more than 100%. The mixed number, $2\frac{1}{2}$ is equal to 250%. Percent expressions can be mixed numbers, such as the following:

$$^{5.5}/_{100} = 5.5\%$$

CALCULATIONS WITH FRACTIONAL NUMBERS

Reducing Fractions

Data are sometimes obtained in the form of a fraction that is equivalent to a simpler fraction. The simplest expression is preferred for ease of interpretation or further calculations. To reduce a fraction, divide the numerator and the denominator by the same number. (In order for the fraction and its reduced form to remain equivalent, the number used to divide the numerator and denominator must be the same.)

To reduce the fraction 30/750 to its simplest form, find a number that will go evenly into 30 and 750. Both numbers are evenly divisible by 6.

$$\frac{30}{750} = \frac{30/6}{750/6} = \frac{5}{125}$$

Notice that this is not the simplest form of this fraction, because both the numerator and denominator can be further reduced by dividing by 5:

$$\frac{5}{125} = \frac{5/5}{125/5} = \frac{1}{25}$$

To reduce fractions using an electronic calculator, look for the "a‰" function key. Enter the numerator, then press the a‰ function key and then enter the denominator. When the "=" or "exe" key is pressed, the answer will be expressed as the reduced fraction in its simplest form. Press 30, then a‰, then 750 and exe to obtain 1_| 25, for the fraction given earlier.

Common fractions can be added and subtracted from one another as long as the denominators of the fractions involved in the calculation are the same. If the denominators are the same, add or subtract the numerators:

$$\frac{3}{9} + \frac{2}{9} = \frac{5}{9}$$

$$\frac{3}{9} - \frac{2}{9} = \frac{1}{9}$$

If the denominators differ, find the lowest number that is equally divisible by all the denominators involved in the calculation. This is the **least common denominator (LCD)**.

The most straightforward way to find the LCD is to multiply the denominators. Then change the fractions to equivalent fractions with the LCD and add the numerators. To add ½ and ⅓, multiply the denominators 2 × 3 to obtain an LCD of 6. Change ½ to an equivalent fraction of ³⁄₆ and ⅓ to an equivalent fraction of ²⁄₆. The sum of the equivalent fractions is ⁵⁄₆.

 Calculators automatically determine the LCD when any fractions are entered using the "a⅟ₒ" key.

Addition and Subtraction of Decimal Fractions

To perform addition or subtraction of decimal fractions, vertically align the decimal points of the addends or subtrahends and minuends. To add 5.6 + 0.07 + 15.00, align the decimal points.

```
   5.6
   0.07
  15.00
  20.67
```

Do the same process for subtraction. To subtract 14.0 – 0.8, align the decimal points.

```
   14.0
 –  0.8
   13.2
```

When multiplying common fractions, multiply the numerators by one another and the denominators by one another.

$$\frac{4}{7} \times \frac{1}{8}$$

$$\frac{4 \times 1}{7 \times 8} = \frac{4}{56}$$

This goes for multiple fractions and complex fractions as well.

$$\frac{4}{7} \times \frac{1}{8} \times \frac{½}{¾} =$$

$$\frac{4 \times 1 \times ½}{7 \times 8 \times ¾} = \frac{2}{42} = \frac{1}{21}$$

Alternatively, convert complex fractions to proper or improper fractions before performing the multiplication.

$$\frac{½}{¾} = \frac{1}{2} \times \frac{4}{3} = \frac{4}{6}$$

$$\frac{4 \times 1 \times 4}{7 \times 8 \times 6} = \frac{16}{336} = \frac{1}{21}$$

When multiplying decimal fractions, use standard multiplication. To place the decimal point in the answer, count the number of places to the right of the decimal point in the multiplier and multiplicand. Place the decimal point in the product so that the number of digits to its right is the sum of the number of digits to the right of the multiplicand and multiplier.

$$
\begin{array}{r}
0.\,4 \\
\times\ 2.\,3 \\
\hline
1\ \ 2 \\
8 \\
\hline
0.\,9\ 2
\end{array}
$$

To divide common fractions, invert the divisor fraction and multiply. When a fraction is inverted, the resulting value is a **reciprocal number**. The reciprocal of 2 (²⁄₁) is ½. The reciprocal of ¼ is 4 (⁴⁄₁). Reciprocal numbers are used when fractions or proportional parts are divided into other numbers. When a number is converted to its reciprocal, the division function becomes multiplication.

$$½ \div ⁴⁄₃ = \frac{1}{2} \times \frac{3}{4} = \frac{3}{8}$$

 Division of decimal fractions is frequently performed using a calculator. Decimal fractions are entered and divided using the "÷" key, just as for whole numbers.

ORDER OF CALCULATIONS

When more than one mathematical function is applied to a group of numbers, there is a defined order in which the calculations are performed.

Numbers may or may not be separated by parentheses: ( ). When parentheses are absent, multiplications and divisions are performed first, and then additions and subtractions.

$$5 + 15 \times 3 - 2$$

Multiplication is performed first:

$$5 + (15 \times 3) - 2 = 5 + 45 - 2$$

Addition and subtraction are then performed:

$$5 + (45) - 2 = 50 - 2 = 48$$

Numbers may be grouped in layers using sets of braces, brackets, and parentheses arranged in the following order: {[()]}.

$$(8 + 20 \times 7 - 10) \div [3 + (6 \times 4) - 1] =$$

$$\frac{8 + 20 \times 7 - 10}{3 + (6 \times 4) - 1} =$$

$$\frac{8 + 140 - 10}{3 + 24 - 1} = \frac{148 - 10}{27 - 1} = \frac{138}{26} = 5.3$$

Work from inside out:

$$\{47 + [9 \times (3 \times 6)]\} - 50 =$$
$$\{47 + [9 \times 18]\} - 50 =$$
$$\{47 + 162\} - 50 =$$
$$209 - 50 = 159$$

Electronic calculators will automatically order calculations. They also have parenthesis keys "(" and ")" which can be used to represent parentheses, brackets, and braces by pressing the left or right parenthesis multiple times. In the foregoing example, the numbers would be entered as follows: (, 47, +, (, 9, ×, (, 3, ×, 6,),),), –, 50. Pressing the "=" or "exe" key should give the answer: 159.

ROUNDING OFF NUMBERS

When a value is written as a decimal fraction, the number of digits preceding and/or following the decimal point is an indication of the confidence in that number. The number 2.0345 shows certainty to 10-thousandths of units, whereas 2.03 shows certainty to hundredths of units. When making mathematical calculations, numbers with many digits may result. It is important not to use more digits than is achievable by the laboratory test. A test that measures the number of red blood cells in a unit volume of blood provides a result in the range of millions of cells per microliter. A report of a normal red blood cell count may be 5,200,000 per unit volume. A report of 5,217,891 per unit volume would suggest confidence in the number of cells down to single cells. The methods used to count cells may not provide this level of confidence, so such a detailed number would be misleading. A subsequent count will differ by tens to hundreds of cells, which may give the false impression of an increase or decrease in cell count.

To indicate a value without overstating confidence, numbers are delimited in a process called **rounding off**. To round off numbers, determine the decimal place to which there is confidence in the number. Then drop the digits after this number. If the number immediately to the right of the last retained number is more than 5, add 1 to the last retained number. If the number immediately to the right of the last retained number is less than 5, do not change the last retained number. If the number immediately to the right of the last retained number is 5, make the retained number even. That is, the last retained number is an odd number, add 1 to it. If the last retained number is an even number and the digit immediately to its right is 5, do not change it. To round off the number 5.55 to one place to the right of the decimal point (one decimal place), the rounded off number would be 5.6. Note the following relationships:

Number	Rounded Off
3.19	3.2
3.12	3.1
3.15	3.2
3.25	3.2
3.35	3.4

The purpose of rounding off 5 to the even number is to balance error. Numbers greater than 5 are closer to the next higher number than the next lower number, whereas numbers less than 5 are closer to the next lower number. Numbers ending in 5 may be actually closer to either the next higher or next lower number. Without knowing which, moving to the even number, which will be up half of the time and down half of the time, will not generate bias to the higher number (when the actual number may be closer to the lower number) or to the lower number (when the actual number may be closer to the higher number).

SIGNIFICANT FIGURES

A number expressed as 3.75298 indicates confidence in its accuracy ±0.000005, whereas a number expressed as 3.8 indicates confidence ±0.05. If the method, equipment, or instrument cannot accurately and reproducibly measure values to ±0.000005, then 3.75298 should not be reported.

Protocols may require numbers reported to specified levels of confidence or **significant figures**. If a number is to be reported to three significant figures, three digits will be used. The significance of zeroes and nonzero numbers is interpreted differently. All nonzero numbers are considered significant. Zeroes may or may not be significant, depending on their relationship with the decimal point and other nonzero numbers. The following rules apply to significance of zeroes.

1. Zeroes to the right of a nonzero number are significant on either side of the decimal point. For large numbers ending in zeroes, not all the zeroes may be significant, but they have to be included in the number. In this case, a bar, ‾, over a number marks the last number retained. The numbers, 10$\bar{0}$ and 0.10$\bar{0}$ and 10, $\bar{0}$00 all have three significant figures.

2. Zeroes to the right of the decimal point are not significant if there is no nonzero number to their left. The number 0.00152 has three significant figures.

3. Zeroes between nonzero numbers are significant. The numbers 1,001 and 0.1001 have four significant figures.

The following numbers are all expressed to three significant figures.

$$1.23$$
$$0.123$$
$$0.00000123$$
$$1.02$$
$$12.3$$

Values with different numbers of significant figures are often used for calculations. When expressing the answer, retain the smallest number of figures found among the terms given. Because electronic calculators, spreadsheets, or other specialized software are often used for laboratory mathematics, the figure retention during the computational process is automatic. The final answer can then be rounded off to the appropriate number of significant figures, that is, the smallest number of figures among the terms entered for the calculation. The answer to the calculation,

$$(0.02 \times 7.228)/0.279 = 0.14456/0.279 = 0.5181362 = 0.52$$

has two significant figures. For practice problems, round off the final answer at the end of the calculation.

BASIC CONCEPTS

Certain basic concepts are important when working with numbers and numerical results. Attention to these concepts will help to avoid errors and miscommunication in the laboratory or with others outside of the laboratory.

1. Consider each result critically. Judge the result and consider the expected value. If a readout of a concentration for a diluted substance is more than that for the undiluted substance, then a miscalculation or misreading must have taken place, and the test or calculations should be repeated (Fig. 1-3). Some unexpected results may be correct, but a

careful reassessment is still useful, especially if an explanation of the unusual value must be provided.

2. Use the proper numerical nomenclature or unit values when reporting results. There are different ways to express the same value. The expressions ½, 0.5, ⁵⁄₁₀, 50%, ½, or "50 in 100" all represent the same mathematical value; however, only one may be appropriate for a test result. Use of the wrong nomenclature can result in misinterpretation of the test results. For example, after a bone marrow transplant, measurement of engraftment of donor bone marrow in recipient patients is reported in percent (for instance, 90% donor). The raw data are measured as 0.90. A report of 0.90 may be interpreted as 0.90% donor, a number that has very different clinical implications from 90% donor.

3. Handwritten data are still prevalent in the laboratory, so write clearly when manual notation is required. If you find that a manual entry is not clearly written, request clarification or redo the calculation. Avoid writing over, erasing, or using correction fluid. Instead, cross out the erroneous or unclear writing and rewrite the correct value legibly.

4. Computer-generated results are clearly expressed; however, clerical errors in transferring these data may occur (Fig. 1-4). When numbers or letters are miskeyed into a laboratory instrument, calculator, or computer, the resulting answer will be incorrect. Such clerical errors can generate disastrous results for patients. A misplaced decimal point changes the reported value at least 10-fold depending on how far away

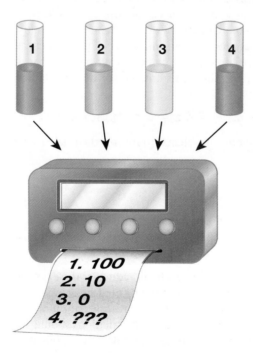

Figure 1-3 A readout shows high values associated with color intensity for samples 1 to 3. Based on the visible color intensity, the expected reading for sample 4 should be similar to that of sample 1. If it is lower than that of sample 2, then a misreading or error may have occurred.

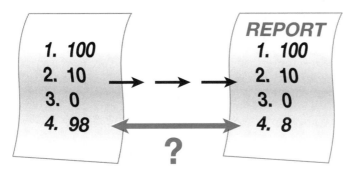

Figure 1-4 Transcription errors can occur when data are transferred from instrument readings to final reports.

the decimal point is from its proper place. To avoid errors, consider the estimated result and redo the calculations, if an error is suspected. At least two people should review manually entered test results before their release. Laboratory information systems include rules automatically applied in response to instrument data. These systems will initially perform a check on the data and offer options to the technologist to review the results if a potential error is flagged. These systems may still require comparison of rules with laboratory recommendations and periodic review.

5. Check any manual calculations performed, such as preparation of a reagent or calculation of how much of a mixture is required for a certain number of samples. Most calculations can be performed in more than one way. A good check is to perform the same computation using an alternative mathematical process to see whether the same value results. If no alternative method is available, work the process backward from the result to see whether the original values are produced.

PRACTICE PROBLEMS

Fundamental Concepts

1. A test result is reported in increasing units of color with the degree of pigment in the sample. A darkly pigmented sample yields a result value lower than that of a lightly pigmented sample. Is this expected? (See Fig. 1-3.)

2. If a handwritten test result has a value of 1 crossed out with a value of 2 written below it, what is the result?

3. A sample is diluted 1/10. The test reading of the diluted sample is 10 times less than the original undiluted substance. Is this correct?

4. Test results for substance A are reported as 40%, 10%, 60%, and so forth. Is a result of "0.50" correctly reported?

5. Scientist A makes a quick mental calculation on how much reagent is required for a test. Because the amount calculated is conveniently the same amount of reagent available, the scientist proceeds with the test. Is this correct?

6. A small amount of salt weighs more than a larger amount of the same substance. Is this acceptable without reviewing the process?

7. Your calculator gives an unexpected value. Is this necessarily correct, because you used your calculator?

8. True or False: When handwritten values for a repetitive protocol are illegible, the values most frequently observed in previous tests should be assumed.

9. Your automatic pipet is set to pick up a volume twice as large as a volume previously pipetted; however, the amount in the pipet tip looks smaller than the amount previously pipetted (Fig. 1-5). Which pipetted amount is likely incorrect, the previous amount (1) or the current amount (2), or both?

10. If a calculation calls for division of a whole number into another number, should the answer be greater or smaller than the divided number?

Numerals

Perform the following mathematical exercises.

11. $\frac{1}{2} + \frac{3}{4}$

12. $5\frac{1}{2} + 3\frac{1}{4}$

13. $\frac{2}{3} - \frac{1}{2}$

14. $\frac{7}{8} + \frac{1}{9} - \frac{2}{3}$

15. $\frac{3}{7} \times \frac{2}{3}$

16. $6\frac{1}{4} \times 2\frac{1}{3}$

17. $7 \times (3\frac{1}{2} + \frac{3}{7})$

18. $(\frac{6}{4}) / \frac{1}{2}$

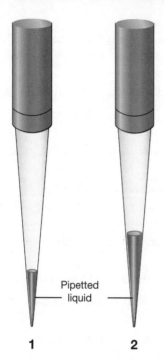

1   **2**   **Figure 1-5** Visual comparison of liquid drawn into pipets.

19. $(5\frac{2}{3}) / 7\frac{1}{3}$

20. $\{[(\frac{4}{5})/(\frac{2}{3})] \times \frac{1}{4}\} + 100$

Express the following numbers in decimal fractions and percentages.

21. $\frac{7}{10}$

22. $\frac{3}{6}$

23. $\frac{1}{3}$

24. $\frac{1}{5}$

25. $2\frac{2}{3}$

26. $\frac{5}{100}$

27. $1\frac{7}{9}$

28. $\frac{24}{52}$

PRACTICE PROBLEMS *cont.*

29. $\dfrac{505}{100}$

30. $\dfrac{466}{1,000}$

Write the reciprocal of the following numbers.

31. 98

32. $\dfrac{1}{7}$

33. $\dfrac{6}{10}$

34. x

35. $\dfrac{a}{b}$

Use common and decimal fractions to solve the following problems.

36. How many units comprise $\dfrac{1}{2}$ of 50 units?

37. If you make five aliquots of a 3-ounce sample, how many ounces would be in each aliquot?

38. One tenth of the sum of 4 parts plus 2 times 3 parts is how many parts?

39. What is 0.5 of 0.25?

40. How many parts are in $\dfrac{1}{4}$ of a $\dfrac{1}{3}$ aliquot of 30 parts?

Round off the following values and express in three significant figures.

41. 1.754

42. 0.86237

43. 0.001747

44. 100.96

45. 1,531.2

46. 0.0115

47. 0.0125

48. 124.7

49. 1,111,111

50. 0.000999

APPLICATIONS

Laboratory Inventory

A procedure uses 10 units of reagent per sample. Two runs are performed every week. Each run consists of 22 patient specimens, two controls, and a reagent blank consisting of the reagent and other test components, without the substance being tested (target analyte). The reagent costs $500.00 per package of 1,000 units. The shelf life of the reagent requires reorder every month. How many packages of reagent must be ordered to last for 1 month (4 weeks)?

Hematology

The white blood cell count (total leukocyte count) is a standard measurement of blood analysis for almost any condition. White blood cells are not all the same, and the number of different types of white cells is also frequently reported as the differential count, that is, the number of each type of cell. Many laboratories report a **relative differential** expressed as percent along with the white blood cell count. The cell count is reported in numbers of cells per unit volume (microliters).

```
Total white blood cells 6,000 per microliter
Segmented neutrophils                56%
Banded neutrophils                    3%
Lymphocytes                          28%
Monocytes                             7%
Eosinophils                           4%
Basophils                             2%
                                    100%
```

The **absolute differential** is the number of each type of leukocyte per unit volume. Multiply the total white blood cell count (6,000) by the decimal fraction represented by the relative percentage of each cell type to determine the absolute differential values.

Reporting Confidence

An analytical balance was used to measure the amount of dry powder reagent added to a fixed volume of water. An aliquot of this mixture measured by a liquid handler was placed into a reaction chamber along with the patient's sample.

Analytical balance reading: 5.7482 milligrams
Pipet measurement: 2.55 milliliters
Final reading from reaction chamber: 25.019257 units

What value (how many significant figures) should be reported?

Continued

APPLICATIONS cont.

Chemistry

The concentrations of positive ions or cations in serum should equal the concentration of negative ions or anions (electrolyte balance). Electrolyte balance is measured by the anion gap, which is the difference between the sum of the most concentrated cations, sodium (Na^+) and potassium (K^+), and the sum of the most concentrated anions, chloride (Cl^-) and bicarbonate ion (HCO_3^-):

(Na^+ concentration + K^+ concentration) − (Cl^- concentration + HCO_3^- concentration)

These electrolytes are measured in automated laboratory systems and are reported as an electrolyte profile. Calculate the anion gap for a patient with the following electrolyte profile:

Na^+ 138
K^+ 4.0
Cl^- 101
HCO_3^- 23

The anion gap normally ranges between 10 and 20.

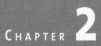

ALGEBRA

THE EQUATION

Algebra is a method of solving problems by using different expressions of equal value (Box 2-1). These expressions are placed on either side of an equal sign (=), forming an **equation**. Thus, an equation has two equal parts (Fig. 2-1). Each part contains one or more **terms** or numerical expressions. The terms are placed on opposite sides of the equal sign, as shown here:

$$6 \times 30 = 90 \times 2$$

An equation may be used to find the value of an **unknown**. The unknown is usually denoted by x; however, any non-numerical expression may be used for the unknown. When an equation has multiple unknowns, different letters are used for each unknown. Three unknowns in the same equation could be expressed as x, y, and z (Box 2-2).

There are different types of equations, depending on the number and/or exponents of unknowns that appear in each term of the equation. Most laboratory math problems are solvable with **linear,** or **first degree,** equations. The following are linear equations:

$$2x = 5$$
$$x + 5y = 8$$
$$-x + 2y - 3z = 20$$

In these equations, unknowns are represented by x, y, or z. Each number with an unknown component or term in the equations has a single unknown (e.g., $2x$). Terms can have more than one unknown, such as $2xy$.

Box 2-1   Historical Background

The term *algebra* originated in the 9th century from a textbook containing the word "al-jabr" as a way to solve practical problems in terms of equations.

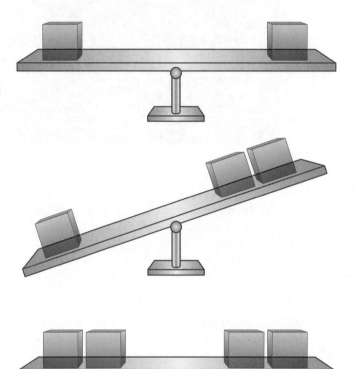

Figure 2-1 An equation must remain balanced. If one side of the equation is changed (two blocks added), the other side must be equally changed.

Box 2-2   Second Degree Equations

Second degree equations have two unknowns in a term or an unknown with an exponent other than 1. The following are second degree equations:

$$3xy = 17$$
$$7x^2 - 5 = y$$

In these equations, two unknowns appear in the term $3xy$, and an unknown with an exponent different from 1 appears in the term $7x^2$.

SOLVING EQUATIONS FOR THE UNKNOWN VARIABLE

First Degree Equations With One Unknown

Fundamental arithmatic is used to solve an equation for the unknown, "*x*". Equations, by definition, demand equal values on both sides of the equal sign. To solve for an unknown, manipulate the equation so that the unknown is isolated on one side of the equal sign. Consider the equation:

$$x + 5 = 27$$

Isolate the unknown *x* on one side of the equation by subtracting 5 from both sides. This will keep both sides equal:

$$x + 5 - 5 = 27 - 5$$

After subtraction:

$$x + 0 = 22 \text{ or}$$
$$x = 22$$

Many problems with numerical values can be solved with an equation. Suppose you have six bottles of reagent in one room of the laboratory (Room A) and you find that there are 18 bottles in another room (Room B). You want to have an equal number of bottles of reagent (18 bottles) stocked in each of the two areas. The reagent bottles are supplied in packages of two. How many packages of reagent are required to add to the six bottles in room A in order to have 18 bottles? This problem can be expressed as a numerical equation asking what number (*x*) when multiplied by 2 and added to 6 is equal to 18. This can be written as:

$$(2 \text{ bottles/package times } x \text{ packages}) + 6 \text{ bottles}$$
$$= 18 \text{ bottles}$$

or

$$2x + 6 = 18$$

To solve the equation for the unknown, first isolate the unknown (*x*) on one side of the equation. In doing this, remember that both sides of the equation must remain equal in value so that whatever is done to one side must be done to the other. Subtract 6 from both sides of the equation.

$$2x + 6 - 6 = 18 - 6$$
$$2x = 18 - 6$$
$$2x = 12$$

Divide both sides of the equation by 2.

$$\frac{2x}{2} = \frac{12}{2}$$
$$x = \frac{12}{2}$$

Box 2-3   Check by Substitution

After solving an equation, one can arithmetically verify that the result is correct with a check by substitution. Substitute the solution of the equation for the unknown in the original equation. If the solution is the correct value of x, both sides of the equation should be the same.

$$2x + 6 = 18$$
$$2(6) + 6 = 18$$
$$12 + 6 = 18$$
$$18 = 18$$

Then solve the right side of the equation to find the value of x.

$$x = \frac{12}{2} = 6$$

The value of the unknown, x, in this equation is 6. Six packages of two bottles must be provided to stock 18 bottles of reagents in Room A (Box 2-3).

First Degree Equations With Multiple Unknowns

Terms in first degree equations have single unknowns (e.g., x). There can be, however, different unknowns (e.g., x or y) in separate terms in the same equation. When an equation contains more than one unknown, the value of the unknowns cannot be determined unless there are additional equations expressing the same unknowns. One may encounter such an equation, for instance, when designing a test method. The time it takes to mix the samples and test reagents (x minutes) and analyze the result (y minutes), also called hands-on time, is intended to be 30 minutes. This can be expressed as follows:

$$x + y = 30$$

Infinite values can be added together and sum to 30, even with reasonable limits on how fast one can mix reagents or analyze results. Therefore, this equation cannot be solved for a single value of either unknown. If, however, it is known that it takes twice as long to mix reagents (x) as it does to analyze the results (y), another equation can be made:

$$x = 2y$$

Expressing both unknowns differently, only one value for x and one value for y can satisfy both equations. A set of equations considered together in the same problem is called a **system of simultaneous equations** or a **system of equations**. The previous example is a system of two linear equations in two unknowns. Alternative methods can be used to solve for the unknowns.

Use the two equations to solve for the unknowns by the **method of substitution**. First, express one unknown in terms of the other using one of the equations. One equation is already expressed with isolated x in this example; however, either unknown may be used.

$$x = 2y$$

Substitute $2y$ for x in the second equation, so that the equation has only one unknown.

$$x + y = 30$$
$$2y + y = 30$$

Solve the equation for the single unknown.

$$3y = 30$$
$$\frac{3y}{3} = \frac{30}{3}$$
$$y = 10$$

Use the value of the found unknown, y, to solve for the remaining unknown, x, using either equation.

$$x = 2y$$
$$x = 2 \times 10$$
$$x = 20$$

Using these equations, it should take 20 minutes to mix the samples and reagents and 10 minutes to analyze the result.

Either of the two original equations may be used to verify that the results are correct with the check by substitution method.

$$x + y = 30$$
$$20 + 10 = 30$$
$$30 = 30$$

An alternative way to solve for two unknowns is the **method of comparison**. Rearrange one or both equations so that one unknown is expressed in the same way in both equations. In the example, x is expressed as x in both equations, so no rearrangement is required. Subtract one equation from the other, thus eliminating that unknown.

$$x = 2y$$
$$x - 2y = 2y - 2y$$
$$x - 2y = 0$$

The equations can then be subtracted, in this case, to eliminate x:

$$\begin{array}{r} x + y = 30 \\ - \underline{(x - 2y = 0)} \\ 3y = 30 \end{array}$$

Alternatively, y can be eliminated by rearranging one or the other equation so that y is expressed in a similar way in both equations (y and $2y$).

Equations are applied to a wide variety of problems. Formulae used to convert between units of measure are stated as equations. Increasing or decreasing concentrations or volumes of solutions used in an assay will be done using equations. These processes are so often performed using algebra that they are frequently done without considering that algebraic equations and functions are involved.

EXPONENTS

Laboratory methods and results sometimes involve expressions of very large or very small numbers. For convenience and accuracy, these numbers can be expressed in exponential form, n^a, where n is any number and a is the **exponent**. An exponent is a number denoting how many times a number is multiplied by itself. Exponents provide a shortcut for multiplication. An expression of 3×3 can be expressed as 3^2. Further,

$$3 \times 3 \times 3 \times 3 \times 3$$

can be expressed as 3^5.

The exponent is written as superscript to the right of the number being multiplied, the latter being the **base**. In the term 3^5, 3 is the base and 5 is the exponent.

Base-10 Exponents

In the decimal system, exponential expressions with a base of 10 are practical to use:

$$10 = 10^1$$
$$100 = 10 \times 10 = 10^2$$
$$1{,}000 = 10 \times 10 \times 10 = 10^3$$

For numbers less than 1, exponents are negative. A negative exponent means that the base is the denominator of a fraction, and the fraction is inverted to move the base to the numerator. When the fraction is inverted, the sign on the exponent changes. Using the base 10,

$$0.1 = \frac{1}{10} = \frac{1}{10^1} = \frac{10^{-1}}{1} = 10^{-1}$$

$$0.01 = \frac{1}{100} = \frac{1}{10^2} = \frac{10^{-2}}{1} = 10^{-1}$$

$$0.001 = \frac{1}{1{,}000} = \frac{1}{10^3} = \frac{10^{-3}}{1} = 10^{-3}$$

There are rules for doing calculations with exponents.

- Any number with an exponent of 0 is equal to 1. The exponential numbers 10^0, 2^0, and $1{,}999^0$ are all equal to 1. In general terms:

$$n^0 = 1$$

where n is any number.
- Any number to exponent of 1 is equal to that number: 10^1, 2^1, and $1{,}999^1$ are equal to 10, 2, and 1,999, respectively. In general terms:

$$n^1 = n$$

where n is any number.
- Exponents can be used to multiply and divide numbers **of the same base**.

- To multiply two exponential expressions, add the exponents.

  $n^a \times n^b = n^{a+b}$

  $10^{-1} \times 10^5 = 10^4$

- To divide two exponential expressions of the same base, subtract the exponent of the divisor from that of the dividend.

  $\dfrac{n^a}{n^b} = n^{a-b}$

  $\dfrac{10^5}{10^{-2}} = 10^7$

- To express an exponent of an exponential number, multiply the exponents:

  $(n^a)^b = n^{a \times b}$

  $(10^{-3})^5 = 10^{-15}$

> To enter numbers in exponential form on a calculator, enter the base number and then the y^x or ^. So, for 3^5, enter 3 then the y^x or ^ key, depending on the calculator and then the exponent, 5. The answer should be 243.

In addition to being used for calculations that involve very large and very small numbers, exponents also facilitate the conversions of unit expressions in the laboratory.

SCIENTIFIC NOTATION

Exponents in the base 10 are part of **scientific notation**. For numbers in the base 10 written in exponential form, the exponent is the multiple or **power of 10**. Any number can be expressed in exponential form by first determining the power of 10 in the number. The number 15 is a multiple of one power of 10 (10^1), whereas 5,283 is a multiple of three powers of 10 (10^3), and 597,832 is a multiple of five powers of 10 (10^5).

Scientific notation is the expression of numbers as powers of 10 in the following form:

  $a \times 10^b$

where a is the **coefficient** (also called the mantissa) expressed as a number between 1 and 10 and b is the **base** written as powers of 10 in exponential form.

To express numbers in scientific notation, move the decimal point so that the number to be expressed is between 1 and 10. For expression of 150 in scientific notation, move the decimal point two places to the left to produce a coefficient between 1 and 10 (1.50).

  150.

  ← ←

  1.50

Write that number times 10 to the power of the original number (150). This is also the number of decimal places the decimal point was moved (to the left for numbers greater than 1). The scientific notation for 150 would then be:

$$150 = 1.50 \times 10^2$$

The decimal was moved two places to the left, so the exponent of 10 is 2.

The numbers 5,283 and 897,832 would be:

$$5{,}283 = 5.283 \times 10^3$$

$$897{,}832 = 8.97832 \times 10^5$$

The same rules apply to numbers less than 1. Move the decimal point to the right until the resulting number is between 1 and 10. For the number 0.0015, move the decimal point three places to the right:

0.0015

$$\rightarrow \rightarrow \rightarrow$$

1.5

Because the decimal is moved to the right (from higher to lower value), the exponent of 10 will be negative.

$$0.0015 = 1.5 \times 10^{-3}$$

Alternatively, count the number of zeroes to the right of the decimal point, add 1, and change the sign to obtain the negative exponent. The number 0.0015 has two zeroes to the right of the decimal point. Add $1 + 2$ to obtain the exponent of 10 (3), then change the sign (-3).

Similarly, 0.15 is 1.5×10^{-1} (no zeroes plus 1) and 0.000000000015 is 1.5×10^{-11} (10 zeroes plus 1). The latter number illustrates how exponential form can simplify expressions.

Follow these rules for determining the exponent of 10 to be used in scientific notation:

- For numbers greater than one, the exponent is the number of digits to the left of the decimal point minus 1.
- For numbers less than one, the exponent is the number of zeros to the right of the decimal point plus 1, with a negative sign.

The rules for rounding off and significant figures apply to the coefficient in scientific notation. If the following numbers were to be expressed in scientific notation as three significant figures, the numbers would be:

$$15.0 = 1.50 \times 10^1$$

$$5{,}283 = 5.28 \times 10^3$$

$$897{,}832 = 8.98 \times 10^5$$

To convert numbers in scientific notation, $a \times 10^b$, to common numbers, perform the expressed multiplication.

$$6.973 \times 10^4 = 6.973 \times 10{,}000 = 69{,}730$$
$$5.129 \times 10^{-3} = 5.129 \times 0.001 = 0.005129$$

On a calculator, use the EXP or EE key. For 1.5×10^3, enter (1.5), then EXP (or EE), and then 3. On pressing the EXE or = key, the answer 1,500 should appear. Note that the EE or the EXP key is not used if the base is other than 10. After numbers are entered, calculations proceed with the +, −, ×, and ÷ keys. The result is expressed in nonexponential terms.

CALCULATIONS IN SCIENTIFIC NOTATION

Expression of numbers in scientific notation, $a \times 10^b$, greatly simplifies mathematical calculations of very large and very small values. Certain points must be considered.

For addition and subtraction, numbers must be in the same power of 10. To add

$$(5.85 \times 10^5) + (3.67 \times 10^5)$$

sum the coefficients. The answer will have the same power of 10 as the two addends.

$$(5.85 \times 10^5) + (3.67 \times 10^5) = 9.52 \times 10^5$$

To add

$$(5.85 \times 10^5) + (3.67 \times 10^4)$$

convert either number to match the power of 10 of the other by moving the decimal point in the coefficient left or right and adjusting the exponent of 10 accordingly (add one to the exponent for each place moved to the left and subtract one from the exponent for each place moved to the right):

$$5.85 \times 10^5 \rightarrow 58.5 \times 10^4$$

Moving the decimal point one place to the right in the coefficient lowers the exponent of the base or power of 10 by 1 from 5 to 4. The two numbers can then be added with decimal points aligned:

$$\begin{array}{r} 58.5 \times 10^4 \\ + \ 3.67 \times 10^4 \\ \hline 62.17 \times 10^4 \end{array}$$

Moving the decimal point one place to the left in the coefficient of the sum raises the exponent by 1 and restores the coefficient to a number between 1 and 10.

$$62.17 \times 10^4 \rightarrow 6.217 \times 10^5 = 6.22 \times 10^5$$

For numbers less than 1, moving the decimal point will have the same effect on the exponent. To add

$$(7.98 \times 10^{-7}) + (3.27 \times 10^{-8})$$

convert one number to match the power of 10 of the other. Moving the decimal point one place to the right will lower (subtract 1 from) the exponent

$$7.98 \times 10^{-7} = 79.8 \times 10^{-8}$$

The two numbers can then be added with decimal points aligned:

$$\begin{array}{r} 79.8 \times 10^{-8} \\ + \; 3.27 \times 10^{-8} \\ \hline 83.07 \times 10^{-8} \end{array}$$

Moving the decimal point one place to the left in the coefficient raises the value of the exponent by 1 and restores the coefficient to a number between 1 and 10.

$$83.07 \times 10^{-8} \rightarrow 8.307 \times 10^{-7} = 8.31 \times 10^{-7}$$

An alternative method is to convert numbers in scientific notation to decimal numbers and add.

$$5.854 \times 10^5 = 585,400$$
$$3.67 \times 10^4 = 36,700$$
$$\begin{array}{r} 585,400 \\ + \; 36,700 \\ \hline 622,100 \end{array}$$
$$622,100 = 6.22 \times 10^5$$

The same rules are used for adding more than two addends.

For subtraction in scientific notation, use the same process:

$$(8.75 \times 10^7) - (7.32 \times 10^6)$$
$$7.32 \times 10^6 = 0.732 \times 10^7$$
$$\begin{array}{r} 8.75 \times 10^7 \\ - \; 0.732 \times 10^7 \\ \hline 8.02 \times 10^7 \end{array}$$

Multiplication of numbers in scientific notation does not require the same power of 10. Multiply the coefficients and then add the base exponents. Multiply (2.5×10^9) times (3.0×10^2):

$$(2.5 \times 10^9) \times (3.0 \times 10^2)$$

The coefficient of the product is $2.5 \times 3.0 = 7.5$. The exponent of 10 is the sum of the exponents in the multiplier and multiplicand:

$$(2.5 \times 10^9) \times (3.0 \times 10^2) = (2.5 \times 3.0) \times (10^9 \times 10^2)$$
$$= 7.5 \times 10^{11}$$

Division in scientific notation is performed by dividing the coefficients and subtracting the exponents of 10. Divide (5.2×10^7) by (4.0×10^3):

(5.2 ÷ 4.0) = 1.3

10^7 ÷ 10^3 = 10^4

(5.2 x 10^7) ÷ (4.0 x 10^3) = 1.3 x 10^4

On the calculator, enter the multiplier and multiplicand in exponential form as described in the previous section using the EXP or EE key. To perform the calculation shown, enter 5.2EXP7, then the division key, and then 4EXP3. After pressing the = or EXE key, the answer will be expressed as 13,000 in nonexponential form.

USE OF EQUATIONS IN RATIO AND PROPORTION

Ratio is the relative amount of one component to another (Fig. 2-2). It is expressed as the ratio of component A *to* component B, or A:B. If a solution or substance consisted of two components—3 units of component A and 6 units of component B, the ratio of component A to component B would be 3:6 or 1:2. Ratio can describe more than two components. A substance consisting of five components of equal amounts would be described by a ratio of 1:1:1:1:1. The substance or solution could contain any number of units of each component as long as it has the same number of units of the other components.

Proportion describes the relative amount of one component to the total amount of substance or solution (see Fig. 2-2). It is expressed as the proportion of component A *in* the total substance or A/total. In the previous examples,

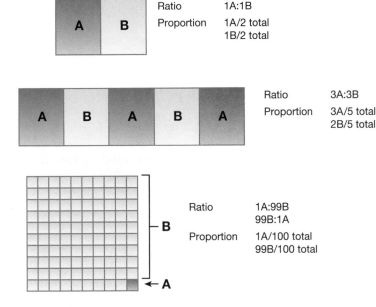

Figure 2-2 *Top:* Ratio is the number of parts A to parts B. Proportion is parts in total parts. *Bottom:* When the proportion is minimal with regard to total (1/100), ratio and proportion are similar (1/100 ~ 1:99). When the proportion is large with regard to the total (1/2), ratio and proportion are not the same (1:1 ≠ 1/2).

a 1:2 ratio would be a 1/3 proportion of component A and a 2/3 proportion of component B in the total mixture. A 1:1:1:1:1 ratio would be a 1/5 proportion of each component. Preparation of specimens and reagents often requires adjustment of component volumes and concentrations. The degree of adjustment is indicated by a statement of ratio or proportion.

Ratio and proportion are flexible expressions applicable to any total amount of a substance or solution made up of separate parts. Equations are used to convert volumes. When reagents are prepared in different amounts, say, for batches of different numbers of specimens, procedures may be written using ratio, rather than exact amounts. This allows adjustment to the required amount of reagent.

For instance, a mixture of substance A and substance B has a ratio of 1 unit A:4 units B. Use ratio and proportion to determine how much substance A and substance B would be required to increase the volume of this mixture from 5 to 50 volumetric units.

The ratio of A:B is 1:4. The total volume is $1 + 4 = 5$
The proportion of A in the mixture is 1/5
The proportion of B in the mixture is 4/5

For substance A, set up an equation expressing equal values (proportions) of A on both sides for 5 and 50 volumetric units:

$$\frac{1}{5} = \frac{x}{50}$$

Solve the equation for x:

$$\frac{(1 \times 50)}{5} = x$$

$$x = 10$$

Similarly, for substance B,

$$\frac{4}{5} = \frac{x}{50}$$

$$\frac{(4 \times 50)}{5} = x$$

$$x = 40$$

To make 50 volumetric units, use 10 units A and 40 units B.

PRACTICE PROBLEMS

Equations
Which of the following pairs of values would comprise two sides of the same equation?

1. $2 + 4, 3 + 3$

2. $5 \times 6, \dfrac{300}{10}$

3. $\dfrac{3}{9}, \dfrac{1}{6}$

4. $2 \times 0.5, 2.5$

5. $0.2, \dfrac{100}{200}$

6. $(\frac{1}{5}) \times 4, \dfrac{80}{100}$

7. $3x, 6x - 3x$

8. $x, [\dfrac{(250 - 240)}{10}] x$

9. $0.2x, \dfrac{x}{2}$

10. $3x + 3y, (5x + 2y) - (2x - y)$

Solving for the Unknown Variable
Solve the following equations for x.

11. $3x + 3 = 9$

12. $5x + 1 = 400 - 394$

13. $\dfrac{x}{2} = 0.25$

14. $\dfrac{(5x)}{3} = \dfrac{90}{9}$

15. $(x - 27) = 1{,}000$

Use the method of substitution to solve for x and y.

16. $x - 2y = 8; x + y = 11$

17. $x - y = -22; 0.5x + y = 25$

18. $3x = 5y + 30; 2x + 2y = 36$

19. $4x + 8y = 17; \dfrac{(32x + 2y)}{2} = 6$

20. $\dfrac{(3x)}{4} = 2y; \dfrac{(3x + 3y)}{3} = 11$

Use the method of comparison to solve for x and y.

21. $2x - 3y = 12; x + y = 11$

22. $3x + y = 23; (x + y) \times 0.2 = 0.6$

23. $\dfrac{x}{2} + 10 = y - 85; \ y = 5x + 50$

24. $2x - 3y = 33; 2x + y = 21$

25. $1{,}000x + 2y = 1{,}900; x + y = -48$

Exponents
Convert the following exponential terms to real numbers.

26. 3^1

27. 10^1

28. a^0

29. 50^{-1}

30. 100^{-2}

31. 10^{-4}

Express the following numbers in exponential form.

32. 25 (base 5)

33. 64 (base 2)

34. 100,000 (base 10)

35. 0.001 (base 10)

36. 1 (any base a)

Continued

PRACTICE PROBLEMS   *cont.*

Perform the following calculations.

37. $3^2 \times 3^3$

38. $8^2 \times 8^{10}$

39. $3^2 \times 2^3$

40. $3^2 + 3^3$

41. $5^2 - 3^2$

42. $\dfrac{(10^2)}{(10^3)}$

43. $\dfrac{(7^9)}{(7^3)}$

44. $\dfrac{(10^{-2})}{(10^3)}$

45. $\dfrac{(10^2)}{(10^{-3})}$

46. $\dfrac{(10^{-1})}{(10^2)}$

47. $\dfrac{(10^2 \times 10^{-2})}{(10^3)}$

Express the following numbers in scientific notation.

48. 237

49. 415,000

50. 60,000,000

51. 0,175

52. 0.000327

Convert the following ratios (A to B) to proportion (A in total/B in total).

53. 1:2

54. 5:20

55. 9:1

APPLICATIONS

Laboratory Automation

1. Reagents supplied for a new instrument are to be adjusted before use. The instrument requires a reaction mix made of three supplied reagents in a total of 10 mL. The directions call for a mixture of 3.0 parts reagent A plus 2.0 parts reagent B plus 5.0 parts reagent C. What are the ratio and proportion of reagents A, B, and C?

2. The total volume of the mix must be at least 5.0 parts. You find that there is only half (1 part) of the amount of reagent B available. Is it still possible to make this reaction mix? How much of reagents A and C would be used? What are the ratio and proportion of reagents A, B, and C in this case?

Computer Maintenance

1. A new software package works with 1 megabyte (1,000,000 bytes) of random access memory, or RAM. The computer you are using has a capacity of 512 kilobytes (512,000 bytes) but is upgradeable. How much memory in bytes must you add to the computer?

2. Memory for the computer is supplied in 512 kilobyte modules. How many of these are required to achieve the proper memory?

CHAPTER 3

SYSTEMS OF MEASUREMENT

TYPES OF MEASUREMENT

The nature of a substance can be described by its **properties**. Properties are non-numerical (qualitative) or numerical (quantitative). Qualitative observations do not have numerical descriptions, whereas quantitative observations include amounts. Qualitatively, milk is a white, opaque liquid. We can also describe milk in quantitative amounts such as pints and quarts. Laboratory results are descriptions of qualitative and quantitative properties of substances being analyzed. Qualitative results are reported as yes/no or positive/negative or by other textual descriptions. In microbiology, a Gram stain is a way to classify bacteria into two types, Gram-positive or Gram-negative. The blue appearance of bacteria under the microscope (Gram-positive) is a qualitative result. If the cells under the microscope are counted with regard to the number of bacteria per unit volume of sample, the result is quantitative.

Results may be measured quantitatively but reported as relative to a previous or reference amount, as an approximation of the actual result, or in a qualitative manner. These are semiquantitative results. In molecular diagnostics, loss or gain of gene copies is reported relative to a control, rather than in absolute numbers of gene copies. A test for panel reactive antibodies, performed before an organ transplant, results in identification of antibodies in the blood and an approximation of the level of these antibodies. Some tests are reported as positive if quantitative levels are above a set (clinically important) level and negative below that level.

SUBSTANCE PROPERTIES

Quantitative and qualitative properties are physical and chemical. **Physical properties** include mass or weight (Box 3-1), length (or area or volume), temperature, boiling or freezing point, thermal or electrical conductivity, odor,

LEARNING OUTCOMES
- Define and differentiate among quantitative, qualitative, and semiquantitative measurements.
- List examples of physical and chemical properties of substances.
- State the general difference between a physical property of a substance and its chemical properties.
- Define systems of measurement including the metric and SI systems.
- List and define prefixes used with basic and primary units.
- Define temperature.
- Compare and contrast the three temperature scales: Celsius, Fahrenheit, and Kelvin.
- Convert temperatures to equivalent values in the three scales.

Box 3-1	Weight and Mass

Note that mass and weight are used interchangeably in this text. Technically, mass is the actual amount of substance, and weight is the mass under the force of gravity. Because all weight measurements made in earthly laboratories are under the same force of gravity, mass may be expressed as weight and vice versa.

hardness, malleability, color, density, and refractive index (Table 3-1). These characteristics can be measured by physical means, such as using a thermometer to determine temperature or a scale to determine mass. Although physical properties may change with the surrounding environment, observation or measurement does not change them. The physical property of water is liquid above its freezing point and below its boiling point, but taking the temperature of a sample of liquid water does not change the property of "liquid."

Table 3-1	Physical Properties	
Property	Observation	Examples of Laboratory Application
Mass or weight	Amount of a substance	Preparing reagents; determining organ size (in pathology)
Length (or area or volume)	Distance from one point to another, measured in one, two, or three dimensions	Size of a bacterium, cell, or other structure under the microscope; distance of migration of nucleic acid in electrophoresis
Temperature	Warmness or coldness	Storage conditions of test specimens and reagents; laboratory procedures performed in containers held at temperatures optimal for the method to work
Boiling or freezing point	Temperatures at which substances transition from solid to liquid to gaseous states	Freezing point of body fluids, depending on the amount of dissolved particles
Thermal conductivity	Ability to transfer heat	Thin-walled tubes designed to transfer heat rapidly in reactions where the temperature of the substance must be changed, as in the polymerase chain reaction (PCR)
Electrical conductivity	Ability to carry a current	Electrophoresis of proteins or nucleic acids
Odor	Detectable scent caused by molecules emitted or released from a substance	Useful in identification of organisms, such as *Proteus vulgaris* which emits a distinctive odor
Hardness	Resistance to deformation or scratching	Microscope lenses and filters or quartz cuvettes used in spectrophotometry cleaned with special cloths to avoid scratching

Continued

Table 3-1   Physical Properties—cont'd

Property	Observation	Examples of Laboratory Application
Malleability	Ability to accept changes by molding or shaping	Tissue specimens may be described by their malleability; calcifications, such as a kidney stone
Color	Reflection of light at a specific wavelength	The color of pH indicators; color tests for specific substances
Density	Mass per unit volume of a substance	Densities of commercial preparations, such as hydrochloric acid, used to determine the volume required to deliver a certain mass
Refractive index	The extent to which light is bent or refractive when traveling through the interface of two substances	Serum protein concentration measured in a refractometer

Chemical properties determine how substances will react with each other in a given physical environment. Chemical properties include ionization potential, solubility, electronegativity, and oxidation state (Table 3-2). Unlike physical properties, if a chemical reaction is used to measure a chemical property, the reaction may change the property in the process. In chemistry, electronegativity may be measured by combining a negative compound with a positive compound, or oxidation state may be measured by testing the degree of reduction of one compound by another.

Table 3-2   Chemical Properties

Property	Observation	Examples of Laboratory Application
Ionization potential	Tendency to dissociate	Complete or partial dissociation of acids in solution
Solubility	Ability to dissolve in water or another solvent	Injected medications, not easily soluble in water, mixed with a solubilizing agent to facilitate their activity in the body
Electronegativity	Attraction to a positive pole	Electrophoretic migration to the positive pole by negatively charged particles, such as nucleic acids
Oxidation state	The charge of an ion or compound resulting from the relative number of associated electrons	Ferrous iron converted to ferric iron by ferritin; serum ferritin levels measured in iron studies for anemia

SYSTEMS OF MEASUREMENT

Measurement is expressed as a numerical description of properties in units, or **units of measure**. A unit of measure defines the dimension or magnitude of something. In blood analysis, a red blood cell can be described in terms of its diameter, or a blood sample may be described in terms of the number of red blood cells per unit volume.

There are seven basic dimensions: amount (number of units), mass, length, time, temperature, electric current, and luminosity (luminous intensity). A group of units measured together is a **system of measure**. The most commonly used systems of measure are the metric system, the Systeme Internationale (SI), the United States customary system (USCS), and the British imperial system (BIS). Although the metric system is used for most laboratory applications, the USCS and the BIS may also be encountered in laboratory work, as when reagents are supplied by the gallon or pound. Because of the complex and often confusing nature of these systems, their use is not frequent in scientific applications. A list of these units and a comparison with metric units are shown in Appendix G.

In 1960, the Conférence Générale des Poids et Mesures (CGPM) adopted the International System of Units or **SI system**, measured in metric units. Originally designed for physics, modifications to the SI system are allowed to make its use more practical for clinical work.

Properties of the SI System

The SI system consists of **basic properties** and **derived properties**. There are seven basic properties of the SI system (Table 3-3). Basic properties, such as mass and length, are not calculated from other properties; they are directly measured. In contrast, the derived properties, such as density and concentration, are multiples or ratios of basic properties (Box 3-2).

Table 3-3	Basic and Derived Properties of the SI System		
Property	Symbol	Unit	Unit Symbol
Basic Properties			
Mass	M, m	Kilogram	kg
Length	L, l	Meter	m
Time	T, t	Second	s
Current		Ampere	A
Temperature	T,	Kelvin	K
Luminous intensity	I, J	Candela	Cd
Amount	N, n	Mole	Mol
Derived Properties			
Volume	V	Cubic meter, liter	m³, L

Continued

Table 3-3	**Basic and Derived Properties of the SI System—cont'd**		
Property	Symbol	Unit	Unit Symbol
Area	A	Square meter	m^2
Units		International unit	Int. unit, IU
Mass density	Δ	Kilograms per liter	kg/L
Mass rate	$\Delta m/\Delta t$	Kilograms per second	kg/s
Catalytic activity	z	Katal	kat, mol/s
Concentration (molarity)	c	Moles per liter	mol/L
Content (molality)	n_c/m_s	Moles per kilogram	mol/kg
Osmolarity	OsM	Osmoles per liter	osmol/L
Number of entities	N	Unity	1, 2, 3, ...
Pressure	P	Pascal	Pa, Pa/m^2

Box 3-2	**Basic and Derived Properties**

The liter, which is a primary unit of the metric system, is not a basic property in the SI system. Rather, the liter is a derived property in the SI system because it is volume derived from cubic distance (centiliter^3). The mole (6.023×10^{23} molecules) is a basic property, whereas concentration in moles/liter is a derived property in the SI system.

The Metric System

The metric system is designed to work with decimal notation. It is composed of primary units and prefixes. The primary units of the metric system are the **gram** for mass, **meter** for length, and **liter** for volume. These primary units are comparable to but distinct from the basic units of the SI system discussed earlier. The SI system basic unit of weight is a kilogram, rather than a gram. The liter is a derived unit in the SI system. The meter is the same in both systems. Prefixes to the primary units of the metric system are used to conveniently express a wide range of measurements (Table 3-4).

The terms in Table 3-4 more than cover the range of measurements in the clinical laboratory. Common laboratory procedures require practical knowledge of numbers from the pico- to the tera- range (Box 3-3). Liquids are frequently measured in milliliters or $\frac{1}{1,000}$ of a liter. More precise liquid delivery pipets can measure microliters or $\frac{1}{1,000,000}$ liter volumes. The higher multiple prefixes are used with automated systems and high-speed computers to express increasing amounts of information processed per second. Gigabytes (1,000,000,000 bytes) and terabytes (1,000,000,000,000 bytes) are now common terms. Clinical laboratory tests now include genomic analyses. Three billion units of information (nucleotides) are present in the human genome. Advanced

Table 3-4 SI Prefixes Used With the Metric System

SI Prefix	Symbol	Value	Power of 10	Name
Novena, Xenno		1,000,000,000,000,000,000,000,000,000	10^{27}	Octillion
Yotta		1,000,000,000,000,000,000,000,000	10^{24}	Septillion
Zetta		1,000,000,000,000,000,000,000	10^{21}	Sextillion
Exa	E	1,000,000,000,000,000,000	10^{18}	Quintillion
Peta	P	1,000,000,000,000,000	10^{15}	Quadrillion
Tera	T	1,000,000,000,000	10^{12}	Trillion
Giga	G	1,000,000,000	10^{9}	Billion
Mega	M	1,000,000	10^{6}	Million
Kilo	K	1,000	10^{3}	Thousand
Hecto	H	100	10^{2}	Hundred
Deca	Da	10	10^{1}	Ten
No Prefix		$10^{0} = 1$	10^{0}	Primary units, no prefix
Deci	D	0.1	10^{-1}	Tenth
Centi	C	0.01	10^{-2}	Hundredth
Milli	M	0.001	10^{-3}	Thousandth
Micro	μ	0.000001	10^{-6}	Millionth
Nano	N	0.000000001	10^{-9}	Billionth
Pico	P	0.000000000001	10^{-12}	Trillionth
Femto	F	0.000000000000001	10^{-15}	Quadrillionth
Atto	A	0.000000000000000001	10^{-18}	Quintillionth

Box 3-3 Terms for Large Numbers

In the European system, 10^{9} is a milliard, 10^{12} is a billion, 10^{15} is a billiard, 10^{18} is a trillion, 10^{21} is a trilliard, 10^{24} is a quadrillion, and 10^{27} is a quadrilliard. To avoid confusion in expressing these numbers, the SI prefixes are preferred.

technologies used to determine the order of these nucleotides generate terabytes of data that are analyzed using powerful computer systems. A related type of study involves metagenomics, which involves determining all genes in all microbes in an environment. In this application, there are much shorter genomes but millions of genomes to be determined (Box 3-4).

Box 3-4 The Largest Number

Mathematically, numbers can exceed those indicated in Table 3-4. The highest number that can be physically represented is 10^{80}, which is the number of protons in the universe. There is no largest counting number because any large number can be exceeded by adding 1 to it. The largest named number is the googolplex, which is 10 to the googol power. A googol is 10^{100}.

Box 3-5 Obsolete Terms

In older procedures, one may find references to lambda (λ), gamma (γ), and micron (μ). Lambda is an old term for microliter (10^{-6} liter). In an unrelated application, lambda is also used as a term meaning wavelength. Gamma is an old term for microgram (10^{-6} gram). Mu, or micron, is an old term for micrometer (10^{-6} meter). These terms are no longer used. Instead, express units using the micro- prefixes. A practice that should be avoided is the use of more than one prefix. It is confusing to express units with millimicro- prefixes when nano- means the same thing.

Another unit of measure in the metric system is the **angstrom** (Å). The angstrom is one-tenth nanometer or 10^{-10} meter. This unit is used in expressions of wavelengths, electron microscopy, and crystallography. In molecular diagnostics, nucleic acid concentrations are determined by reading absorbance of light at a wavelength of 260 nm (2,600 Å), whereas proteins absorb light at 280 nm (2,600 Å). This level of measurement is also used in subcellular analysis. A ribosome (the cellular organelle where proteins are made) measures about 250 angstroms or 25 nanometers in diameter (Box 3-5).

TIME

A measurement frequently made in the laboratory is time. The second is a basic property of the SI system, used with prefixes (milliseconds, microseconds). Seconds with prefixes are also used in the metric system. Measures of time in minutes, hours, and days are used with the metric system, but without prefixes.

In the laboratory, reactions occur in seconds, minutes, or hours. Enzyme activity can be measured by the accumulation of the product of the enzyme reaction over time. The amount of substance in a solution is also measured by the accumulation of product over time as it is altered by an enzyme. In the SI system, enzyme activity is measured by the **international unit** (IU). One IU of enzyme activity is defined as the amount of an enzyme that will catalyze the reaction of 1 micromole of substrate in 1 minute (with optimal temperature, pH, and substrate concentration).

Time is also a useful way to identify specimens. Electronic records identify specimens by the date of accession using the **Julian Day Calendar** system, in which each day of the year is designated as a number from 1 to 365 (366 in leap years). A specimen accession number may include the year, the day, and the number of the sample received that day as a unique identifier. Days measured in this way facilitate calculation of time periods by subtraction. If a test is received on day 165 of the year, and another sample is received on day 358, the time between tests in days is quickly determined:

$$
\begin{array}{r}
358 \\
-\ 165 \\
\hline
193 \text{ days}
\end{array}
$$

Spreadsheets and automated laboratory systems can convert days to weeks or months, if required.

Laboratories measure the time from sample accession to result reporting (turnaround time) as a performance metric. Turnaround time can be in minutes for some chemistry tests to weeks for genomic analyses. Culturing of pathogens may take days. Physicians may ask for an estimate of turnaround time to know when to schedule patient visits.

TEMPERATURE AND HEAT

Heat may be defined as the energy in matter that results in motion of particles within it. This form of heat is also called **thermal energy**. The tendency of matter to gain or lose thermal energy, sensed as coldness or warmness, is **temperature**. Thermal energy will always move from warmer matter to cooler matter. Different types of materials transfer energy at different rates.

Temperature is a quantitative characteristic of substances. In the laboratory, temperature is measured in many applications. The storage temperatures of reagents, reaction temperatures, and instrument block and chamber temperatures, and also room temperature, are monitored in the medical laboratory. Temperature is important for the reliable performance of reagents as well as for integrity of specimens. Material stored or used at the wrong temperature can result in erroneous results. If a chemical conversion of a substrate proceeds at optimal rate at room temperature, and the room temperature in the laboratory is outside an acceptable range, the resulting products of the reaction may not reflect the actual amount of substrate. Specimens containing temperature-sensitive substances are held at refrigerator temperature and should not be exposed to room temperature for extended times. The effect on such substances occurs more quickly in small samples because they will come to the higher temperature more quickly than samples in larger volumes. It is therefore very important to recognize temperature requirements and to understand the differences in temperature readings, which are often on different scales.

Temperature Scales

Three temperature scales are commonly encountered in U.S. laboratories. All three scales are measured in thermal energy units or **degrees**. In the metric system, temperature is expressed in degrees **Celsius** (also once called centigrade). In the English system, the **Fahrenheit** scale is used. The **Kelvin** scale is used in the SI system. Most procedures encountered in the clinical laboratory are in degrees Celsius, although some Fahrenheit measurements may be found. The Kelvin scale is preferred in physics. The size of degree units is the same in the Celsius and Kelvin scales. The degrees in Fahrenheit are smaller than Celsius or Kelvin degrees. The **zero point** of all three scales is also different, based on the definition of 0 degrees in the three systems:

Zero degrees Kelvin is defined as the theoretical temperature at which matter has no more thermal energy to lose, also referred to as **absolute zero.**

Zero degrees Celsius is defined by the point that pure water freezes.

Zero degrees Fahrenheit is the lowest temperature attainable in a salt and ice mixture.

The three systems of temperature measurement are displayed in Figure 3-1. Absolute zero is 0 Kelvin, −273.15° Celsius, and −459.67° Fahrenheit. Neither the term "degree" nor the degree symbol "°" is used with the Kelvin scale. The freezing point of pure water is 0° Celsius, 32° Fahrenheit, and 273 Kelvin (rounded off). The boiling point of pure water is 100° Celsius, 212° Fahrenheit,

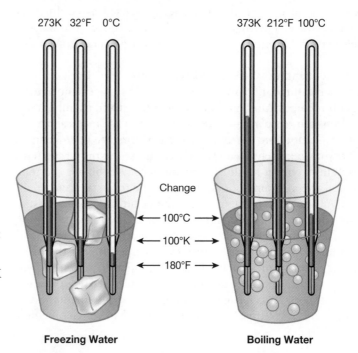

273K 32°F 0°C   373K 212°F 100°C

Change

← 100°C →
← 100°K →
← 180°F →

Figure 3-1 Degrees K, C, and F are defined in different ways. The range of temperatures from freezing water to boiling water is 273 to 373 K (100 degrees K), 0 to 100°C (100°C), and 32 to 212°F (180°F). As a result, there are $^{180}/_{100}$ or $^9/_5$ degrees F for each K or C degree.

Freezing Water   **Boiling Water**

and 373 Kelvin. The normal temperature of the human body is 37° Celsius, 98.6° Fahrenheit, and 310 Kelvin. Human pathogens are often cultured at body temperature for laboratory analysis.

Temperature Conversions

Although the metric Celsius temperature degrees are preferred for most clinical laboratory applications, any of the three temperature systems may be encountered and it will become necessary to convert from one temperature scale to another. There are several ways to do this. The simplest way is to use computer and calculator programs in which the input temperature is automatically converted to the desired scale. Another simple method is to use conversion tables that can be found in many text and reference books.

If electronic and tabular conversion data are not available, temperatures can be converted by calculation. Celsius and Kelvin scales are based on the same degree unit, so conversion between these two scales is straightforward. Zero degrees Celsius is 273 Kelvin (absolute zero is 0 Kelvin, −273° Celsius), so to convert Kelvin to Celsius, subtract 273° from the Kelvin temperature. To convert Celsius to Kelvin, add 273.

```
Celsius degrees = Kelvin - 273
       C = K - 273
Kelvin = Celsius degrees + 273
       K = C + 273
```

10°C converted to Kelvin would be:

```
K = C + 273
K = 10 + 273 = 283 K
```

380 K converted to °C would be:

```
C = K - 273
C = 380 - 273 = 107°C
```

At the freezing point of water, which is 0°C, the Fahrenheit reading is 32°. Water boils at 100°C, which is 212°F. The range from boiling to freezing of pure water is 100° − 0° = 100 in degrees Celsius and 212° − 32° = 180 in degrees Fahrenheit. Fahrenheit degrees are thus 1.8 times smaller than Celsius (and Kelvin) degrees; that is, one degree Celsius (or Kelvin) is equal to 1.8 Fahrenheit degrees. The relationship between Fahrenheit and Celsius degrees is therefore:

```
180/100 = 1.8 = 9/5
```

Every Celsius degree is equivalent to ⅑ or 1.8 Fahrenheit degrees (Box 3-6).

To convert Celsius to Fahrenheit, start by multiplying the Celsius reading by 1.8 or ⅑. Because 0°C is 32°F, add 32 to obtain the final number of Fahrenheit degrees, thus producing the following formula:

```
°F = [ (9/5) x °C ] + 32°
```

Conversely, every Fahrenheit degree is equivalent to ⅟₁.₈ or ⁵⁄₉ Celsius degree. To convert Fahrenheit to Celsius, start by subtracting 32° from the Fahrenheit reading, and then multiply the adjusted Fahrenheit reading by 0.556 or ⁵⁄₉.

$$°C = (°F - 32°) \times 5/9$$

Another conversion formula can be derived from this equation:

$$°C = (°F - 32°) \times 5/9$$
$$9 \times °C = (°F - 32°) \times 5$$
$$9 \times °C = 5 \times °F - 160°$$

or

$$9C = 5F - 160°$$

The latter formula is preferred by some laboratorians, as it does not involve the fractional expressions, ⁵⁄₉ and ⁹⁄₅ that might lead to error.

To convert Fahrenheit degrees to Kelvin degrees, first convert the Fahrenheit reading to Celsius and then add 273. Thus, **73°F** would be:

$$°C = (°F - 32°) \times 5/9$$
$$°C = (73° - 32°) \times 5/9$$
$$°C = (41°) \times 5/9 = 22.8°C$$
$$22.8°C + 273 = 295.8 \text{ K}$$

To convert Kelvin to Fahrenheit degrees, reverse the process. Subtract 273 from the Kelvin reading to obtain degrees Celsius, and then convert the Celsius reading to Fahrenheit. **373 K** would be:

$$°C = K - 273$$
$$°C = 373 - 273 = -100$$
$$°F = [(9/5) \times °C] + 32°$$
$$°F = [(9/5) \times 100] + 32°$$
$$°F = [180] +32 = 212$$

Box 3-6	Quick Temperature Comparisons

When comparing equivalent temperatures in the Celsius and Fahrenheit scales, consider landmark temperatures such as 0°C = 32°F or 100°C = 212°F. The higher reading will be the Fahrenheit reading.

PRACTICE PROBLEMS

Types of Measurement

Indicate whether the following results are quantitative or qualitative.

1. The presence or absence of a color
2. White cells per μL blood
3. Glucose levels in blood
4. Bacterial colony morphology
5. Blood alcohol content

Types of Properties

Indicate whether the following properties are physical or chemical.

6. Mass
7. Odor
8. Solubility
9. Length
10. Ionization potential
11. Oxidation state
12. Freezing point
13. Density
14. Temperature
15. Electronegativity

Systems of Measure

16. List the three primary units of the metric system for mass, length, and volume. What unit symbol is used with each unit?

For the following SI units:

   a. Indicate whether the unit is basic or derived
   b. Give the unit and unit symbol for each of the units

17. Volume
18. Mass
19. Time
20. Density
21. Current
22. Concentration
23. Luminous intensity

Continued

24. Pressure

25. Temperature

Give the unit and unit symbol for each of the units in questions 16 to 25.

Prefixes
Name the prefix, symbol, and power of 10 for the following orders of magnitude.

26. 0.000001

27. 1,000,000

28. 1,000,000,000

29. 0.1

30. 0.001

31. 1,000

32. 0.000000001

33. 0.000000000001

34. 1,000,000,000,000

35. 100

36. 1

37. Write the expression of an angstrom in meters.

38. A millimeter is how many meters?

39. A microliter is how many liters?

40. A kilogram is how many grams?

Heat

41. Temperature is what type of substance property: physical or chemical)?

42. Motion of particles in matter is _____ energy.

43. True or False? Heat will always move from the cooler to the warmer object.

Give the basis for zero degrees for each of the temperature scales.

44. Fahrenheit

45. Celsius

46. Kelvin

Temperature Scales

47. Which of the three temperature degrees are equal in scale?

48. 0°C is what temperature on the Fahrenheit scale?

PRACTICE PROBLEMS *cont.*

49. 0°F is what temperature on the Celsius scale?

50. 0 K is what temperature on the Celsius scale?

51. 0°C is what temperature on the Kelvin scale?

Temperature Conversions

Convert to Celsius.

52. 100°F

53. 25.0°F

54. 150°F

55. −25.0°F

56. 212°F

57. 50.0 K

58. 500 K

59. 75.0 K

60. 100 K

Convert to Kelvin.

61. 150°C

62. −100°C

63. 25.0°C

64. 500°C

65. 22.0°F

66. 212°F

67. −10.0°F

68. 100°F

69. 0°F

70. −55.0°F

Convert to Fahrenheit.

71. 23.0°C

72. −50.0°C

73. 37.0°C

74. 3.56°C

75. −29.0°C

76. 20.0 K

Continued

PRACTICE PROBLEMS *cont.*

77. 250 K

78. 100 K

79. 350 K

80. 0 K

81. The laboratory room temperature reads 32.0°C. Is this too warm, too cool, or correct for room temperature (72°F–75°F)?

82. A hot plate is set to 100°F. Will this boil water?

83. Cultures of yeast (optimal growth temperature, 30°C) are placed in an incubator set at 303 K. Is this correct?

84. Water-ice mixtures freeze at

  a. 500 K
  b. 0°C
  c. –32°F
  d. 100°C

85. Will heat-loving (thermophilic) bacteria collected from a 100°C oceanic heat vent grow optimally at 300 K?

86. A body thermometer reads 37°C. Is this normal?

87. The freezer is set to 20°C. If water freezes at 32°F, is this correct?

88. A water bath in the laboratory is set at 50°F. The protocol calls for a water bath set at 50°C. Should the bath temperature be adjusted up or down?

89. The freezer alarm has sounded. The freezer was set at –80°C. The temperature inside the freezer must have risen above:

  a. 193 K
  b. –20 K
  c. 0 K
  d. –273 K

90. Infectious bacteria grow at human body temperature (98.6°F). Will human cell cultures grow at 310 K?

APPLICATIONS

Hematology

Red blood cell (RBC) indices (also called erythrocyte indices or corpuscular indices) are used to identify types of anemias and other blood disorders. In addition to the RBC count, RBC indices include the RBC size, weight, and hemoglobin (Hb) concentration. Hb contains iron and is the oxygen-carrying protein that is responsible for the color and shape of the RBC. Hb is assessed as weight (hemoglobin, Hb) or by volume (hematocrit, Hct). When both are measured, the Hct in percent should be approximately three times the Hb value.

The overall RBC volume is the mean corpuscular volume (MCV). It is based on the Hct and the RBC count. Normal MCV values for an adult range between 80 and 98 fL. The average weight of the Hb contained in one RBC is the mean corpuscular hemoglobin (MCH). MCH is the quotient of the weight of the Hb (× 10) divided by the RBC count:

$$MCH = \frac{Hb\ (g/dL)\ \times\ 10}{RBC\ count/L}$$

Normal adult values for MCH are 27 to 31 pg.

1. What is the estimated Hct if the Hb is measured at 15.5?
2. What is the estimated Hb value if the Hct is 41%?
3. What is the MCH if the RBC count is 5,000,000 RBC/µL and the Hb is 15 g/dL?

Enzymology

International units (IU) are terms of measure of enzyme activity. IU are measured in terms of amount of substrate (µmol), time of exposure to enzyme (minutes), and reaction volume (mL or L). Adjustments for pH and temperature may also be made if a test reaction is to be carried out under conditions different from those defined by the IU reference. Results for a given reaction are reported in IU/mL or IU/L.

Other types of units may be converted to IU by converting the terms of expression involved. If an enzyme activity is measured in µmol substrate/min/dL, the dL term must be divided by 100 to convert dL to mL or multiplied by 10 to convert dL to L. Activity measured in mg substrate/min/mL is converted to IU by using the atomic weight of the substrate to calculate the number of µmol in 1 mg:

$$1\ mg = 1,000\ \mu g$$

$$\frac{1,000\ \cancel{\mu g}}{(number\ of\ \cancel{\mu g}/\mu mole)} = \mu mole$$

If unit activity of an enzyme is meaured as the amount of enzyme that will hydrolyze 1 µmole substrate in 1 hour in a reaction volume of 1 mL, how many IU would be in 1,500 of these units?

CHAPTER 4

DILUTIONS

A **solution** is the mixture of one substance (**solute**) into another (**solvent**). A **dilution** reduces the concentration of the original solute(s) in the solution. To make a dilution, solvent or other substance, called a **diluent**, is mixed with a solution to decrease the concentration of the solute. Dilutions are quite common in laboratory work. Reagents are often made, shipped, and/or stored in high concentrations that must be adjusted down (diluted with water or other diluent) before use. For example, in molecular diagnostic methods, a buffer used for isolation and purification of nucleic acids is supplied in 3-mL aliquots. Each aliquot is mixed with 27 mL reagent alcohol before use. It is more convenient and cost-effective to ship and store 3 mL of stable reagent than 30 mL of the alcohol mixture, which would evaporate on long storage.

EXPRESSIONS OF DILUTIONS

The preferred way to describe a dilution is by the number of parts of the substance in the *total* number of parts of the final diluted solution. This differs from describing a mixture as a ratio. A ratio is the relative amount of one component to another. Ratio is a more general term and does not designate total volume (see Fig. 2-2).

A dilution can be specifically defined if a volume of the diluted material is given. If 1 mL of a reagent is mixed with 4 mL diluent (total volume, 5 mL), the dilution is defined as 1 mL reagent/5 mL total volume (or 4 mL solvent/5 mL total volume).

The ratio of component parts in a dilution can be determined from the information describing the dilution (Box 4-1). A 3/10 dilution of serum in saline defines a ratio of 3 parts serum:7 parts saline (or 7 parts saline:3 parts serum). The actual volume is not indicated by the ratio. A ratio of 3 parts to 7 parts could be 3 gallons to 7 gallons (total volume 10 gallons), 300 mL to 700 mL (total volume 1,000 mL), or 3 μL to 7 μL (total volume 10 μL).

LEARNING OUTCOMES

- Define expressions of dilutions.
- Calculate the concentration of substance in a mixture after adding other substances to the mixture.
- Describe a dilution in terms of the relative amounts of its component parts.
- Calculate the absolute amount and concentration of a diluted substance.
- Determine the amount of a substance required to make a given volume of its dilution.
- Diagram how to make a series of dilutions.
- Calculate the amount of diluted substance in each step of a dilution series.
- Describe how to make serial fold-dilutions.
- Show applications of dilution series for standards, antibiotic resistance, and antibody titers.

Box 4-1 | **Expressing Ratios and Dilutions**

When writing dilution expressions, a ratio is indicated by a colon ":", whereas a dilution is indicated by a slash "/". When expressing or asking for equivalent ratios, a double colon "::" is used, whereas an equal sign "=" is used for equivalent dilutions.

Consider a mixture of 1 mL serum plus 19 mL saline:

The serum-to-saline ratio (serum:saline) is 1:19
The saline-to-serum ratio (saline:serum) is 19:1

Contrast this with dilutions:

The serum in saline dilution (serum/total) is 1/(1 + 19) = 1/20
The saline in serum dilution (saline/total) is 19/(1 + 19) = 19/20

Dilutions are relative terms, that is, they do not necessarily define the units or the total volume, which can vary, such as making just enough of a mixture of diluted stock solutions to perform the required number of analytical tests. Instructions may read: mix 2 parts reagent A to 3 parts reagent B. If the final volume required was 5 mL, then 2 mL of reagent A would be mixed with 3 mL of reagent B. If the final volume required was 25 mL, then 10 mL reagent A would be mixed with 15 mL reagent B. We can write:

2 parts reagent A / 5 total parts = 10 parts reagent A in 25 total parts.

That is, 2/5 is equivalent to **10/25.**

In contrast to ratios, dilutions define the total amount (or multiple of) components (Box 4-2). Expression of a dilution implies bringing one reagent *up to the final volume* with the other component(s) in the mixture. Procedures that call for a 2/5 dilution of reagent A in reagent B indicate the total volume and the amount of reagent A, but not the amount of reagent B. One would bring 2 mL reagent A up to 5 mL total volume with reagent B. For 25 mL, bring 10 mL reagent A up to 25 mL with reagent B. In practice, dilutions may be prepared by adding a substance, such as serum, and diluents, such as

---

Box 4-2 | **Distinguishing Between Ratios and Dilutions**

It is important to distinguish ratio from dilution when performing a procedure. The difference becomes small when the dilution or ratio is large. A 1/1,000 dilution is not much different from a 1:1,000 ratio (which is a 1/1,001 dilution). In contrast, a 1/2 dilution is a decrease in concentration of the diluted substance by half (1 part in a final volume of 2 parts), whereas a 1:2 ratio is a concentration decrease by two-thirds (1 part in a final volume of 3 parts). A 1:1 ratio is equivalent to a 1/2 dilution of each component. A 1/1 dilution means the substance is not diluted at all.

saline together. The amount of diluent is determined by subtracting the volume of serum from the total volume.

CALCULATING CONCENTRATIONS OF DILUTED SUBSTANCES

To calculate the concentration of a substance in a mixture after dilution, multiply the starting concentration of the substance (before dilution) by the dilution.

Starting concentration x Dilution = Diluted concentration

Starting with 6.0 μg glucose/mL, a 1/10 dilution of this material would be:

6.0 *μg/mL* x 1/10 = 0.60 *μg/mL*

A 1/100 dilution of the original substance would contain 0.060 μg glucose/mL or 60 ng glucose/mL:

6.0 *μg/mL* x 1/100 = 0.06 *μg/mL* = 60 ng/mL

It may be necessary to determine the amount of a substance required to make a dilution. The absolute amount of the substance will depend on the total volume of diluted substance to be prepared. Suppose a procedure required 50 mL of the 0.60 mg/mL glucose solution. One way to find the volume of undiluted glucose required is first to determine the absolute amount (mass) of glucose contained in the 50 mL. The mass of glucose required is calculated by multiplying the diluted concentration by the desired volume (50 mL):

0.60 *μg/mL* x 50 mL = 30 *μg*

The volume of the 6.0 μg/mL glucose solution is determined by dividing the absolute amount (mass) of glucose required by 6.0 mg/mL:

30 *μg* /(6.0 *μg/mL*) = 5.0 mL

It would therefore take 5 mL of the undiluted glucose solution to make 50 mL of the diluted glucose solution. To make the dilution, bring 5.0 mL of the 6.0 μg/mL solution to 50 mL with water.

Use a reverse of this process to determine how much of a diluted substance can be made from a given volume of undiluted substance. Suppose only 2.0 mL of the 6.0 μg/mL glucose solution is available. How much of the 0.60 μg/mL dilution can be made? To find out, first calculate the mass of glucose in the 2.0 mL. To find this, multiply the concentration of the undiluted substance times the available volume.

6.0 *μg/mL* x 2.0 mL = 12 *μg*

To determine the volume of the dilution that can be made, divide the amount available (12 μg) by the diluted concentration:

12 *μg*/(0.60 *μg/mL*) = 20 mL

To make 20 mL of the 0.60 μg/mL glucose, bring the 2.0 mL of the 6.0 μg/mL glucose to 20 mL with water.

An alternative way of determining the dilution volumes is to use ratio and proportion. Because a 1/10 dilution will yield a 0.60 µg/mL glucose solution. For a volume of 50 mL, therefore, find an equivalent fraction to $\frac{1}{10}$ with a denominator of 50:

$$\frac{1}{10} = x/50$$

Solve for x:

$$x = \frac{50}{10} = 5.0$$

5.0 mL of the 6.0 µg/mL solution plus 45 mL (50 mL – 5 mL) of diluent will make 50 mL of the 0.60 µg/mL solution.

Use the reverse process to determine how much diluted solution that could be made from a given amount of the 6.0 µg/mL solution. If 2 mL of the stock solution is available, what total volume of 0.60 µg/mL solution can be made? An equivalent fraction to $\frac{1}{10}$ in this case would have 2 in the numerator:

$$\frac{1}{10} = 2/x$$

Solving for x,

$$x/10 = 2.0$$

$$x = 20$$

2.0 mL of the 6.0 µg/mL solution can make 20 mL of 0.60 µg/mL solution.

COMPONENT PARTS OF DILUTIONS

Increasing the volume of a solution using a diluent is the simplest form of dilution. As shown in the previous section, the resulting dilution contains the same amount (mass) of the substance at a concentration that is lower (and a volume that is higher) than the original solution. Instructions may read: "Dilute 2 mL of serum with 8 mL of saline." This is carried out by adding 8 mL of saline to 2 mL of serum (or adding 2 mL serum to 8 mL saline) in a tube or other vessel that can hold 10 mL.

$$2 \text{ mL serum} + 8 \text{ mL saline} = 10 \text{ mL diluted serum}$$

The serum in total dilution is:

$$\frac{2 \text{ mL serum}}{10 \text{ mL total}} = \frac{1}{x}$$

$$2x = 10$$

$$x = 5$$

$$\frac{2 \text{ mL serum}}{10 \text{ mL total}} = \frac{1}{5}$$

This is a 1/5 dilution of the serum.

What is the dilution of plasma when 3.0 mL plasma is added to 27 mL diluent?

$$\frac{3.0 \text{ mL plasma}}{30 \text{ mL total}} = \frac{1}{x}$$

$$3x = 30$$

$$x = 10$$

$$\frac{3.0 \text{ mL serum}}{30 \text{ mL total}} = \frac{1}{10}$$

A dilution containing 3.0 mL plasma mixed with 27 mL diluent is a 1/10 dilution of the plasma.

The amount of substance in a specified volume of a diluted mixture can be determined by the following formula:

Total volume of dilution x Specified dilution = Volume of substance

Using this formula, the **amount of serum** in 3.0 mL of a 1/5 dilution (1.0 mL serum in every 5.0 mL total volume) can be calculated:

$$3.0 \text{ mL} \times \frac{1.0 \text{ mL serum}}{5.0 \text{ mL total mixture}} = 0.60 \text{ mL serum}$$

This mixture is also a 4/5 dilution of saline in serum. The amount of saline in 3.0 mL of the 4/5 dilution of saline in serum is:

$$3.0 \text{ mL} \times \frac{4.0 \text{ mL saline}}{5.0 \text{ mL total mixture}} = 2.4 \text{ mL saline}$$

Alternatively, the amount of diluent required is the total volume minus the volume of serum:

$$3.0 \text{ mL total volume} - 0.60 \text{ mL serum}$$
$$= 2.4 \text{ mL of saline diluent}$$

Dilution Volumes

Dilutions are prepared by starting with a certain amount of substance in a volumetric container, then bringing that substance up to the final volume with diluent. When making a dilution, rather than mixing the indicated ratio of substances together (e.g., a measured 500 mL volume of substance mixed with a measured 1,500 mL volume of diluent to make 2,000 mL of a 1/4 dilution), the best approach is to place the substance to be diluted in a volumetric container and then add the diluent to the final desired volume. With some substances, the method of mixing the two measured volumes first will not result in the correct volume and concentration (Fig. 4-1). A mixture of 0.5 L alcohol with 0.5 L of water (1:1 ratio or 1/2 dilution of alcohol in water) will not yield 1 L (0.5 + 0.5). This is because the alcohol and molecules arrange themselves so that the final

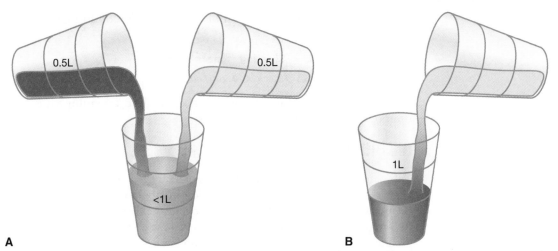

Figure 4-1 Mixing of a substance and diluent with measured volumes of 0.5 L each may not produce a mixture with a total volume of 1 L (A). To ensure that the mixture will be 1 L, measure 0.5 mL of the substance, and bring the mixture to 1 L with the diluent (B).

volume is less than 1 L. The dilution of alcohol will then be 1 in less than 2. To make this alcohol dilution, start with 0.5 L of alcohol, and add water up to 1 L.

Dilution Concentrations

The concentration of a dilution is the product of the original concentration and the dilution, or the quotient of the original concentration of a substance divided by the **dilution factor** (Box 4-3). The dilution factor is the *reciprocal of the dilution.* (Refer to Chapter 1 on reciprocals.) A dilution of 1 mL into a total volume of 5 mL is a 1/5 dilution and has a dilution factor of 5. A dilution of 3 mL in a total volume of 10 mL is a 3/10 dilution and has a dilution factor of 10/3.

The final concentration of a diluted substance is determined using the dilution factor. Divide the starting concentration of the substance by the dilution factor.

Starting concentration / Dilution factor = Dilution concentration

Box 4-3	Expressing Concentrations

Concentrations are expressed in a variety of ways. Substance concentrations are expressed as percent, units of weight/units of volume, molarity, molality, or osmolality. Complex biological fluids, such as urine, bile, blood, serum, or plasma, are considered undiluted, 100%, or 1/1.

To calculate the concentration of a 1/10 dilution of 20 mg/mL sodium chloride:

20 mg/mL = Starting concentration

(20 mg/mL) /10 = 2.0 mg/mL

Dividing by the dilution factor is an alternative to multiplying by the dilution, as described earlier.

DILUTIONS AS CORRECTION FACTORS

Substance concentrations in biological materials can vary widely. The most efficient range of concentrations of detection in laboratory assays, however, may be relatively narrow. If an instrument accurately measures concentrations up to 500 mg/dL, then solutions with concentrations above this range may not be accurately measured. Laboratory test methods are designed to be sufficiently sensitive to low levels of analyte (the substance measured), but, as a result, they may have measurement ranges that do not include high concentrations. To measure a substance with a high concentration of analyte accurately, the substance must be diluted such that the diluted concentration is within the measurement range. Once the analyte concentration in the diluted sample is determined, the original concentration can be calculated by multiplying the diluted concentration by the dilution factor. The dilution factor represents the number of times the original sample was diluted, so it is "undiluted" by multiplication.

Diluted concentration x Dilution factor = Starting concentration

Suppose a 1/20 dilution (dilution factor = **20**) of a plasma sample was made before measurement of analyte A, and a reading of 25 mg/dL resulted. The concentration of analyte A in the plasma is:

25 mg/dL x 20 = 500 mg/dL

For many assays, a dilution factor is included in the protocol. Some instrument software programs automatically multiply by the dilution factor to yield the original concentration, after reading from the dilution. A dilution factor may be entered before the reading or set as a default if the same dilution factor is always used. For new assays or highly variable samples, the dilution required may not be known. In this case, depending on the availability of sample and diluents, multiple dilutions may be made, starting with one dilution, reading it, and determining from the reading whether a higher or lower dilution is required.

Dilution factors may also be used to correct for sample adjustments, if allowed by the procedure. Suppose a protein assay requires 5.0 mL of sample, but only 3.0 mL of sample is available. The technologist can perform the assay by bringing the 3.0 mL of sample to 5.0 mL with the appropriate diluent. Suppose the test result of the diluted specimen is 28.0 μg/mL. To find the original concentration, multiply by the dilution factor. In this case, the dilution is 3.0 mL sample in 5.0 mL total or 3/5. The dilution factor is **5/3**. The protein concentration in the sample is:

28.0 μg/mL x 5/3 = 46.7 μg/mL

When correcting or adjusting concentrations in this way, the correction (dilution factor) will always be more than 1. The corrected or adjusted concentration will always be greater than the concentration of the diluted specimen.

DILUTION SERIES

There are two ways to make a dilution series (Fig. 4-2). One way is to make independent dilutions of the original substance (dilution series). The other way is to make one dilution from the original substance, and use that dilution to make a second dilution, and then use the second dilution to make a third dilution (serial dilution).

Independent Dilutions

Some laboratory procedures call for different concentrations of the same substance or for extremely dilute concentrations. Both are achieved by making a series of dilutions. In a dilution series, the concentration of the diluted substance decreases as the dilution increases.

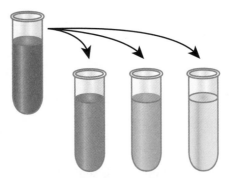

Independent Dilution Series

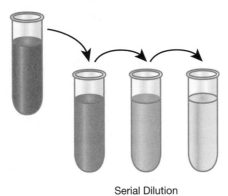

Serial Dilution

Figure 4-2 A set of dilutions may be prepared by making a series of independent dilutions (*top*) or by making a serial dilution (*bottom*).

Here is an example of making independent dilutions. Suppose a protocol requires reagent A diluted 1/2, 1/10, and 1/20. No volume is specified, so the simplest way to make these independent dilutions is to vary the volumes of diluent. Using three tubes, add 1 mL substance to each of three separate tubes, and bring the first tube up to 2.0 mL, the second tube up to 10 mL, and the third tube up to 20 mL.

$$\text{For each dilution:} \quad \frac{1 \text{ mL substance}}{\text{Total volume of dilution}}$$

$$\text{For the } 1/2 \text{ dilution:} \quad \frac{1.0 \text{ mL reagent A}}{2.0 \text{ mL total}} = \frac{1}{2}$$

$$\text{For the } 1/10 \text{ dilution:} \quad \frac{1.0 \text{ mL reagent A}}{10 \text{ mL total}} = \frac{1}{10}$$

$$\text{For the } 1/20 \text{ dilution:} \quad \frac{1.0 \text{ mL reagent A}}{20 \text{ mL total}} = \frac{1}{20}$$

If the procedure calls for 50 mL of each dilution, then ratio and proportion can be used to determine the amount of reagent A for each dilution.

$$\text{For the } 1/2 \text{ dilution:} \quad \frac{x \text{ mL reagent A}}{50 \text{ mL total}} = \frac{1}{2}$$

$$x \text{ mL} \times 2 = 1 \times 50$$

$$x = 25 \text{ mL reagent A}$$

$$\text{For the } 1/10 \text{ dilution:} \quad \frac{x \text{ mL reagent A}}{50 \text{ mL total}} = \frac{1}{10}$$

$$x \text{ mL} \times 10 = 1 \times 50$$

$$x = 5 \text{ mL reagent A}$$

$$\text{For the } 1/20 \text{ dilution:} \quad \frac{x \text{ mL reagent A}}{50 \text{ mL total}} = \frac{1}{20}$$

$$x \text{ mL} \times 20 = 1 \times 50$$

$$x = 2.5 \text{ mL reagent A}$$

Add 25 mL, 5 mL, and 2.5 mL of reagent A respectively to each of three tubes, and bring the volume in each tube to 50 mL with diluent.

Suppose the procedure calls for 1.0 mL of each dilution, rather than 50 mL. This requires calculating how much reagent A will be required to bring the volume to 1.0 mL.

$$\text{For the } 1/2 \text{ dilution:} \quad \frac{x \text{ mL reagent A}}{1.0 \text{ mL total}} = \frac{1}{2}$$

$$x \text{ mL} \times 2 = 1.0 \times 1$$

$$x = 0.50 \text{ mL reagent A}$$

$$\text{For the } 1/10 \text{ dilution:} \quad \frac{x \text{ mL reagent A}}{1.0 \text{ mL total}} = \frac{1}{10}$$

$$x \text{ mL} \times 10 = 1.0 \times 1$$

$$x = 0.10 \text{ mL reagent A}$$

$$\text{for the 1/20 dilution: } \frac{x \text{ mL reagent A}}{1.0 \text{ mL total}} = \frac{1}{20}$$

$$x \text{ mL} \times 20 = 1.0 \times 1$$

$$x = 0.050 \text{ mL reagent A}$$

To make the 1/2, 1/10, and 1/20 dilutions, add 0.50 mL, 0.10 mL, and 0.25 mL of reagent A, respectively, and bring each volume to 1.0 mL.

Serial Dilutions

Independent dilution series are not used as frequently as serial dilutions, especially when the amounts of substance to be diluted and diluent are limited (Box 4-4). In the serial dilution method, the original substance is diluted, and subsequent dilutions are made using each previous dilution to make the next.

Using the volumes and dilutions (1/2, 1/10, and 1/20) in the previous examples, a serial dilution is made by bringing 1.0 mL reagent A to 2.0 mL, followed by bringing 1.0 mL of that 1/2 dilution to 10 mL, and finally bringing 1 mL of the 1/10 dilution to 20 mL. Note that this method uses 1 mL of reagent A, whereas the independent dilution series uses 3.0 mL reagent A. The serial method yields dilutions up to 1/400, compared with 1/50 for the example dilutions series shown earlier.

$$\frac{1.0 \text{ mL reagent A}}{2.0 \text{ mL total}} = \frac{1}{2}$$

$$\frac{1.0 \text{ mL (1/2 reagent A)}}{10 \text{ mL total}} = \frac{1}{2} \times \frac{1}{10} = \frac{1}{20}$$

$$\frac{1.0 \text{ mL (1/20 reagent A)}}{20 \text{ mL total}} = \frac{1}{2} \times \frac{1}{10} \times \frac{1}{20} = \frac{1}{20} \times \frac{1}{20} = \frac{1}{400}$$

If the procedure calls for a specified volume (e.g., 50 mL) of each dilution, then ratio and proportion may be used to determine the amount of reagent A and diluted reagent A required, as described earlier.

$$\text{for the first dilution: } \frac{x \text{ mL reagent A}}{50 \text{ mL total}} = \frac{1}{2}$$

$$x = 25 \text{ mL reagent A in 50 mL}$$

$$\text{for the second dilution: } \frac{x \text{ mL (1/2) reagent A}}{50 \text{ mL total}} = \frac{1}{10}$$

$$x = 5 \text{ mL (1/10) diluted reagent A in 50 mL}$$

Box 4-4 Serial Dilutions

An independent dilution of 1/400 would require 399 mL of diluent to 1 mL reagent A. It would also produce 400 mL of diluted reagent A, which may be a larger volume than required. The serial dilution method produces the desired concentration using less diluent and in a small, more practical volume (20 mL in the example given).

$$\text{for the third dilution:} \quad \frac{x \text{ mL (1/10) reagent A}}{50 \text{ mL total}} = \frac{1}{20}$$

$$x = 2.5 \text{ mL (1/10) diluted reagent A in 50 mL}$$

Using this approach, **25 mL** reagent A, **5 mL** of (1/2 reagent A dilution), and **2.5 mL** of (1/10 reagent A dilution) would be brought to 50 mL for each of the dilutions.

$$\frac{25 \text{ mL reagent A}}{50 \text{ mL total}} = \frac{1}{2}$$

$$\frac{5 \text{ mL (1/2 reagent A)}}{50 \text{ mL total}} = \frac{1}{2} \times \frac{5}{50} = \frac{5}{100} = \frac{1}{20}$$

$$\frac{2.5 \text{ mL (1/20 reagent A)}}{50 \text{ mL total}} = \frac{1}{20} \times \frac{2.5}{50} = \frac{2.5}{1,000} = \frac{1}{400}$$

The resulting dilutions from the serial method remain 1/2, 1/20, and 1/400, but with 50-mL volumes.

DEFINITIONS

A set of dilutions is defined by the volume and concentration of the diluted substance and total dilution required for the application. It is therefore helpful to define terms used to characterize a dilution series.

Consider the following dilution series of substance A (Fig. 4-3): One milliliter of substance A (100 µg/mL) is brought to 10 mL in tube #1. One milliliter of the tube #1 dilution is brought to 5.0 mL in tube #2. Two milliliters of the tube #2 is brought to 20 mL in tube #3.

Amount transferred: the volume of substance or dilution taken from the previous tube and placed in each tube in the series. In Figure 4-3, the amounts transferred are:

    Tube #1   1.0 mL
    Tube #2   1.0 mL
    Tube #3   2.0 mL

Total volume before transfer: the sum of the substance or amount transferred and diluent used in each tube in the series. In Figure 4-3, the total volumes are:

    Tube #1   1.0 mL + 9.0 mL = 10 mL
    Tube #2   1.0 mL + 4.0 mL = 5.0 mL
    Tube #3   2.0 mL + 18 mL = 20 mL

Total volume after transfer: the total volume in each tube minus the amount taken out to make the next dilution. This volume will be the

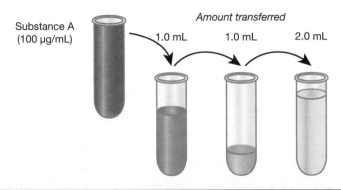

Substance A
(100 µg/mL)

Amount transferred

1.0 mL   1.0 mL   2.0 mL

Tube#	1	2	3
Total volume (before transfer)	10 mL	5.0 mL	20 mL
Total volume (after transfer)	9.0 mL	4.0 mL	20 mL
Tube diltuion	1/10	1/5	2/20 (= 1/10)
Solution diltuion	1/10	1/50	1/500
Substance volume	1.0 mL	0.10 mL	0.04 mL
Substance volume after transfer	0.90 mL	0.96 mL	0.04 mL
Substance concentration	10 µg/mL	2.0 µg/mL	0.20 µg/mL

Figure 4-3 Each dilution in a series has a characteristic volume, tube dilution, sample dilution, substance volume, and substance concentration. Tube dilution, total volume, and amount transferred can be adjusted according to the procedure being used. Availability of substance and diluent may limit volume selections.

amount of each dilution available for use in an assay or application. In Figure 4-3, the total volumes after transfer are:

Tube #1   10 mL - 1.0 mL = 9.0 mL

Tube #2   5.0 mL - 1.0 mL = 4.0 mL

Tube #3   20 mL

Because nothing is transferred from the last dilution (tube #3), the total volume after transfer is the same as the total volume before transfer for that tube.

Tube dilution: the dilution of the original substance or a previous dilution of the original substance in a particular tube that was made *in that tube*. Tube dilutions are chosen as part of the design of the dilution series. In Figure 4-3, the tube dilutions are:

Tube #1   1/10

Tube #2   1/5

Tube #3   2/20 = 1/10

Sample dilution: the dilution of the original substance in each tube. The sample dilution is the product of all previous tube dilutions. For a tube dilution of a substance that has already been diluted, multiply the dilutions together to obtain the sample dilution. The sample dilution is used to determine the substance concentration in each dilution. In Figure 4-3, the sample dilutions are:

```
Tube #1    1/10 (tube dilution made in tube #1)

Tube #2    1/10 x 1/5 = 1/50 (tube #1 dilution x
           tube #2 dilution)

Tube #3    1/10 x 1/5 x 1/10 = 1/500 (product of all
           previous dilutions) or

           1/50 x 1/10 = 1/500 (sample dilution present
           in tube #2 x tube #3 dilution)
```

Substance volume: the amount of the original substance delivered to each tube. The substance volume is the product of the amount transferred times *its* sample dilution, starting with 1.0 mL of undiluted sample (1/1) added to tube #1. In Figure 4-3, the substance volumes are:

```
Tube #1    1.0 mL x 1/1  = 1.0 mL

Tube #2    1.0 mL x 1/10 = 0.10 mL

Tube #3    2.0 mL x 1/50 = 0.04 mL
```

Substance volume after transfer: the total volume in each tube minus the amount used for the next dilution. In Figure 4-3, the substance volumes after transfer are:

```
Tube #1    1.0 mL  - 0.1 mL  = 0.90 mL

Tube #2    0.10 mL - 0.04 mL = 0.96 mL

Tube #3    0.04 mL
```

Because nothing is removed from tube #3, the substance volume remains the same.

Substance concentration: the final concentration of the original substance in each tube.

The substance concentration is the product of the concentration of the original substance times the sample dilution. In Figure 4-3, the substance concentrations are:

```
Tube #1    100 µg/mL x 1/10  = 10 µg/mL

Tube #2    100 µg/mL x 1/50  = 2.0 µg/mL

Tube #3    100 µg/mL x 1/500 = 0.20 µg/mL
```

All these terms and procedures are used in designing a dilution series or determining the amount or concentration of substance in each dilution. The example in Figure 4-3 yields 20 mL of a 0.20 µg/mL solution of substance A. The same solution can be made using a different dilution series, such as a 1/10 dilution in tube #1, 1/5 dilution in tube #2, and 1/10 dilution in tube #3. Another alternative would be 1/2 dilution in tube #1, 1/5 dilution in tube #2, and 1/50 dilution in tube #3. In fact, there are infinite ways to make a 0.20 µg/mL substance A from a 100 µg/mL solution of substance A. In determining the best series to use, take into account the amount and concentration of the final dilution required, the amount required for transfer from each tube, and the amounts of the original substance and dilutant available. If only 0.50 mL of the 100 µg/mL substance is available, then the first dilution could be 0.50 mL brought to 5.0 mL (1/10 dilution) because a 0.50/5.0 dilution is equivalent to a 1/10 dilution. If 50 mL of the 0.20 µg/mL substance is required, the dilution into tube #3 will require all 5 mL of the tube #2 dilution.

FOLD SERIAL DILUTIONS

The **fold dilution** is a type of serial dilution in which all tube dilutions are the same. A twofold dilution means that a 1/2 dilution is carried out in each tube. A 10-fold dilution means that a 1/10 dilution is carried out in each tube. Fold dilutions are usually made with equal volumes transferred for convenience.

Consider the following threefold dilution of a 90-mg/dL solution (Fig. 4-4). For each 1/3 dilution, 1.0 mL is transferred from each tube and brought to 3.0 mL total volume.

Total dilution volume before transfer:

Tube #1	3.0 mL
Tube #2	3.0 mL
Tube #3	3.0 mL

It is convenient but not required that you use the same total volume for all the dilutions.

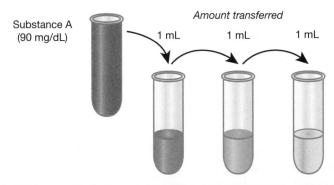

Tube#	1	2	3
Total volume (before transfer)	3.0 mL	3.0 mL	3.0 mL
Total volume (after transfer)	2.0 mL	2.0 mL	3.0 mL
Tube diltuion	1/3	1/3	1/3
Solution diltuion	1/3	1/9	1/27
Substance volume	1.0 mL	0.33 mL	0.11 mL
Substance volume after transfer	0.67 mL	0.22 mL	0.11 mL
Substance concentration	30 mg/dL	10 mg/dL	3.3 mg/dL

Figure 4-4 In a fold dilution, all tube dilutions are the same. In a threefold serial dilution, all tube dilutions are 1/3. In the series shown, all total volumes are the same, but that is not required as long as the tube dilution is 1/3. A 1/3 tube dilution could be made by bringing 2 mL to 6 mL with diluent.

Amount transferred:

Tube #1	**1.0 mL**
Tube #2	**1.0 mL**
Tube #3	**0 mL**

Total dilution volume after transfer:

Tube #1	**3.0 mL − 1.0 mL = 2.0 mL**
Tube #2	**3.0 mL − 1.0 mL = 2.0 mL**
Tube #3	**3.0 mL (nothing transferred)**

Tube dilution:

Tube #1	**1/3**
Tube #2	**1/3**
Tube #3	**1/3**

Note that the tube dilutions for a fold dilution are all the same.
Sample dilution:

Tube #1	**1/3**
Tube #2	**1/3 x 1/3 = 1/9**
Tube #3	**1/3 x 1/3 x 1/3 = 1/27**
	or 1/9 x 1/3 = 1/27

Substance volume before transfer:

Tube #1	**1.0 mL**
Tube #2	**1/3 x 1 mL = 0.33 mL**
Tube #3	**1/9 x 1 mL = 0.11 mL**

Substance volume after transfer:

Tube #1	**1.0 mL − 0.33 mL = 0.67 mL**
Tube #2	**0.67 mL − 0.22 mL = 0.56 mL**
Tube #3	**0.22 mL (nothing transferred)**

Substance concentration:

Tube #1	**1/3 x 90 mg/dL = 30 mg/dL**
Tube #2	**1/9 x 90 mg/dL = 10 mg/dL**
Tube #3	**1/27 x 90 mg/dL = 3.3 mg/dL**

Fold dilutions provide a series of similar dilutions that can be used for standard curves or for titrations.

These definitions are important to convey protocols and avoid error. A serial dilution is described by the tube dilutions and total volumes in each tube. The sample dilutions are determined by multiplying the tube dilutions. The sample dilutions are used to determine the substance concentrations, which should be appropriate for use in the assay. In some cases, all dilutions in the series may be used. In other cases, only the final dilution is used.

The volume of each dilution before and after transfer is important because adequate volume (after transfer) should be available for use. If this is not the case, then the total volume planned for the each tube dilution can be increased (or decreased). Small volumes may not provide enough dilutions for use, whereas large volumes will result in waste of substance and diluent.

Dilution series are used for a variety of applications. In the laboratory, a set of reference solutions of different concentrations may be required for instrument calibration, or test validation, or a test specimen of unknown starting concentration may require dilution to fall within the measurement range of an assay.

APPLICATIONS OF DILUTIONS

Standard Curves

Many laboratory protocols require a **standard curve**, that is, determination of a relationship between amount of substance and a measured signal, such as turbidity, color, fluorescence, radiation, or any measurable signal. For a standard curve, serial dilutions are made of the measured substance (referred to as the standard), and each dilution is measured for signal. Suppose a color reaction is used to determine the concentration of a substance. The color intensity of the substance in solution is measured on an instrument. To convert the color intensity as detected by the instrument to actual concentration, a standard curve is prepared of known concentrations. A set of decreasing substance concentrations is made through serial dilution of the substance in water. By adjusting the number of tubes and their tube dilutions, sample dilutions and substance concentrations are produced that cover a desired range, such as 10 to 250 mg/dL.

A graph is then drawn to establish the relationship between concentration and signal. This graph can be used for determining the concentration of unknowns by reading the signal. Standard curves are further discussed in Chapter 10.

Titrations

A **titer** is the smallest concentration of a substance that will give a measurable response, such as prevention of bacterial growth, neutralization of an acid or a base, or generation of a detectable signal. The titer concentration is determined by **titration,** or testing of dilutions of the substance for the dilution of lowest concentration that will still produce the effect, such as antibiotic activity. The titer may be expressed as that dilution, or the reciprocal of that dilution, as is done with antibody titers.

Antibiotic Resistance

A common titration performed in microbiology is the determination of a microorganism's sensitivity to antibiotics. Microorganisms may develop resistance to commonly used antibiotics. This is the basis for the development of new formulations of antibiotics. With a variety of available treatments, antibiotic resistance tests are performed to determine the most effective drug to use.

Antibiotic titers can be performed in solution or on solid agar. For solution analysis, an isolated colony of a pathogenic microorganism is obtained from the patient's specimen. A quantity of microorganisms is then suspended into solution. The isolate is inoculated into serial dilutions of antibiotics and incubated. The higher the concentration of antibiotic in which the isolate grows, the more resistant the organism is to the antibiotic. Using turbidity as an indication of bacterial growth, if isolate A is turbid in a 1/10 dilution of ampicillin and isolate B is turbid only in a 1/10,000 dilution of antibiotic, then isolate A is 1,000 times more resistant to the drug than isolate B (Fig. 4-5A). The titer of the antibiotic for isolate A can be expressed as 1/10 or the reciprocal, 10. The titer of the antibiotic for isolate B can be expressed as 1/10,000

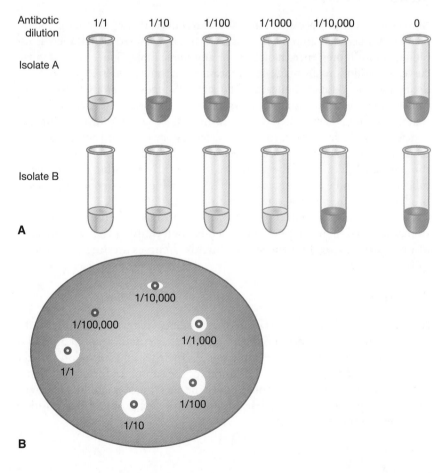

Figure 4-5 Antibiotic resistance tests may be performed in solution (*A*) or on solid agar (*B*). In solution, antibiotic is diluted, and the dilutions are added to equal inocula in liquid culture. The turbidity is compared to an identical culture without antibiotic (0). In this example, isolate A shows more resistance to the antibiotic than isolate B. The titer for isolate A is 10 or 1/10 compared with the titer for isolate B, which is 10,000 or 1/10,000.

or 10,000. Although the antibiotic may be very effective against isolate B, the amount that would have to be used to be effective against isolate A would be very high, possibly causing undesirable side effects. An alternative drug must be used against isolate A.

Antibiotic resistance may also be measured by spreading a suspension of bacteria from a pure culture on an agar plate (Fig. 4-5B). Small discs containing different dilutions of antibiotics (or different antibiotics) are placed on the plate. The plate is then incubated to allow the bacteria to grow. If the antibiotic is effective, a clear area (zone of inhibition) will surround the disc. The diameter of the zone is measured to further define the level of resistance. According to the Clinical and Laboratory Standards Institute (CLST) the diameter of zones of inhibition of sensitive bacteria should fall within specified limits. If the antibiotic is not effective, the bacteria will grow up to the edges of the disc. Results are reported as resistant, intermediate, or susceptible.

In an example, discs containing undiluted antibiotic (1/1) and 10-fold serial dilutions of antibiotic are placed on a lawn of bacteria. After a 16- to 18-hour incubation, a 200-mm zone of clearance appears around the undiluted 1/10 and 1/100 discs. The zone around the 1/1,000 disc is 20 mm, and no zone is seen around the 1/10,000 and 1/100,000 discs. If effectiveness of the antibiotic is defined as a zone of 20 mm in diameter, then the resistance of the bacterium is expressed as 1/1,000 or 1,000. If effectiveness is defined as no zone of clearance, then the resistance of the bacterium is expressed as 1/10,000 or 10,000.

The definition of antibiotic resistance titers depends on the way the antibiotic is administered to the patient, its side effects, and how it is metabolized. Resistance protocols provide information to determine the effective levels of antibiotics.

Antibody Titers

Antibodies in body fluids are informative targets for clinical tests. The presence of antibodies to specific bacteria or viruses is an indication of current or previous infection by that organism. Antibody titers can also be used to determine whether immunity has been developed after a vaccination. Autoimmune diseases are the result of antibodies generated against one's own body, with consequent degradation of tissues or cellular dysfunction.

A serum sample is diluted 1/2, 1/4, 1/8, 1/16, and 1/32. Each serum dilution is tested for reaction to antigen (Box 4-5). If no reaction is detected in the 1/16 and 1/32 dilutions, but a reaction is detected in the 1/8 tube, then

---

Box 4-5 **Antibody Titer Measurements**

Antibody titers are measured using a variety of methods including enzyme-linked immunosorbent assays (ELISA), indirect fluorescent antibody (IFA) tests, and agglutination tests. Each test has a defined signal or result indicating the presence of antibody.

the antibody titer of this serum is 1/8 or 8. Thus the quantity of antibodies present is determined by how much the serum can be diluted while still showing a measurable reaction to antigen. A titer of 1/32 or 32 is a high antibody titer because the concentration of antibody is such that even diluted to 1/32, it is high enough to produce a reaction. A titer of 1/2 or 2 is a low antibody titer because the antibody concentration is low enough such that dilution by 1/2 lowers it below detection.

Half-Life

Many biologically active substances lose activity during storage. When this happens, **specific activity** or the activity per unit weight or volume decreases over time. For less stable substances, a half-life, or the time it takes to lose half of the remaining activity, is provided. If a specific number of active units is required for a procedure, the half-life is used to determine the current specific activity of the substance. After 1 year of storage, an enzyme with a specific activity of 10 units/μL and a half-life of 6 months will have a specific activity of:

$$10 \times 1/2 \times 1/2 = 2.5 \text{ units}/\mu L$$

(One year = two half-lives.)

Therefore, if a procedure calls for 10 units of enzyme, where 1 μL of fresh enzyme would be used, after 1 year of storage, 4 μL of the enzyme would have to be added to the reaction mix to provide the same 10 units of enzyme activity.

Radioactive substances emit energetic particles (radiation). This radiation is used and measured in the laboratory in some applications (Box 4-6). Because radioactive materials lose particles with each emission, radioactivity decreases over time. The half-life for a radioactive substance is the amount of time it takes for that substance to lose half of its radioactivity. Radioactive half-life ranges from nanoseconds to thousands of years. The graph in Figure 4-6 shows the relationship between the number of half-lives and the amount of radiation remaining.

Half-life is also useful in handling and disposal of the radioactive substances. Although use of these agents is increasingly being replaced by nonradioactive methods, some procedures (or instruments) still require the use of isotopes such

---

Box 4-6   Half-Lives of Radioactive Seeds

Radioactive (iodine-125 or palladium-103) seeds are used as a treatment for cancer in a method called brachytherapy. The radioactive seeds are implanted in and around a tumor under ultrasound for guidance. The implants remain in place permanently, and because the iodine-125 has a half-life of 60 days and palladium-103 has an even shorter half-life of 17 days, the seeds become biologically inert (no longer useful) after 5 to 12 months. This technique allows a high dose of radiation to be delivered to a tumor with limited damage to surrounding tissues.

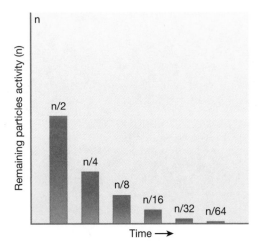

Figure 4-6 Half-life is the time required for decay or loss of half of starting or remaining activity of a substance. A half-life can be nanoseconds to thousands of years long, depending on the substance and the activity. With each half-life, half again of the substance activity is lost. So, after six half-lives, only $1/64$ of the original activity remains.

as radioactive phosphorus (^{32}P or ^{33}P) for detection of target molecules in certain laboratory procedures. The half-life of ^{32}P is 2 weeks. Every 2 weeks, the amount of radiation in the preparation decreases by one-half. Safety recommendations require storage for at least seven half-lives before radioactive phosphorus waste can be discarded. Note the relative amount of starting radiation (n) remaining after seven half-lives on the graph in Figure 4-6.

PRACTICE PROBLEMS

Dilutions and Ratios

1. What is the total number of parts in a 1 part in 10 part dilution?

2. What is the total number of parts in a 1 part to 10 part ratio?

3. When substance A is diluted $\frac{2}{5}$, how many parts of substance A are in 10 parts total?

4. When the substance A:water ratio is 2:5, how many parts of substance A are in 10 parts total?

5. When the substance A:water ratio is 2:5, how many parts of substance A are in 14 parts total?

6. A $\frac{1}{10}$ dilution of serum in saline has a ratio of how many parts saline to serum?

7. A $\frac{1}{10}$ dilution of serum in saline has a ratio of how many parts serum to saline?

8. A 1:10 ratio of serum to saline has how many parts saline to serum?

9. A 1:2 ratio of serum to saline has how many parts serum in 3 parts total?

10. A 1:2 ratio of serum to saline has how many parts serum in 2 parts total?

Amount of Substance in a Dilution

11. Calculate how many milliliters of substance A are in 100 mL of the following dilutions of substance A in diluent.

    a. $\frac{1}{20}$

    b. $\frac{1}{3}$

    c. $\frac{1}{30}$

    d. $\frac{1}{1,000}$

    e. $\frac{9}{10}$

12. What is the total volume of a solution in the following dilutions in milliliters?

    a. $\frac{1\,mL}{10\,mL}$

    b. 1 mL:4 mL

    c. $\frac{1\,mL}{20\,mL}$

    d. 1 mL:9 mL

    e. $\frac{5\,mL}{10\,mL}$

13. Prepare 50 mL of $\frac{1}{5}$ substance A in water.

14. Prepare 1 L of $\frac{70}{100}$ ethanol in water.

15. What volume of saline is required to make 0.10 mL of a $\frac{1}{10}$ serum in saline dilution?

Continued

PRACTICE PROBLEMS *cont.*

16. What volume of undiluted reagent is required to make 100 mL of a $\frac{1}{25}$ dilution in water?

17. How much plasma is required to make 1.0 mL of a $\frac{1}{50}$ dilution of plasma in saline?

18. The linear range of an instrument requires a $\frac{1}{100}$ dilution of normal serum for accurate readings of a test analyte. How much serum is required per test if each test takes 10 mL total diluted serum?

19. How much diluent is in 100 mL of a $\frac{1}{200}$ dilution?

20. What is the volume of water in 500 mL of a in a 250 mL/L dilution in water?

21. What is the final dilution if 1 mL of a $\frac{1}{10}$ dilution is brought to 10 mL?

22. What is the final dilution if 2 mL of a $\frac{1}{5}$ dilution is brought to 20 mL?

23. What series of three dilutions would make a $\frac{1}{1,000}$ dilution? (Note: There are multiple answers; provide one.)

24. What series of three dilutions would make a $\frac{1}{5,000}$ dilution? (Note: There are multiple answers.)

25. What series of four dilutions would make a $\frac{1}{20,000}$ dilution? (Note: There are multiple answers.)

Dilution Factors

26. What is the dilution factor if 2 mL substance is brought to 10 mL total volume?

27. What is the dilution factor if 0.5 mL substance is brought to 1.0 mL total volume?

28. What is the dilution factor if 5 mL substance is brought to 15 mL total volume?

29. What is the dilution factor if 10 mL substance is brought to 20 mL total volume?

30. What is the dilution factor if 0.01 mL substance is brought to 2.00 mL total volume?

Dilution Series

For the following set of dilutions, list:

   a. The tube dilution made in each flask or tube
   b. The resulting sample dilution in each flask or tube
   c. The substance concentration in each flask or tube
   d. The dilution factor for each flask or tube

31. Five milliliters of a 1,000 mg/dL glucose solution is brought to 50 mL with water in flask A, 2 mL of the 1,000 mg/dL glucose solution is brought to 50 mL with water in flask B, and 1 mL of the 1,000 mg/dL glucose solution is brought to 50 mL with water in flask C.

32. Three milliliters of 10 μg/mL calcium chloride is brought to 30 mL with water in flask A, 2 mL of 10 μg/mL calcium chloride is brought to 60 mL with water in flask B, and 1 mL of 10 μg/mL calcium chloride is brought to 100 mL with water in flask C.

33. Four milliliters of 50 ng/mL dye solution is brought to 5 mL with saline in tube A, 2 mL of the 50 ng/mL dye solution is brought to 5 mL with saline in tube B, 1 mL of the 50 ng/mL dye solution is brought to 5 mL with saline in tube C, and 0.5 mL of the 50 ng/mL dye solution is brought to 5 mL with saline in tube D.

Serial Dilutions

For the following set of dilutions, list:

  a. The tube dilution made in each flask or tube
  b. The resulting sample dilution in each flask or tube
  c. The substance concentration in each flask or tube
  d. Total volume in each flask or tube after transfer

34. Consider the following dilution series of a 100 μg/mL solution: 1 mL of the solution is brought to 2 mL in tube A, 1 mL of diluted solution in tube A is brought to 10 mL in tube B, and 5 mL of diluted solution in tube B is brought to 10 mL in tube C.

35. A 5,000 mg/L solution is diluted in the following series: 0.1 mL is brought to 1 mL in tube A, 0.5 mL of the diluted solution in tube A is brought to 10 mL in tube B, and 5 mL of diluted solution in tube B is brought to 50 mL in flask C.

36. Fifty microliters of 100 μg/mL magnesium chloride solution is brought to 5 mL with water in tube A, 1 mL of the dilution in tube A is brought to 10 mL with water in tube B, and 5 mL of dilution in tube B is brought to 10 mL with water in tube C.

37. One hundred microliters of 580 mg/dL is brought to 10 mL with water in tube A, 1 mL of the dilution in tube A is brought to 100 mL with water in flask B, and 50 mL of dilution in tube B is brought to 200 mL with water in flask C.

38. Fifty microliters of 10,000 μg/mL is brought to 50 mL with water in tube A, 2 mL of the dilution in tube A is brought to 10 mL with water in tube B, 5 mL of dilution in tube B is brought to 10 mL with water in tube C, and 2 mL of the dilution in tube C is brought to 10 mL with water in tube D.

Design of a Dilution Series

39. A method for preparing an antibody solution requires 10 mL of a $\frac{1}{10,000}$ dilution, made with tube dilutions of $\frac{1}{20}$, $\frac{1}{50}$, and $\frac{1}{10}$ in buffer. Only 0.5 mL of antibody solution is available. How can the method be adjusted to achieve the proper dilution?

40. With 20 mL buffer and 1 mL plasma, how would you prepare 1 mL of a $\frac{1}{10,000}$ dilution of plasma in buffer?

Fold Dilutions

41. What is the tube dilution in the fifth tube of a fivefold serial dilution?

42. What is the tube dilution in the 10th tube of a twofold serial dilution?

43. What is the sample dilution in the fifth tube of a 10-fold serial dilution?

44. What is the sample dilution in the 10th tube of a twofold serial dilution?

45. Starting with 1 mL pure substance and making 1 mL transfers, what is the substance volume in the fourth tube of a fivefold serial dilution?

46. Starting with 0.5 mL of a 40 g/L solution in 10 mL (first tube), what is the concentration in the second tube of a 20-fold serial dilution?

47. What is the substance concentration in percent in the fourth tube of a $\frac{1}{5}$ serial dilution?

Continued

Corrections for Dilutions

48. A $\frac{1}{10}$ dilution of a substance is determined to have a concentration of 10 mg/dL. What is the concentration of the undiluted substance?

49. A $\frac{1}{100}$ dilution of nucleic acid is determined to have a concentration of 55 μg/mL. What is the concentration of the undiluted substance?

50. A procedure requires 5 mL volume for concentration reading. Accidentally, 2 mL of the solution is spilled. The remaining 3 mL is brought back to 5 mL with diluent to have adequate volume for the detection device. The reading is 17.0 mg/dL. What is the concentration of the undiluted substance?

51. A method to detect concentration of a serum protein is designed for analysis of $\frac{1}{10}$ dilution of serum, so that the final reading is automatically adjusted to account for the dilution. The serum sample is diluted $\frac{1}{20}$ by mistake. The reading is 20.5 μg/mL. What is the concentration of the serum?

52. A procedure calls for 0.5 mL plasma in 1.0 mL saline for determination of concentration of a plasma component. The final reading is automatically adjusted to account for the dilution. Instead of 0.5 mL, 1.0 mL of undiluted plasma is used. The reading is 3.6 μg/mL. What is the concentration in the plasma?

Standard Curves

53. Four 10-fold dilutions of a 500 mg/dL glucose solution are prepared. What is the concentration of each dilution?

54. Three twofold dilutions of a 20.0 mg/dL reference standard are prepared. What is the concentration of each dilution?

Antibiotic Resistance

55. Three 10-fold dilutions of antibiotic are added to bacterial cultures. The bacteria grow in the third dilution, but not the first two. What is the antibiotic titer?

56. Five twofold dilutions of antibiotic are added to bacterial cultures. The bacteria grow in all dilutions except the first. What is the antibiotic titer?

57. A bacterial strain is spread on an agar plate. Discs imbued with antibiotic at diluted $\frac{1}{5}, \frac{1}{25}, \frac{1}{50}, \frac{1}{100}$, and $\frac{1}{250}$ are placed on the spread. A clear zone of no growth appears only around the disc with the $\frac{1}{5}$ dilution of antibiotic. What is the antibiotic titer?

Half-Life

58. The half-life of an enzyme (specific activity 1,000 units/mL) is 10 days. What is the effective specific activity after 30 days?

59. The half-life of ^{32}P is 2 weeks. What is the effective specific activity of a 100 μCi/mL ^{32}P-labeled probe after 14 weeks?

60. The half-life of ^{32}P is 2 weeks. What is the effective specific activity of waste containing a total of 10 mCi of ^{32}P probe after 16 weeks?

APPLICATIONS

Molecular Diagnostics

1. A molecular biology method requires a reaction mix having several components. One of these components is a reagent supplied at a concentration of 100 μM. The procedure calls for a 2.5-μM working stock of this reagent.
   a. What is the dilution required to prepare the 2.5-μM working stock from the 100-μM reagent?
   b. Each sample is tested in a 50-μL reaction mix containing 1 μL of the working stock. What is the final concentration of the reagent in the reaction mix?
   c. For multiple samples, the reaction mixes are prepared together in one master mix. How much of the stock must be added to 1 mL of master mix, sufficient for 20 samples? If you adjusted the setup procedure to require 2.0 μL of this component/50-μL mix, how would you dilute the 100-μM stock to provide the same reagent concentration in the final reaction mix?
2. A DNA sample is to be analyzed by capillary gel electrophoresis. Detection on the capillary instrument is very sensitive. Before loading, 5 μL of specimen were brought to 20 μL with water. Then 1 μL of the diluted specimen was brought to 20 μL with formamide. The results of the run showed that the diluted sample was still too concentrated. The results will be improved by further diluting the sample 1/2 and 1/5. Give examples of how to adjust the specimen or diluent volumes to make 1/2 and 1/5 further tube dilutions of the sample with the final dilution in 20 μL formamide.

Hematology

Normal blood contains 5,000 to 10,000 white blood cells (WBCs)/μL. Cells are manually counted in a specialized slide chamber called a hemocytometer. The WBCs are counted in 10 0.1-μL volumes. For accurate counts, each 0.1-μL chamber volume must contain between 50 and 100 cells.

1. A patient with an acute infection may have an elevated WBC count that is double the normal value. Based on the normal blood count, find the dilution of the blood specimen from this patient that will yield the appropriate concentration of WBCs for accurate counting on the hemocytometer.
2. Use this factor to determine the WBC count for this patient.

Radiation Safety

Radioactive elements (radionuclides or radioisotopes) emit energy in the form of alpha particles, beta particles, or gamma rays originating from the atomic nucleus. The rate of emission of radioactivity (decay) is measured in Becquerel or disintegrations per second (dps). The number of dps depends on the amount of the radioisotope present. Each radionuclide has a characteristic half-life or the amount of time for half of its radioactivity to decay. A radioisotope of phosphorus (^{32}P) is used in a procedure, generating waste measured at 7,500 dps. The half-life of ^{32}P is 14 days. What percent of the radioactivity will be present after 98 days? What will be the dps at that time?

Continued

APPLICATIONS cont.

Molecular Diagnostics

A set of dilutions was prepared using a commercial reference solution of DNA molecules. The starting reference concentration was 250 nM. The molecular weight of the DNA molecule was 24,532 g/mol. The set of seven 10-fold dilutions and the undiluted reference solution were read on a spectrophotometer. The sixth dilution when tested generated a positive signal, whereas the seventh dilution produced no signal.

a. What was the sample dilution in the sixth tube?
b. What was the lowest detectable molar concentration in this assay?
c. If the reaction volume is 20 μL, what is the lowest absolute number of molecules detected in this assay?

CHAPTER **5**

EXPRESSIONS OF CONCENTRATION

SOLUTIONS AND THEIR COMPONENTS

A solution is a mixture of two or more substances. Although premixed commercial preparations of solutions are used with increasing frequency in the clinical laboratory, knowledge of the nature of the components of solutions and how they are made is still important. Almost all chemical reactions studied in the clinical laboratory occur in solutions. If the solution is not correctly prepared, erroneous results may occur. Such critical errors negatively affect patients and impair optimal treatment. For example, a solution with proper magnesium concentration is required for enzymatic reactions that detect viral infections. If the magnesium concentration is incorrect, an inaccurate low or negative reading may result. This could lead to inadequate treatment of a critically infected patient.

A solution consists of two components, the **solute** (dispersed phase) and the **solvent** (dispersing phase). The solvent is usually liquid, although the solute can be gas, liquid, or solid. The solute is dissolved (dispersed) in the solvent.

> ❗ **CAUTION:** Some substances become unstable with changes in temperature or in the presence or absence of other substances. Before mixing chemicals, read the safety information found on the labels and the material safety data sheets (MSDSs). Wear proper protective equipment (goggles or safety glasses, gloves, protective gown) as indicated.

TYPES OF SOLUTIONS

The nature of a solution depends on the physical and chemical characteristics of the solute and solvent (Fig. 5-1; Box 5-1). In homogenous solutions, the solute particles are less than 1 nm in size. Examples of such solutions

LEARNING OUTCOMES

- Define solutions and their components.
- Compare and contrast different types of solutions.
- Describe concentration expressions.
- Define density and show how it is used in preparing solutions.

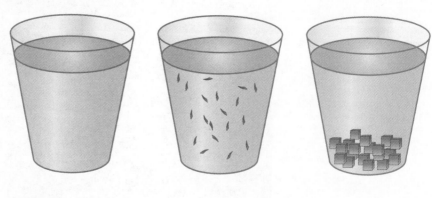

Figure 5-1 In solutions (*left*), solute is completely dissolved in solvent. Colloid solutions (*center*) are thick or gel-like as a result of the larger solute particles. Particles in suspension are so large that they can settle to the bottom of the container unless the suspension is agitated (*right*).

Box 5-1 **Types of Solutions**

In 1861, Thomas Graham described substances based on the degree of diffusion of solute, crystallinity (three-dimensional order of component atoms), and ability to pass through a parchment barrier. He classified these substances as either crystalloids, made of smaller particles, or colloids, composed of much larger particles. When mixed with solvent, Graham's crystalloids formed what he called true solutions.

---

are glucose in water and sodium chloride in water. **Colloid solutions** contain solute particles 1 to 200 nm in size. Examples of substances that form colloid solutions are glue, gelatin, starch, and long-chain nucleic acids. If the solute particles are larger than 200 nm, the solution is a **suspension**. Examples of suspensions are beads (silica, Sepharose, glass) in liquid for use in various procedures. To keep the particles suspended homogeneously, agitation is required before sampling.

When two substances in solution spontaneously mix, the solute is said to be **soluble** (capable of being dissolved) in the solvent. In this solution, solute will move within the solvent from areas of high concentration to areas of lower concentration by the process of **diffusion**. A given solvent can hold only so much solute. When the solvent holds the maximum amount of solute, the solution is **saturated**. Adding more solute makes the solution **supersaturated**. A supersaturated solution requires temperature and pressure conditions that keep the solution intact. If these factors change, the supersaturated solvent will easily lose excess solute. Carbonated beverages are examples of supersaturated solutions of carbon dioxide in liquid. While the solution is contained under pressure in the can or bottle, the carbon dioxide remains dissolved in the liquid. Opening the container and releasing the pressure allow the gas to escape from the liquid in the form of bubbles. The blood of deep-water divers is also supersaturated with gases under the pressure of the deep water. Surfacing or release of the pressure too quickly results in the release of gases, with adverse physical effects ("the bends").

True and colloid solutions are composed of **miscible** components; that is, they combine to form a stable mixture. When substances do not combine to form a stable solution, they are said to be **immiscible**. Immiscible mixtures separate into phases (Fig. 5-2). Immiscible mixtures form **emulsions** on agitation. Emulsions can be stabilized by adding other chemicals or stabilizers to the mixture (Box 5-2). Whole milk is an example of a stable emulsion.

The degree of immiscibility of substances also changes with environmental conditions such as temperature, humidity, and air pressure. This fact is well known to bakers and candy makers whose products can be affected by the altitude, humidity, and barometric pressure of the area in which they are prepared.

EXPRESSIONS OF CONCENTRATIONS

The **concentration** of a solution is the amount of solute contained in a given amount of solvent. Working with solutions requires description of the concentration of an existing solution or prediction of the amount of solute required if the solution is to be prepared. Components of a solution are indicated in most expressions of concentration.

The most accurate expression of concentration is weight of solute in weight of solution, or **w/w**, such as 10 g of sodium chloride (NaCl) dissolved in 1,000 g of water. Weight (mass) is more accurate than other means of measuring because it is not affected by temperature or pressure. Ten grams of NaCl will weigh 10 g regardless of the temperature and atmospheric pressure in the laboratory. The most common expression of concentration is weight solute in volume of solution (**w/v**). This expression is less accurate because

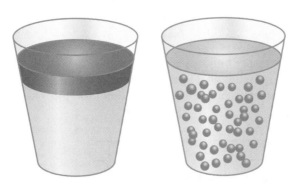

Figure 5-2 Two immiscible liquids will form phases when mixed together (*left*). Each phase will be homogenous, one floating on the other. If the mixture is agitated, an emulsion will form, in which one phase will break into "bubbles" within the other phase (*right*).

Box 5-2   **Water-in-Oil Emulsions**

Hydrophobic (oily) and hydrophilic (water-loving) substances mixed together can form aqueous droplets suspended in the oily phase. When they are adequately stabilized, independent chemical reactions can be performed in each aqueous droplet suspended in one emulsion, a method used in some advanced medical laboratory procedures capable of simultaneously testing hundreds of thousands of targets.

volume can change with temperature or pressure. For example, 10 g of solute dissolved in 100 mL solvent measured at high temperature will yield a lower concentration than if the 100 mL solvent is measured at low temperature. A third expression of concentration is volume of solute in volume of solution (**v/v**). This is the least accurate expression because both solute and solvent can change with temperature or pressure variation. When mixing two volumes together, the volume of solute should be brought up to the total volume with solvent.

Parts

Parts per Million and Parts per Billion

Parts expressions, such as parts per million (ppm) or parts per billion (ppb), are a general way to express concentration without using units. For example, a concentration of 0.001 parts arsenic per million parts of water does not use units, such as grams or milliliters. It simply says that there is 1 part arsenic for every 1,000,000,000 parts of water in a sample of any size (Fig. 5-3). Ppm and ppb are expressions used for extremely dilute or high-volume solutions. Though any volume can be used, one ppm$^{w/v}$ in practice means one microgram per liter of solution. In environmental monitoring, chloride levels in drinking water may range from 2 to 200 ppm. These terms are not used frequently in the clinical laboratory because most measurements of analytes and solute concentrations are well above these levels. Ppm and ppb are used more frequently in environmental or geological sciences, in which trace levels of substances are measured or high volumes are tested.

Parts per Hundred (Percentage)

Parts per hundred parts are frequently used in the laboratory as percent. Percent is indicated by the symbol, %, meaning per 100. Many clinical test results are reported in units per deciliter (100 mL), which is the same as percent. In

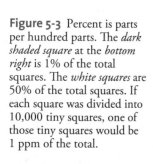

Figure 5-3 Percent is parts per hundred parts. The *dark shaded square* at the *bottom right* is 1% of the total squares. The *white squares* are 50% of the total squares. If each square was divided into 10,000 tiny squares, one of those tiny squares would be 1 ppm of the total.

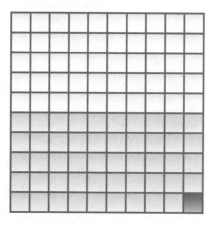

clinical chemistry, a metabolic panel report may include an albumin result of 4.5 g/dL, blood urea nitrogen ranging from 6 to 20 mg/dL, a calcium level of 9.0 mg/dL, a glucose concentration of 100 mg/dL, a total bilirubin of 0.5 mg/dL, and a total protein of 7.0 g/dL, among other results.

Molarity

As defined in Chapter 3, a **mole** of any substance is 6.023×10^{23} molecules of that substance. A mole is a count similar to the expression of a dozen, which is 12 units of something. The weight of a mole of any compound is the sum of the atomic weights of the atoms that make up the substance. Atomic weights (atomic masses) are included in the information found in periodic tables. Using NaCl as an example:

22.99 g (Na atomic weight) + 35.45 g (Cl atomic weight)
= 58.44 g

This means that 1 mole of NaCl weighs 58.44 g, or NaCl has 58.44 g/mole.

Molarity is the number of moles of substance in 1 L of solution. To express molarity, the atomic weight of the substance (g/mole) must be known. If 58.44 g of NaCl were dissolved in 1 L of water, the resulting solution would be 1.0 mole/L or 1.0 **molar** NaCl (1 molar NaCl = 1.0 mole/L NaCl). If 29.22 g NaCl (the weight of ½ mole) were dissolved in 1 L of water, the resulting solution would be 0.50 molar NaCl.

Molar expressions are used with the prefixes of the metric and SI systems. If 58.44 mg of NaCl (1 millimole of NaCl) were dissolved in 1 L of water, the resulting solution would be 1 millimole/L, or 1 millimolar NaCl (1 mM NaCl). If 58.44 ng (1 nanomole) of NaCl were dissolved in 1 L of water, the resulting solution would be 1 nanomolar NaCl, or 1 nM NaCl. The terms millimolar, micromolar, and nanomolar refer to 1 L of solvent. That is, 1 L of solvent will contain millimolar, micromolar, or nanomolar amounts of solute.

Molarity of Hydrates

Molecules of some salts chemically combine with molecules of water (Box 5-3). Compounds with associated water molecules are called **hydrates**. The associated water molecules change (increase) the amount of hydrated compounds required to achieve a specified concentration of the salt, compared with the same compound without any water molecules (**anhydrous** compounds). Calcium chloride ($CaCl_2$) is often used as a hydrate. The molecular weight of anhydrous $CaCl_2$\(110.98 g/mole) is less than that of its hydrate. Because of this a greater weight of the hydrate would be required to achieve the same concentration of $CaCl_2$.

Compounds with one water molecule per molecule of substance are **monohydrates**, those with two water molecules per molecule of substance are **dihydrates**, and those with three water molecules per molecule of substance are **trihydrates**. A compound may have as many as 10 (decahydrate) or more associated water molecules. Formulae of hydrates are written with

> **Box 5-3** | **Hygroscopic Compounds**
>
> Anhydrous compounds can be **hygroscopic**, that is, they can attract and bind water from the surrounding atmosphere. The results are sticking and clumping, and the material can liquefy. Therefore, hydrates, which are less hygroscopic, are often stocked in the laboratory.

the formula of the compound and then the number of water molecules (H_2O). Thus, the anhydrous version of calcium chloride is $CaCl_2$. Calcium chloride monohydrate is written $CaCl_2 \cdot H_2O$. Calcium chloride dihydrate is written $CaCl_2 \cdot 2H_2O$. Calcium chloride decahydrate is written $CaCl_2 \cdot 10H_2O$.

To calculate molecular weights of hydrates, add 18.01 g/mole—the molecular weight of water—to the molecular weight of the compound for each water molecule. Cupric sulfate, $CuSO_4$, is another compound frequently used as a hydrate. The molecular weight of $CuSO_4$ is 159.62 g/mole. Cupric sulfate monohydrate, $CuSO_4 \cdot H_2O$, has the following molecular weight:

$$159.62 \text{ g/mole} + 18.01 \text{ g/mole} = 177.63 \text{ g/mole}$$

A 1-molar solution of anhydrous cupric sulfate would contain 159.62 g of $CuSO_4$, whereas a 1-molar solution of cupric sulfate monohydrate would contain 177.63 g of $CuSO_4 \cdot H_2O$.

Attention to the type of compound available is important when making solutions according to a protocol. If a procedure describes making 1 L of a 0.1^0 molar $CaCl_2$ solution by bringing 11.0 g anhydrous $CaCl_2$ to 1 L and the laboratory has only calcium chloride decahydrate ($CaCl_2 \cdot 10H_2O$) available, the amount of $CaCl_2$ will have to be adjusted. More than 11.0 g of the decahydrate compound will be required to make the 0.1^0 molar solution. The molecular weight of the decahydrate is approximately:

$$110.98 \text{ g/mole} + 180.10 \text{ g/mole} = 291.08 \text{ g/mole}$$

The 0.1^0-molar solution would then require 29.1 g of the decahydrate:

$$291.08 \text{ g/\cancel{mole}} \times 0.1 \text{ \cancel{moles}/liter} = 29.1 \text{ g/L}$$

Molality

Molality is based on mass in kilograms, rather than on volumes in liters. A 1-molal solution contains one mole of substance in 1 kg (rather than 1 L) solvent. To make a 1-molal solution of NaCl, for instance, bring 58.44 g NaCl to 1 kg with solvent. Molality is the most precise measurement of concentration because, unlike volume, weight is not affected by environmental conditions.

Molal solutions are not frequently used in routine laboratory work. It is less convenient to weigh solutions than to use volumetric vessels. The relatively minor increase in precision does not warrant the increased effort required to make the weighed solutions. If, however, a protocol calls for molal concentrations, then mass should be used.

Normality

In contrast to molarity and molality, which are based on molecular weight, normality is based on **equivalent weight**. One equivalent is the amount of a substance that can replace or combine with 1 mole of hydrogen (valence). Equivalent weight is determined by dividing the molecular weight of a substance by its valence or the number of **equivalents (Eq)** in the compound. In a monovalent compound such as sodium hydroxide (NaOH), Na^+ can replace 1 mole of hydrogen (H^+) or OH^- can combine with 1 mole of H^+, that is, NaOH has one equivalent and therefore the molecular weight and equivalent weight are the same, 40.00 g/Eq. Compare this with sulfuric acid, H_2SO_4, which has two H^+ equivalents, or $SO_4^=$ can combine with two H^+ equivalents. Its equivalent weight is

$$98.08 \text{ g/mole (molecular weight)/ 2 Eq/mole} = 49 \text{ g/Eq}$$

The equivalent weight is always equal to or less than the molecular weight.

    Normal solutions are expressed in equivalents per liter. For a divalent compound like sulfuric acid, a 1-N solution contains 49.04 g/L H_2SO_4, rather than the 98.08 g/L in a 1-M solution. In this case, 1 N H_2SO_4 is the same as 0.5 molar H_2SO_4. In contrast, the molecular weight and the equivalent weight of NaOH are approximately 40.00 g/mole. Because the equivalent weight of a monovalent compound such as NaOH is the same as its molecular weight, a 1-N solution is the same as a 1-molar solution, or 40.00 g/L in this case. The grams per liter concentration of a normal solution is always equal to or less than the grams per liter concentration of a molar solution. This means that *an expression of normality is always equal to or more than the expression of molarity, given the same number of grams of compound.*

    Normality is used where equivalent positively or negatively charged particles can neutralize one another. An acid compound such as, hydrochloric acid (HCl) releases hydrogen ions (H^+) that combine with negatively charged hydroxyl ions (OH^-) released by a base such as NaOH. Each H^+ is one equivalent, and each hydroxyl ion is one equivalent. In these applications, the number of equivalents has functional importance.

Osmolarity and Osmolality

Osmolarity is the number of particles in solution. It is based on the number of dissociable particles in a substance. The concentration of particles has osmotic effects that influence the physical properties of solutions and the movement of fluids across membranes (Fig. 5-4; Box 5-4). The concentration of dissolved ions and molecules can direct this movement. Fluids move from a low osmolar concentration to a high osmolar concentration until the concentrations are equal or equilibrated. In physiology, osmolarity affects fluid movements through body compartments and therefore is an important clinical measurement.

    The osmolar weight is equal to the molecular weight divided by the number of particles formed on dissociation of the compound, or **osmoles**. If the compound does not dissociate, then the number of osmoles is equal to the

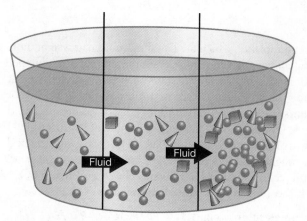

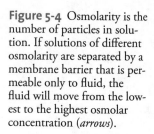

Figure 5-4 Osmolarity is the number of particles in solution. If solutions of different osmolarity are separated by a membrane barrier that is permeable only to fluid, the fluid will move from the lowest to the highest osmolar concentration (*arrows*).

Box 5-4 | Osmolarity

Blood cells placed in a dilute (hypotonic) solution swell and burst from the fluid moving into the cells where the osmolarity is higher than in the surrounding solution. Cells placed in solution with a high osmolarity (hypertonic) shrivel as fluid moves from the cells into the surrounding more concentrated solution. Blood samples are therefore most often collected in a solution with similar osmolarity as the cells (isotonic). Hypotonic solutions may be used in the laboratory to swell and lyse cells purposely for procedures read under a microscope, such as chromosome analysis.

---

number of moles divided by 1; that is, osmolarity is equal to the molarity. In contrast to normality, the number of dissociable particles is not based on valence. Compared with moles and equivalents, described earlier, NaOH dissociates into 2 particles or osmoles; therefore, the osmolar weight of NaOH is:

$$\frac{40.00 \text{ g/mole}}{2 \text{ particles/mole}} = 20.00 \text{ g/osmole NaOH}$$

In contrast, glucose is a compound that does not dissociate; therefore, the osmolar weight of glucose is:

$$\frac{180.16 \text{ g/mole}}{1 \text{ particle/mole}} = 180.16 \text{ g/osmole glucose}$$

Sulfuric acid has 3 dissociable particles (osmoles). Therefore, a 1-osmolar solution of sulfuric acid would contain approximately

$$\frac{98.08 \text{ g/mole}}{3 \text{ particles/mole}} = 32.69 \text{ g/osmole } H_2SO_4$$

A 1-osmolar solution of H_2SO_4 contains 32.69 g/L H_2SO_4, compared with the 98.08 g/L in a 1-molar solution. In this case, 1 osmolar H_2SO_4 is the same as 0.33 molar H_2SO_4. The grams per liter concentration of an osmolar solution is always equal to or less than the grams per liter concentration of a molar solution. This means that *osmolarity is always equal to or more than molarity, given the same number of grams of compound.*

In the clinical laboratory, **osmolality** is measured in physiological fluids such as urine or plasma (Box 5-5). These are complex solutions with many dissociated and undissociated components. For these measurements, it is not possible to count the dissociated particles directly; rather, a physical effect of the particles in solution is used, and that is the depression of **freezing point**. Freezing point is the temperature at which a liquid transitions to a solid state at atmospheric pressure. Water freezes at 0°C. It is a familiar observation that when salt is added to water, the water-salt solution will freeze at a lower temperature than water alone. The higher the salt concentrations (particles), the lower the freezing point. This characteristic can be applied to complex mixtures by using the effect on freezing point to measure osmolality.

One osmole lowers the freezing point of 1 kg of water by 1.86°C; that is, a 1-osmolar solution (of any compound) will have a freezing point of −1.86°C. For physiological levels, this measurement is often expressed in milliosmoles. One milliosmole lowers the freezing point of 1 kg water by $0.00186°C = 1.86 \times 10^{-3}$ °C.

Use ratio and proportion of the freezing points to determine osmolality. Suppose the freezing point, measured in an osmometer, of a urine specimen is −0.69°C. The osmolar concentration is:

$$\frac{1 \text{ osmole}}{-1.86°C} = \frac{x \text{ osmole}}{-0.69°C}$$

$$x = -0.69/-1.86 = 0.37 \text{ osmolar} = 370 \text{ mOsmolar}$$

Conversely, the freezing point of a solution can be predicted based on its osmolality. A 0.25-osmolar salt solution in water has a freezing point below 0°C. The freezing point is calculated using ratio and proportion:

$$\frac{1 \text{ osmole}}{-1.86°C} = \frac{0.25 \text{ osmole}}{x°C}$$

$$x = -1.86 \times 0.25$$

$$x = -0.46°C$$

Freezing point: −0.46°C

If solutions of different osmolar concentrations are mixed, the effect on freezing point is additive. Suppose 135 mOsmoles of glucose (24.3 g glucose) were

---

Box 5-5 Physiological Osmolality

Serum and urine osmolality are measured to determine the body's water balance. Sodium ions (Na^+), glucose molecules, and other natural particles affect how fluids move through the kidneys and into the urine. Abnormally high or low levels of these particles not only change the concentration of the substances themselves but also affect the volume of fluid in different body compartments.

added to a 250-mOsmolar salt solution, the resulting mixture would have a combined milliosmolarity of 385 mOsmolar. The freezing point would be:

$$\frac{1 \text{ osmole}}{-1.86°C} = \frac{0.385 \text{ osmole}}{x°C}$$

$$x = -0.716°C$$

Freezing point: −0.716°C

DENSITY

Density is the amount of matter per unit volume of a substance. Density is a property of all substances. The density of water is close to one. At 23°C, 1 L of water weighs approximately 1 kg (997.54 grams); 1 mL of water weighs approximately 1 g (0.99754 g). For purposes of calculations, the density of water is rounded to 1.000.

A related property of substances is **specific gravity**. Specific gravity is the mass of a substance divided by the mass of an equal volume of water. If 5 mL of a liquid weighs 7.46 g, then the specific gravity is:

$$\frac{7.460 \text{ g/} 5.000 \text{ mL}}{5.00 \text{ g/} 5.00 \text{ mL water}} = 1.49$$

Specific gravity is a characteristic of concentrated commercial liquids (Table 5-1). Specific gravity of commonly used substances can be found on the package label or from various references. Labels and references to specific gravity also provide **assay** or **percent purity**. The formula weight (60.05 g/mole), specific gravity (1.04 g/mL), and assay or purity (99.5%),

Table 5-1	Specific Gravity, Assay, and Purity of Common Commercial Preparations	
	Specific Gravity	Purity (%)
Acetic acid (glacial)	1.05	99.8
Formic acid	1.20	90.5
Hydrochloric acid	1.19	37.2
Hydrofluoric acid	1.18	49
Lactic acid	1.2	85
Nitric acid	1.42	70
Perchloric acid	1.67	70.5
Phosphoric acid	1.70	85.5
Sulfuric acid	1.84	96.0
Potassium hydroxide	1.46	45
Sodium carbonate	1.10	10
Sodium hydroxide	1.54	50.5

for instance, are provided on the label of a bottle of glacial acetic acid. These numbers determine the weight of a substance per mL of liquid (w/v).

When preparing a solution from a commercially preparation, use the percent purity and specific gravity to determine the volume of the concentrated solution required to deliver the desired weight of the substance. To find the weight (number of grams) of substance in a unit volume (mL) (i.e., the specific gravity of the commercial preparation), use the purity in the following way:

Density of the commercial solution (g/mL)
= specific gravity of the solution x purity

For nitric acid (HNO_3) with 71% purity and specific gravity 1.42 g/mL:

Density of the 71% HNO_3 = 1.42 x 0.71 = 1.01 g/mL

To make 100 mL of 10% HNO_3 from this commercial solution, use its calculated density (1.01 g/1 mL) to determine what volume of the commercial preparation will deliver 10 g of HNO_3.

10% = 10 g/100 mL

$$\frac{10 \text{ g}}{101 \text{ g/mL}} = 9.90.\text{mL}$$

Bring 9.90 mL commercial HNO_3 solution to a volume of 100 mL.

> **!** **CAUTION:** Do not add water to strong acid. Start with a volume of water greater than that of the acid (but less than the final volume), and mix it by adding the acid slowly. Then bring the mixture to the required volume.

In preparing normal solutions (Eq/L), remember to use equivalent weights. For example, to make 1 L of 0.50 N HCl, first use the equivalent weight of HCl to determine how many grams of HCl are in 0.50 equivalents:

36.45 g/Eq x 0.50 Eq/L = 18.2 g/L

Then determine the volume of the commercial preparation required to deliver 18.2 g HCl.

Checking the label or other reference, the specific gravity of HCl is given as 1.19, and the percent purity is 37%.

1.19 g/mL x 0.37 = 0.44 g/mL

1 mL of the commercial preparation will provide 0.44 g HCl. To obtain 18.2 g, divide 18.2 by the density of the solution:

$$\frac{18.2 \text{ g}}{0.44 \text{ g/mL}} = 41.4 \text{ mL}$$

Bring 41.4 mL commercial HCl to 1,000 mL. (Start with a few hundred milliliters of water, carefully add the 41.4 mL HCl, and bring the solution to 1,000 mL.)

PRACTICE PROBLEMS

Solutions and Their Components

1. Sodium chloride crystals are dissolved in water. Which is the solute, and which is the solvent?

2. Which of the following will make a solution?
   a. Oil and dilute acetic acid
   b. Glucose and water
   c. Silicate beads and water
   d. Whole milk

3. Gelatin and water in a semisolid state form what type of solution?
   a. Colloid
   b. Suspension

4. If agarose in water forms a gel, what are the diameters of the agarose polymers likely to be?
   a. Less than 1 nm
   b. More than 200 nm
   c. More than 1 micron
   d. Between 1 and 200 nm

5. A solution that loses solute on change in temperature or pressure is _____.

Concentration Expressions

Express the following parts in ppm and percent.

6. 1 part in 100 parts

7. 10 parts in 10,000,000 parts

8. 5 parts to 10 parts

9. 10 parts to 90 parts

10. 1 part in 1,000,000,000 parts

Express the following as molar concentration.

11. 40 g NaOH in 1.0 L (NaOH MW = 40.00)

12. 10 g NaOH in 0.5 L (NaOH MW = 40.00)

13. 58.5 g NaCl in 2.00 L (NaCl MW = 58.44)

14. 1.00 g KCl in 10.0 mL (KCl MW = 74.55)

15. 10.0 mg adenine in 1.00 mL (adenine MW = 135.13)

Express the following as molal concentration.

16. 5.0 g NaOH in 1.0 kg (NaOH MW = 40.00)

17. 20.0 g $MgCl_2$ in 1.0 kg ($MgCl_2$ MW = 95.21)

18. 23.0 g NaCl in 1 L of water (NaCl MW = 58.44)

19. 37.2 mg $CuSO_4$ in 100 mL of water ($CuSO_4$ MW = 159.62)

Continued

PRACTICE PROBLEMS *cont.*

What is the molecular weight of the following hydrates?

20. $CaCl_2 \cdot H_2O$

21. $CaCl_2 \cdot 10H_2O$

22. $Na_3PO_4 \cdot 12H_2O$

Express the following as molar concentration.

23. 10.0 g $CaCl_2$ in 1.00 L of water

24. 10.0 g $CaCl_2 \cdot 5H_2O$ in 1.00 L water

25. 100.0 g $Na_2HPO_4 \cdot 10H_2O$ in 1.0 L water

Use molecular weight to calculate the necessary adjustments.

26. What is the molar concentration of 150 g $CuSO_4 \cdot 10H_2O$ in 0.50 L water? Compare this with the concentration of 150 g anhydrous $CuSO_4$ in 0.50 L water.

27. A procedure calls for a 28.0-mM solution of sodium dihydrogen phosphate prepared by mixing 5.00 g NaH_2PO_4 in 1.50 L water. Only $NaH_2PO_4 \cdot 2H_2O$ is available. How would you prepare the solution?

28. A method calls for a 50.0-mM calcium chloride solution prepared by mixing 14.6 g $CaCl_2 \cdot 10H_2O$ in 1.00 L water. Only $CaCl_2 \cdot 1H_2O$ is available. How would you prepare the solution?

29. Which has more $CuSO_4$, a 9.0% $^{w/v}$ solution of $CuSO_4 \cdot 5H_2O$ or a 9.0%$^{w/v}$ solution of $CuSO_4$?

30. How many grams of $Co(NO_3)_2 \cdot 5H_2O$ are required to make 100 mL of 0.50% $^{w/v}$ $Co(NO_3)_2$? (MW of $Co(NO_3)_2$ is 182.94.)

Determine the normality of the following solutions.

31. 10 g NaOH in 1.0 L water

32. 1.0 g H_2SO_4 in 0.50 L water

33. 30 g H_3PO_4 in 3.0 L water

34. 3.5 g HCl in 0.75 L water

35. 0.50 g KOH in 100 mL water

36. 250 mg $MgCl_2$ in 1 mL water

Determine the osmolarity of the following solutions.

37. 10 g NaOH in 1.0 L water

38. 50 g HNO_3 in 3.0 L water

39. 5.0 g H_3PO_4 in 5.0 L water

40. A 5.0-mL plasma sample with a freezing point of -0.89 °C

41. A 10.0-mL urine sample with a freezing point of -0.65 °C

42. 250 millosmoles glucose (45 g) dissolved in 1 L of a 125-millosmoles NaCl solution

43. 360 millosmoles of (7.2 g) NaOH dissolved in 100 mL water

PRACTICE PROBLEMS *cont.*

Use Table 5–1 on page 94 to answer questions 44 and 45.

44. How many grams of potassium hydroxide are in 2.0 mL of commercial product?

45. What percent phosphoric acid is 3.0 mL commercial reagent in 100 mL water?

How would you prepare the following solutions?

46. 10% potassium hydroxide in 50 mL

47. 0.10 molar HCl in 200 mL

48. 0.20 N H_2SO_4 in 100 mL

49. 0.010 molar formic acid, 0.020 M nitric acid in 500 mL (MW of formic acid = 46.02 g/mole; MW of nitric acid = 63.01 g/mole)

50. A procedure calls for 10 mL of 1.0% phosphoric acid prepared by bringing 100 mg phosphoric acid to 10 mL. How would you prepare this with commercial phosphoric acid solution?

APPLICATIONS

Body Fluids: Renal Tests

Renal clearance is a measure of the rate of removal of material from the blood by the kidneys. It is related to the concentration of substances in the blood. Creatinine and urea levels are measured to test renal clearance. If a blood sample contains 140 mg/dL of creatinine, and 140 mg is passed into urine per minute, then 100 mL of blood has been cleared per minute.

Given the concentration of creatinine in blood and in urine and the volume of urine passed per minute, a formula for renal clearance for an average body surface area can be derived. Because this is a calculation involving volume (urine) and concentration of substance in plasma, the following formula can be used:

$$C \times P = U \times V$$
$$C = U/P \times V$$
$$(or \ C = UV/P)$$

Where C is the clearance per minute, P is the concentration in blood (plasma), U is the concentration in urine, and V is the volume of urine passed per minute.

The formula must be adjusted to compensate for the size of the patient. The adjustment factor is a ratio of the average body surface area ($1.73 \ m^2$) and the body surface area of the test patient (A). (Body surface area can be derived from the patient's height and weight by using a nomogram, computer software, or calculator.)

$$1.73/A$$

The formula then becomes:

$$C = U/P \times V \times 1.73/A$$

Use the formula to determine renal clearance for a male individual with a body surface area, $A = 1.86 \ m^2$ and a urine output of 320 mL/4 hours, blood creatinine concentration of 1.9 mg/dL, and urine creatinine concentration of 140 mg/dL.

Molecular Diagnostics

The concentration of a commercial reference DNA is 25 nM. Tenfold dilutions covering eight orders of magnitude in 25-µL reaction volumes were prepared. The DNA in the seventh dilution was detectable in solution, whereas the eighth dilution produced no signal.

1. What was the lowest detectable molar concentration in this assay?
2. What is the lowest absolute number of molecules detected in this assay?

CHAPTER 6

SOLUTION CALCULATIONS

CALCULATIONS OF CONCENTRATIONS

Calculations of concentrations are central to laboratory procedure. Expressions of concentration are used to determine actual amounts of substances required for solution preparation. Concentration calculations have three applications:

1. Concentration calculations are used to determine the amount of solute or solvent required to prepare a solution of given concentration or to determine the amount of solute or solvent in an existing solution.

2. Convert one expression of concentration to another.

These applications are performed using three basic procedures:

1. Use ratio and proportion when the concentrations of starting and ending solutions are not changed.

2. Use the volume/concentration "VC-VC" method when the concentrations of starting and ending solutions are changed.

3. Use defined formulae.

RATIO AND PROPORTION

Ratio and proportion, utilizing equivalent fractions and algebra, are applied when one has to determine the amount of a substance required to make a solution with a concentration that is proportional to a solution of known concentration (Fig. 6-1). Solution volume and amount of solute are expressed as equivalent fractions, with one unknown.

Suppose a procedure calls for 400 mL of 6%$^{w/v}$ sodium chloride (NaCl). Percent (w/v) refers to grams per hundred milliliters, so 6% is 6 g by weight of solute NaCl per 100 mL solution. If the final solution has a volume of 400 mL, how many grams of NaCl will be required? Three of the terms are

LEARNING OUTCOMES

- List and describe the use of concentration expressions.

- Describe the procedures used for solution calculations: ratio and proportion, $V_1C_1 = V_2C_2$, and formulae.

- Calculate molar, normal, osmolar, and percent concentrations.

- Determine grams per unit volume from molar, normal, osmolar, and percent.

- Convert equivalent orders of magnitude using exponents.

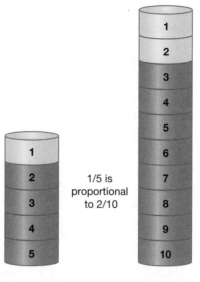

1/5 is
proportional
to 2/10

Figure 6-1 Use ratio and proportion when concentrations remain constant and volume or the amount of solute changes. One part in 5 total parts is equivalent to 2 parts in 10 total parts.

known: 6 g, 100 mL, and 400 mL. A proportion can be established using two ratios. The ratio for 6%$^{w/v}$ NaCl is 6 g/100 mL. The ratio for the 400 mL solution is some unknown x g/400 mL.

$$\frac{6\ g}{100\ mL} = \frac{x\ g}{400\ mL}$$

The equation is then solved for *x*. The result will be in grams:

$$6\ g \times 400\ mL = x\ g \times 100\ mL$$

$$x\ g = \frac{(6\ g \times 400\ \cancel{mL})}{100\ \cancel{mL}}$$

$$x\ g = 24\ g$$

To make 400 mL of 6% NaCl, bring 24 g NaCl to 400 mL.

> **!** **CAUTION:** Some laboratory chemicals are hazardous in pure, highly concentrated form. Chemicals may also become hazardous when mixed with other chemicals. Check the safety data sheets (SDSs) before mixing chemicals together. Use the proper protection equipment (gloves, gown, eye protection) as indicated.

In a similar way, use ratio and proportion when the unknown is expressed as volume.

To make 50 mL of 0.6%$^{v/v}$ serum in saline:

$$\frac{0.6\ mL}{100\ mL} = \frac{x\ mL}{50\ mL}$$

The equation is then solved for *x* mL

$$0.6\ mL \times 50\ mL = x\ mL \times 100\ mL$$

$$x\ mL = \frac{(0.6\ \cancel{mL} \times 50\ mL)}{100\ \cancel{mL}}$$

$$x\ mL = 0.3\ mL$$

Bring 0.3 mL serum to 50 mL with saline. In this example, saline (0.85% NaCl) is used as the solvent. The components of the solvent and their concentrations are not considered because only the solute concentration is being varied.

One can use ratio and proportion to determine an unknown concentration. If 40 mL ethanol is brought to 150 mL with water, what is the percent ethanol?

$$\frac{x\ mL}{100\ mL} = \frac{40\ mL}{150\ mL}$$

Multiply both sides of the equation by 100 to isolate *x*:

$$x\ mL = \frac{(40\ mL \times 100\ \cancel{mL})}{150\ \cancel{mL}}$$

$$x\ mL = 26.7\ mL$$

Expressed as percent, 26.7 mL per 100 mL is 26.7%$^{v/v}$.

Another application of ratio and proportion is to determine how much of a solution of given concentration can be made from a known amount of solute. Suppose 25 mL of 5% NaOH$^{v/v}$ is required for a procedure, but only 1.32 g NaOH is available. Is this enough to make the required amount of 5% NaOH$^{v/v}$? 5% NaOH represents 5 g NaOH/100 mL solvent:

$$\frac{5\ g}{100\ mL} = \frac{1.32\ g}{x\ mL}$$

$$5\ g \times x\ mL = 1.32\ g \times 100\ mL$$

$$x\ mL = \frac{(1.32\ g \times 100\ mL)}{5\ g}$$

$$x\ mL = 26.4\ mL$$

The 1.32 g of NaOH will make 26.4 mL 5% NaOH$^{w/v}$, which is sufficient to make the required amount of solution.

Using Ratio and Proportion With Hydrates

Ratio and proportion adjust for differences in molecular weight (MW) between anhydrous and hydrated compounds. In one of the examples shown in Chapter 5, a protocol calls for dissolving 11.0 g anhydrous $CaCl_2$ in 1.00 L solute. The laboratory, however, only has calcium chloride decahydrate ($CaCl_2 \cdot 10H_2O$) available. Use ratio and proportion to calculate the number of grams of the decahydrate (291.08 g/mole) that are equivalent to 11.0 g anhydrous $CaCl_2$ (110.98 g/mole):

$$\frac{11.0\ g}{110.98\ g/mole} = \frac{x\ g}{291.08\ g/mole}$$

$$x\ g \times 110.98\ g/mole = 291.08\ g/mole \times 11.0\ g$$

$$x\ g = \frac{291.08\ \cancel{g/mole} \times 11.0\ g}{110.98\ \cancel{g/mole}}$$

$$x\ g = 28.7\ g\ of\ decahydrate$$

The 28.7 grams of $CaCl_2 \cdot 10H_2O$ is equivalent to 11.0 g anhydrous $CaCl_2$.

$V_1C_1 = V_2C_2$

In the foregoing examples of ratio and proportion, the starting and ending solution concentrations are the same. When the starting and ending concentrations are different, the $V_1C_1 = V_2C_2$ method is applied (Fig. 6-2). This method is expressed by the formula:

$$V_1 \times C_1 = V_2 \times C_2$$

where V_1 and V_2 are the starting and ending volumes, and C_1 and C_2 are the starting and ending concentrations, respectively. V or C must change and V_1 and V_2 have to be in the same units, as do C_1 and C_2. In addition, three of the four values have to be known.

Suppose a calculation was required to determine how much 2.0 *N* hydrogen chloride (HCl) can be made from 25 mL of 4.0 *N* HCl. The starting volume of HCl is 25 mL (V_1) with a concentration of 4 *N* (C_1); 2.0 *N* is

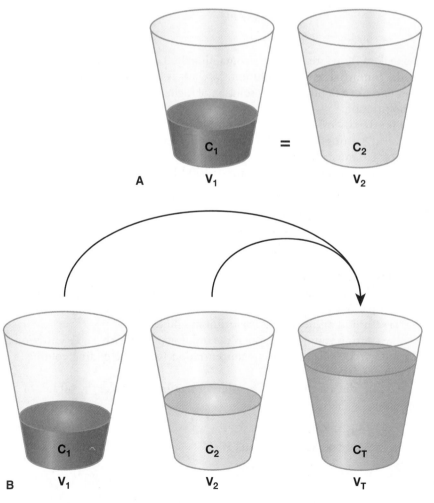

Figure 6-2 $V_1C_1 = V_2C_2$ is used when concentrations change, as when a solution is made from a more concentrated solution (A) or when two solutions of different concentrations of the same solute are mixed together (B). C_T, total concentration; V_T, total volume.

the ending concentration (C_2). The unknown is the volume (V_2) of the 2.0 N solution.

$$V_1 \times C_1 = V_2 \times C_2$$

$$25 \text{ mL} \times 4.0N = V_2 \text{ mL} \times 2.0N$$

$$V_2 \text{ mL} = \frac{(25 \text{ mL} \times 4.0 \text{ N})}{2.0 \text{ N}}$$

$$V_2 \text{ mL} = 50 \text{ mL}$$

The 25 mL 4 N HCl is enough to make 50 mL of 2 N HCl.

How much enzyme supplied in a concentration of 5 units per microliter (μL) is required to make 25 μL of 0.1 unit/μL reaction mix? The starting volume of enzyme (V_1) is unknown. The starting concentration of the enzyme solution (C_1) is 5 units/μL. The desired ending volume (V_2) is 25 μL, and 0.1 unit/μL is the ending concentration (C_2).

$$V_1 \text{ μL} \times 5 \text{ unit/μL} = 25 \text{ μL} \times 0.1 \text{ unit/μL}$$

$$V_1 \text{ μL} = \frac{(25 \text{ μL} \times 0.1 \text{ unit/μL})}{5 \text{ unit/μL}}$$

$$V_1 \text{ μL} = 0.5 \text{ μL}$$

To make a 25-μL reaction mix containing 0.10 unit/μL enzyme, use 0.50 μL of the 5-unit/μL enzyme solution. $V_1C_1 = V_2C_2$ can be used to determine how to make a dilution from a solution of higher concentration to one of lower concentration.

Prepare 100 mL of 1.0-molar solution of reagent A from a 5.0-molar solution. The starting volume of reagent A is the unknown (V_1) with a concentration of 5.0 molar (C_1); 1 molar is the ending concentration (C_2). The ending volume (V_2) of solution is 100 mL (0.100 L).

$$V_1 \text{ L} \times 5.0 \text{ moles/L} = 0.100 \text{ L} \times 1.0 \text{ mole/L}$$

$$V_1 \text{ L} = \frac{(0.100 \text{ L} \times 1.0 \text{ mole/L})}{5 \text{ moles/L}}$$

$$V_1 \text{ L} = 0.020 \text{ L} = 20 \text{ mL}$$

To make this dilution, bring 20 mL 5.0-molar reagent A to 100 mL.

$V_1C_1 = V_2C_2$ calculations determine the amount of solvent required to make a particular dilution. How much saline is required to make 50 mL of 5.0% serum in saline from 25% serum in saline?

The starting volume of saline is the unknown (V_1) with a concentration of 25% (C_1); 5.0% is the ending concentration (C_2). The ending volume (V_2) of saline is 50 mL.

To find the amount of 25% solution required to make the 50 mL of 5% solution:

$$V_1C_1 = V_2C_2:$$

$$V_1 \text{ mL} \times 25\% = 50 \text{ mL} \times 5\%$$

$$V_1 \text{ mL} = \frac{(50 \text{ mL} \times 5\%)}{25\%}$$

$$V_1 \text{ mL} = 10 \text{ mL}$$

Because 10 mL of the 25% solution are serum, subtract 10 mL from the final volume. Thus, the solution requires 40 mL saline.

50 - 10 = 40 mL saline.

The $V_1C_1 = V_2C_2$ equation can be extended to include more than two components (see Fig. 6-2B).

$$(V_1 \times C_1) + (V_2 \times C_2) + (V_3 \times C_3) + \ldots = V_T \times C_T$$

where V_T is the total volume including all components, and C_T is the final concentration of the total mixture.

The expanded equation determines the concentration of a mixture of substances. What is the molar concentration of a mixture of 100 mL 5.0-molar NaCl and 50 mL 2.0-molar NaCl?

$$(V_1 \times C_1) + (V_2 \times C_2) = V_T \times C_T$$

In this example, the total volume (V_T) of the mixture is

100 mL + 50 mL = 150 mL

This leaves only one unknown in the equation:

$$(100 \text{ mL} \times 5 \text{ molar}) + (50 \text{ mL} \times 2 \text{ molar}) = 150 \text{ mL} \times C_T$$

$$\frac{(500 + 100)}{150} = C_T$$

$$C_T = 4.0 \text{ molar}$$

The expanded equation also provides the concentration of one component of a mixture.

What is the concentration of a glucose solution when 80.0 mL are mixed with 30.0 mL of a 0.500-molar solution, yielding a 0.900-molar mixture?

The total volume (V_T) of the mixture is

80.0 mL + 30.0 mL = 110 mL

C_1 is then the unknown in the equation:

$$(80.0 \text{ mL} \times C_1) + (30.0 \text{ mL} \times 0.500 \text{ molar}) = 110 \text{ mL} \times 0.900 \text{ molar}$$

$$(80.0 \times C_1) + 15.0 = 99.0$$

$$(80.0 \times C_1) = 84$$

$$C_1 = \frac{84.0}{80.0} = 1.05 \text{ molar}$$

The volumes of components of a mixture can also be determined with this formula. How much 50-m M manganese chloride (MnCl) must be mixed with 75.0-m M MnCl to make 100 mL of 60-m M MnCl?

$$(V_1 \times C_1) + (V_2 \times C_2) + \ldots = V_T \times C_T$$

To perform this calculation, V_1 and V_2 must be expressed in terms of one unknown.

$$V_1 + V_2 = V_T$$

$$V_1 = V_T - V_2$$

$$V_1 = (100 - V_2)$$

Rearrange and insert the values in the formula:

$$[(100 - V_2) \times 50 \text{ mM}] + (V_2 \times 75 \text{ mM}) + = 100 \text{ mL} \times 60 \text{ mM}$$

$$(5{,}000 - 50 \, V_2) + 75 \, V_2 = 6{,}000$$

$$(-50 \, V_2) + (75 \, V_2) = -1{,}000$$

$$25 \, V_2 = 11{,}000$$

$$V_2 = 40$$

$$V_1 = 100 \text{ mL} - 40 \text{ mL} = 60 \text{ mL}$$

Mix 60 mL of 50-m*M* MnCl with 40 mL of 75-m*M* MnCl to make 100 mL of 60-m*M* MnCl.

FORMULAE

Units of measure are indicators of the mathematical processes required to achieve a particular solution. These units of measure are included in the formulae that describe expressions of concentration. Examples of calculations are listed in Table 6-1.

With the molecular, equivalent, or osmolar weight available from the periodic table or other reference tables, one can determine that amount of a substance (solute) required to make a specific concentration in grams per liter (g/L; Box 6-1).

To make 1 L of 0.60-molar NaOH, first find the molecular weight of NaOH, which is 40.00 g/mole [21.99 (Na) + 16.00 (O) + 1.01 (H)]. The concentration is given as 0.60 mole/L (0.60 molar).

$$\text{g/mole} \times \text{mole/L} = \text{g/L}$$

$$40 \text{ g/\sout{mole}} \times 0.60 \text{ \sout{mole}/L} = 24 \text{ g/L}$$

To make 1 L of 0.60-molar NaOH, bring 24 g NaOH to 1.0 L.

Table 6-1	Formulae Used in Calculating Concentration	
Formula Weight	Concentration	Weight per Unit Volume (1 L)
g/mole	moles/L	g/mole $\times$ moles/L = g/L
g/Eq	Eq/L	g/Eq $\times$ Eq/L = g/L
g/OsM	OsMs/L	g/OsM $\times$ OsMs/L = g/L

Box 6-1	Conversion Factors

Another approach to these calculations is to apply a conversion factor. Such conversion factors are supplied as a reference table. The molarity of a solution of 250 g/L creatinine (MW = 113.12) would be calculated from g/L using the conversion factor 0.008840:

$$250 \text{ g/L} \times 0.008840 = 2.2 \text{ molar}$$

The correct equation is derived from the known units (grams/mole and moles/liter) and the desired units (grams/liter). In this case, the desired units are achieved by multiplying the known units.

Another example: make 500 mL of 0.20 *N* HCl from a commercial HCl preparation. The equivalent weight of HCl is the same as its molecular weight, 36.46 g/mole [1.01 (H) + 35.45 (Cl)]. The concentration given is 0.20 normal or 0.20 equivalents/L.

g/Eq x Eq/L = g/L

36.46 g/Eq x 0.20 Eq/L = 7.3 g/L

Use ratio and proportion to determine the amount of HCl required for 500 mL (1L = 1,000 mL):

7.3 g/1,000 mL = x g/500 mL

x g = $\frac{(7.3 \times 500)}{1,000}$ = 3.6 g

Or, multiply the amount for 1 L by 0.50 L (=500 mL):

7.3 g/L x 0.5 L = 3.6 g

Rearrange the equation to determine molar concentration from weight per unit volume.

Find the molar concentration of a solution of 300 g NaCl in a liter of water. The molecular weight of NaCl is 58.44 g/mole [22.99 (Na) + 35.45 (Cl)]. In this example, the g/L concentration is known; therefore, in the rearranged equation:

moles/L = (g/L)/(g/mole)

moles/L = $\frac{300 \text{ g/L}}{58.44 \text{ g/mole}}$ = 5.2 moles/L NaCl

Find the molarity of a solution of 0.20 g $CaCl_2$ in 1 mL water. Use ratio and proportion to convert 0.20 g/mL to g/L:

0.20 g/1 mL = x g/1,000 mL

x g = 200 g

Then use the formula,

moles/L = (g/L)/(g/mole)

moles/L = $\frac{200 \text{ g/L}}{110.98 \text{ g/mole}}$ = 1.8 moles/L $CaCl_2$

Table 6-2 shows the relationships of different expressions of concentration using formulae. Percent or grams per liter can be converted to molarity using these formulae. Molecular weight (g/mole), valence (Eq/mole), and osmolar particles per mole (osmoles/mole) are readily available from reference tables.

These equations are used to derive expressions in normality, osmolarity, or percent.

To make 150 mL of 0.20 *N* sulfuric acid: The molecular weight of sulfuric acid (H_2SO_4) is 98 g/mole [2.0 (H_2) + 32 (S) + 64 (O_4)].

Table 6-2	Normality, Osmolarity, and Percent From Formula Weight	
Formula Weight		Concentration
(g/mole)/(Eq/mole)= g/Eq		moles/L × Eq/mole = Eq/L
(g/mole)/(osmoles/mole) = g/osmoles		moles/L × osmoles/mole = osmoles/L
(g/L)/10 (dL/L) = g/100 mL = %w/v		% × 10 (dL/L) = g/Lw/v

Because sulfuric acid has two equivalents, the equivalent weight of sulfuric acid is:

$$\frac{(g/\cancel{mole})}{(Eq/\cancel{mole})} = g/Eq$$

$$\frac{98.08 \ g/\cancel{mole}}{2 \ Eq/\cancel{mole}} = 49.04 \ g/Eq$$

The equivalent weight is then used to determine the amount of sulfuric acid required:

$$g/Eq \ x \ Eq/L = g/L$$

$$4904 \ g/\cancel{Eq} \ x \ 0.20 \ \cancel{Eq}/L = 9.8 \ g/L$$

As the volume required is 150 mL, use ratio and proportion to determine the amount of H_2SO_4 required for 150 mL (1 L = 1,000 mL):

$$9.8 \ g/1,000 \ mL \ = \ x \ g/150 \ mL$$

$$(9.8 \ x \ 150)/1,000 \ = \ 1.5 \ g$$

Or, multiply the amount for 1 L by 0.15 L (= 150 mL):

$$9.8 \ g/\cancel{L} \ x \ 0.15 \ \cancel{L} \ = \ 1.5 \ g$$

For 150 mL of 0.20 N sulfuric acid, 1.5 g sulfuric acid will be required (Box 6-2).

Table 6-3 summarizes the conversions among molarity, normality, osmolarity, percent, and concentration in grams per liter. The molecular weight of

---

Box 6-2   Purity and Specific Gravity

For a commercial preparation of concentrated sulfuric acid, the specific gravity of the sulfuric acid preparation determines the volume necessary to deliver 1.5 g (see Chapter 5). If the specific gravity of sulfuric acid is 1.84 and the purity is 96.0%, then the grams per milliliter amount of sulfuric acid in this solution is:

$$1.84 \ x \ 0.96 \ = \ 1.77 \ g/mL \ of \ the \ H_2SO_4$$

$$1.5 \ g/(1.77 \ g/mL) \ = \ 0.85 \ mL \ of \ the \ concentrated$$
$$sulfuric \ acid$$

To provide 1.5 g, 0.85 mL of the concentrated acid is required.

Table 6-3	**Converting Molarity, Normality, and Percent Expressions**	
Molarity × MW = Concentration (g/L)	Normality × EqWt = Concentration (g/L)	Percent × 10 = Concentration (g/L)
moles/L × g/mole = g/L	Eq/L × g/Eq = g/L	g/100 mL × 10 = g/L
[Concentration (g/L)]/MW = Molarity	[Concentration (g/L)]/EqWt = Normality	[Concentration (g/L)]/10 = Percent
(g/L)/(g/mole) = moles/L	(g/L)/(g/Eq) = Eq/L	(g/100 mL)/10 = %
(Percent × 10)/MW = Molarity	(Percent × 10)/EqWt = Normality	
(%× 10)/(g/mole) = moles/L	(%× 10)/(g/Eq) = Eq/L	

EqWt, equivalent weight; MW, molecular weight.

a substance can be used to derive the number of units per unit volume of any desired molarity, normality, osmolarity, or percent.

Here are some examples of using formulae as shown in Table 6-3. Convert 0.85%$^{w/v}$ NaCl to molarity.

$\%^{w/v} \times 10 \text{ (dL/L)} = g/L$

$0.85\%^{w/v} \times 10 = 8.5 \text{ g/L}$

Molarity = moles/L = (g/L)/(g/mole)

$\dfrac{8.5 \text{ g/L}}{58.44 \text{ g/mole}} = 0.14 \text{ moles/L}$

What molarity is 12%$^{w/v}$ potassium chloride (KCl)? (KCl MW = 74.55 g/mole)

$\%^{w/v} \times 10 \text{ (dL/L)} = g/L$

$12\%^{w/v} \times 10 = 120 \text{ g/L}$

Molarity = moles/L = (g/L)/(g/mole)

$\dfrac{120 \text{ g/L}}{74.55 \text{ g/mole}} = 1.61 \text{ mole/L}$

The units in the formula will guide the use of the proper function. Knowing the answer will be moles per liter and the known values are in grams per liter (%$^{w/v} \times 10$) and grams per mole,

$\dfrac{g/L}{g/mole} = \text{mole/L}$

What is the normality of 3.0%$^{w/v}$ potassium carbonate (K_2CO_3)? (K_2CO_3 MW = 138.21 g/mole)

There are two ways to solve this problem. One way is first to convert molecular weight (g/mole) to equivalent weight (g/equivalents) and then determine the normality:

$\%^{w/v} \times 10 \text{ (dL/L)} = g/L$

$3\%^{w/v} \times 10 = 30 \text{ g/L}$

Based on the molecular weight and two equivalents, the equivalent weight of K_2CO_3 is:

$$\frac{138.20 \text{ g/mole}}{2.0 \text{ Eq/mole}} = 69.10 \text{ g/Eq}$$

The formula for normality is then used:

$$\text{(g/L)/(g/Eq)} = \text{Eq/L}$$

$$\frac{30\text{g/L}}{69 \text{ g/Eq}} = 0.43 \text{ Eq/L}$$

Alternatively, solve the problem for molarity and then convert molarity to normality:

$$\%^{w/v} \times 10 \text{ (dL/L)} = \text{g/L}$$

$$3\%^{w/v} \times 10 = 30 \text{ g/L}$$

then

$$\text{(g/L)/(g/mole)} = \text{moles/L}$$

$$\frac{30\text{g/L}}{138.20 \text{ g/mole}} = 0.22 \text{ mole/L}$$

and

$$\text{Eq/L} = \text{mole/L} \times \text{Eq/mole}$$

$$\text{Eq/L} = 0.22 \text{ mole/L} \times 2.0 \text{ Eq/mole}$$

$$= 0.43 \text{ Eq/L}$$

Molecular weight divided by the valence is the equivalent weight, and molarity multiplied by the valence is normality. The units will lead to the proper mathematical function(s) required to solve the problem.

What $\%^{w/v}$ is 3 N H_2SO_4? (H_2SO_4 MW = 98.06 g/mole)
The units are:

$$\text{(g/mole)/(Eq/mole)} = \text{g/Eq}$$

$$\frac{98.08 \text{ g/mole}}{2.0 \text{ Eq/mole}} = 49 \text{ g/Eq}$$

$$3 \text{ Eq/L} \times 49 \text{ g/Eq} = 147 \text{ g/L}$$

Then:

$$\% \times 10 \text{ (dL/L)} = \text{g/L}$$

$$\% = \text{(g/L)/10}$$

$$\frac{147 \text{ g/L}}{10} = 14.7 \text{ g/100 mL} = 14.7\%^{w/v}$$

What is the osmolarity of 10 mg/dL NaOH? (NaOH MW = 40.00)

$$\text{(g/mole)/(osmoles/mole)} = \text{g/osmoles}$$

NaOH separates into two particles.

$$\frac{40.00 \ g/\cancel{mole}}{2.0 \ OsM/\cancel{mole}} = 20 \ g/\cancel{osmole}$$

% x 10 (dL/L) = g/L

10 mg/dL = 0.01g/dL = 0.010%w/v

0.010%w/v x 10 = 0.10 g/L

$$\frac{g/L}{g/osmoles} = osmoles/L$$

$$\frac{0.10 \ g/L}{20 \ g/osmoles} = 0.0050 \ osmoles/L$$

PARTIAL CONCENTRATIONS

Laboratory procedures require standard solutions of elements such as sodium, sulfur, or chlorine. These elements are available in compounds, such as NaCl. Partial concentrations are calculated to determine the concentration of the desired element supplied as part of the compound. The molecular weights of the compound and the component of interest are used to determine the elemental concentration, such as Ca in $CaCl_2$.

For molar concentrations, the molarity of the compound and all of its components are the same. The solutions are then prepared using the molarity of the compound.

How many moles of Ca are contained in 3.0 molar $CaCl_2$?

The molecular weight of $CaCl_2$ is 110.98 g/mole; the molecular weight of Ca is 40.08 g/mole, and the molecular weight of Cl is 35.45.

The molarity of the $CaCl_2$ is given at 3.0 moles/L. This means that the molarity of the Ca is 3.0 moles/L, and the molarity of the Cl_2 is 3.0 moles/L as well.

moles/L = (g/L)/(g/mole)

for $CaCl_2$:

$$3.0 \ moles/L = \frac{x \ g/L}{110.98 \ g/mole}$$

x = 333 g/L

Ratio and proportion shows that the mass of Ca (40.08 g/mole) in the 333 g of $CaCl_2$ is:

$$\frac{333 \ g}{(110.98 \ g/mole)} = \frac{x \ g}{40.08 \ g/mole}$$

x = (333/110.98) x 40 = 120.26 g

Using the formula for molarity,

moles/L = (g/L)/(g/mole)

moles/L = 120/40.08 = 3.0 moles/L Ca

Ratio and proportion also shows that the Cl (35.45 g/mole $\times$ 2) in the 333 g of $CaCl_2$ is.

$$\frac{333 \text{ g}}{110.98 \text{ g/mole}} = \frac{x \text{ g}}{70.90 \text{ g/mole}}$$

x = (333/110.98) x 70.9 = 213

Using the formula for molarity,

moles/L = (g/L)/(g/mole)

moles/L = 213/70.9 = 3.0 moles/L Cl

Therefore, the 3.0 molar $CaCl_2$ is also 3.0 molar Ca and 3.0 molar Cl.

Another example: What is the number of equivalents per liter of chlorine and Ca in 6,500 mg $CaCl_2$ dissolved in 100 mL (1 dL) water? ($CaCl_2$: 110.98 g/mole; Cl: 35.45 g/mole; Ca: 40.00 g/mole)

6,500 mg/dL = 6.5 g/dL = 6.5 g/100 mL = 6.5%$^{w/v}$

6.5%$^{w/v}$ x 10 = 65 g/L

$CaCl_2$ has two equivalents:

$$\frac{110.98 \text{ g/\text{mole} } CaCl_2}{2.0 \text{ Eq/\text{mole}}} = 55.5 \text{ g/Eq } CaCl_2$$

Use the formula,

Eq/L = (g/L)/(g/Eq)

Eq/L = (65 g/L)/(55.5 g/Eq) = 1.2 Eq/L $CaCl_2$

The solution also contains 1.2 Eq/L Cl. Use ratio and proportion to determine the weight of chlorine [(35.45 g/mole $\times$ 2) $\div$ 2 Eq/mole] in the 65 g of $CaCl_2$:

$$\frac{65 \text{ g}}{55.0 \text{ g/Eq } (CaCl_2)} = \frac{x \text{ g}}{35.45 \text{ g/Eq } (Cl)}$$

x = (35.45 x 65)/ 55.5 = 42 g Cl

Eq/L = (g/L)/(g/Eq)

(42 g/L)/(35.45 g/Eq) = 1.2 Eq/L

The number of equivalents per liter of chlorine and $CaCl_2$ is the same. The Ca concentration is also 1.2 Eq/L:

Use ratio and proportion to determine the weight of Ca in the 65 g $CaCl_2$:

$$\frac{65 \text{ g}}{55.5 \text{ g/Eq } CaCl_2} = \frac{x \text{ g}}{40.08 \text{ g/Eq } (Ca)}$$

x g = (40.08 X 65)/ 55.5 = 46 g Ca

Eq/L = (g/L)/(g/Eq)

Eq/L = (46 g/L)/(40.08 g/Eq) = 1.2 Eq/L

By contrast, concentration expressed as percent or g/L will differ among a compound and its components. To find what % chlorine is in 10.0%$^{w/v}$ NaCl

(=10.0 g NaCl/100 mL), use ratio and proportion with the molecular weight to determine how much of the 10.0 g NaCl is chlorine:

$$\frac{10.0 \text{ g}}{58.44 \text{ g/mole NaCl}} = \frac{\text{x g}}{35.45 \text{ g/mole Cl}}$$

$$\text{x} = 6.06 \text{ g Cl}$$

The 10%$^{w/v}$ NaCl contains 6.06 g chlorine in 100 mL or 6.1%$^{w/v}$ chlorine.

A procedure may require an absolute amount of substance. Determine what mass of HNO_3 is required to deliver 0.10 g of nitrogen?

(HNO_3: 63.01 g/mole; N: 14.00 g/mole). Use ratio and proportion to determine the number of grams of nitric acid is equivalent to 0.10 g nitrogen:

$$\frac{\text{x g } HNO_3}{63.01 \text{ g/Eq } (HNO_3)} = \frac{0.10 \text{ g N}}{14.00 \text{ g/Eq } (N)}$$

$$\text{x} = 0.45 \text{ g } HNO_3$$

Therefore, 0.45 g HNO³ will provide 0.10 g nitrogen.

CONVERSIONS OF EXPRESSIONS OF CONCENTRATION USING EXPONENTS

In the metric and SI systems, expression of amounts in units of similar type (volumes: mL to L, or mass: μg to mg) can be interchanged to equivalent expressions using exponents of 10. See Chapter 3, Table 3-4 for the exponents associated with unit prefixes. Simple units are converted by subtracting exponents using the following formula:

Exponent of converted units =
10**Exponent of original units − Exponent of the desired units**

To convert μg (original units, 10^{-6}) to mg (desired units, 10^{-3}), subtract the exponents:

$$(-6) - (-3) = -3$$

A microgram is 10^{-3} mg.

Conversely, to convert mg (10^{-3}) to μg (10^{-6}),

$$(-3) - (-6) = 3$$

A milligram is 10^3 μg.

Convert 3.0 L (10^0) to dL (10^{-1}).

$$(0) - (-1) = 1$$

Three liters is 3.0×10^1 dL = 30 dL.

Convert 45 nL (10^{-9}) to mL (10^{-3}).

$$(-9) - (-3) = -6$$

45 nL is 45×10^{-6} mL = 4.5×10^{-5} mL

CONVERSION OF COMPLEX UNITS

Concentration expressions are complex units. The complex unit mg/dL is a combination of two types of units, weight (or mass), and volume. The complex expression indicates how many units of something are present in a given volume, that is, concentration. Procedures may call for concentrations expressed in different terms, such as micrograms per milliliter or grams per liter.

To convert one expression of concentration to another, both components of the expression must be addressed. For complex units of concentration, use the following formula:

$$\text{Converted units =}$$
$$\text{Original units} \times \frac{10^{\text{Exponent to convert the top unit}}}{10^{\text{Exponent to convert the bottom unit}}}$$

where the exponent to convert the top or bottom units is derived by subtraction as described in the previous formula for conversion of simple units. Convert 65 μg/mL to mg/dL:

Exponent to convert top unit is: $\mu g(-6) - mg(-3) = -3$

Exponent to convert bottom unit is: $mL(-3) - dL(-1) = -2$

Using the formula:

$$10^{-3} \div 10^{-2} = 10^{-1}$$

Using the exponents:

$$(-3) - (-2) = --1$$
$$65 \times 10^{-1} = 6.5$$
$$65 \ \mu g/mL = 6.5 \ mg/dL$$

In another example, convert 1.5 g/mL to ng/μL:

$$g \ (0) - ng \ (-9) = 9$$
$$mL \ (-3) - \mu L \ (-6) = 3$$

Using the formula:

$$10^9 \div 10^3 = 10^6$$

Using the exponents:

$$9 - 3 = 6$$
$$1.5 \times 10^6 = 1,500,000$$
$$1.5 \ g/mL = 1,500,000 \ ng/\mu L$$

Convert 500 ng/μL to μg/L:

$$ng \ (-9) - \mu g \ (-6) = -3$$
$$\mu L \ (-6) - L \ (0) = -6$$

Using the formula:

$$10^{-3} \div 10^{-6} = 10^3$$

Using the exponents:

$$(-3) - (-6) = 3$$

$$500 \times 10^3 = 500{,}000$$

$$500 \text{ ng}/\mu L = 500{,}000 \ \mu g/L$$

Area is measured for laboratory procedures, such as imaging tissues on slides or as a requirement of a minimal cubic volume of tissue for an analysis. To convert units of higher order (e.g., square mm or cubic cm), multiply the derived exponents by 2 for area, or 3 for volume:

To convert 1.5 square mm to square μm:

$$\text{mm } (10^{-3}) \rightarrow \mu \text{m } (10^{-6})$$

$$(-3) - (-6) = 3$$

Multiply this exponent by 2 (for area):

$$3 \times 2 = 6$$

The factor for converting square mm to square μm is 10^6:

$$1.5 \text{ mm}^2 = 1.5 \times 10^6 \ \mu \text{m}^2$$

Convert 3.7 cubic mm to cubic cm:

$$\text{mm } (10^{-3}) \rightarrow \text{cm } (10^{-2})$$

$$(-3) - (-2) = -1$$

Multiply this exponent by 3 (for volume):

$$-1 \times 3 = -3$$

The factor for conversion of cubic mm to cubic cm is 10^{-3}:

$$3.7 \text{ mm}^3 = 3.7 \times 10^{-3} \text{ cm}^3$$

PRACTICE PROBLEMS

Use ratio and proportion for the following calculations.

1. How many grams are in 10 mL of a 6% solution?

2. How many milligrams of solute are in 108 mL of a 25% solution?

3. A manufacturer recommends using 1.5 mL reagent A for every 3.0 mL reagent B. You have only 1.0 mL reagent B. How much reagent A should you use?

4. One milliliter (V_1) of solution A with concentration 0.02 mg/dL (C_1) is equivalent to 10 mL (V_2) of solution B. What is the concentration (C_2) of solution B?

5. A test requires 1.00 L of 0.100%$^{w/v}$ of $CuSO_4$. How do you prepare the proper concentration of $CuSO_4$ using $CuSO_4 \cdot H_2O$?

6. A liquid delivery system requires 500 mL of 1%$^{w/v}$ reagent A. Reagent A is supplied in powder form. How do you prepare the proper concentration of reagent A?

7. A procedure calls for 150 mL of 0.20%$^{w/v}$ KCl. How do you prepare the proper concentration of KCl?

8. Proteins and nucleic acids are separated by sieving through gels. One type of gel is made by mixing powdered agarose in liquid. How do you prepare a 50-mL volume 3%$^{w/v}$ agarose gel?

9. A laboratory method calls for 15.0 g of $CaCl_2$ dissolved in 300 mL water. Only $CaCl_2$ dihydrate is available. How do you prepare the proper concentration of $CaCl_2$?

10. The result of a test was 10.0 mg analyte in 5.00 mL test solution. How much analyte should be added to 45.0 mL of test solution to obtain the same concentration?

Use $V_1C_1 = V_2C_2$ for the following calculations.

11. How do you make 50 mL of 0.25 N NaOH from 5.0 N NaOH?

12. How do you make 5.0 mL of 35 mM NaCl from 2.0 molar NaCl?

13. A procedure calls for 20 mL of 0.10 N HCl. How do you prepare this from 1.0 N HCl?

14. A reagent for use in an instrument is supplied as a 10X concentrate (C_1). What volume of reagent is required to make 250 mL (V_2) of 0.10 $\times$ (C_2) solution?

15. How do you prepare 1,000 mL of 0.05 N H_2SO_4 from a 10%$^{w/v}$ H_2SO_4 solution?

16. How do you prepare 100 mL of 1.0%$^{w/v}$ hydrofluoric acid from a commercial hydrofluoric acid solution? (sp gr $=1.167$ g/mL; purity $= 55\%$)

17. How do you prepare 50 mL of 0.05 N H_2SO_4 from a commercial H_2SO_4 solution (96% pure, sp gr $= 1.84$ g/mL)?

18. How do you prepare 5.0 mL of 0.20 M H_2SO_4 from a 5.0 N H_2SO_4 solution?

19. How do you prepare 10 mL of 2.0 mM NaOH from a commercial NaOH with a specific gravity of 1.54 and a purity of 50%?

20. The recommended concentration of a 50-μL reaction mix is 2.0 mM $MgCl_2$. How much 25 mmoles/L $MgCl_2$ are required to make this reaction mix?

21. What is the concentration of a mixture of 200 mL 60% alcohol plus 50 mL 80% alcohol?

Continued

22. What is the concentration of KCl when 500 mL mixed with 350 mL 10%$^{v/v}$ KCl yields 850 mL of a 25%$^{v/v}$ solution?

23. How much 3-osmolar salt must be mixed with 2-osmolar salt to yield a 10-mL 2.5-osmolar salt solution?

24. What is the final concentration if 10 mL of 2 mg/mL $CuSO_4$ is mixed with 25 mL of 10 mg/mL $CuSO_4$?

25. What is the concentration of a mixture of 20 mL 5-molar $NaCl_2$ plus 30 mL 10-molar $NaCl_2$?

Use formulae to do the following calculations.

26. How many equivalents of NaOH are there in 3 L of 0.6 N NaOH?

27. Convert 0.30 mole/L NaCl to grams per liter.

28. A procedure calls for 1.0 L of 0.50 N HCl. How many grams HCl are required?

29. A solution containing 30 g/L $MgCl_2$ is what molarity?

30. What is the percent concentration of 1.0 osmolar $CuSO_4$?

31. Convert 10%$^{w/v}$ $CaCl_2$ to molarity.

32. Convert 1.0%$^{w/v}$ HCl to normality.

33. Convert 1.0%$^{w/v}$ H_2SO_4 to normality.

34. Is 5.0 mM MnCl more, less, or equally as concentrated as a 1.0% solution?

35. What is the %$^{w/v}$ $CaCl_2$ concentration of 10 mM $CaCl_2 \cdot 10H_2O$?

36. What is the normality of 20.0%$^{v/v}$ nitric acetic acid? (HNO_3: sp gr = 1.42; assay 70.0%)

37. Convert 5.0 osmolar NaCl to molar concentration.

38. Convert 250 mOsmolar glucose to percent$^{w/v}$ concentration.

Perform the following conversions using exponents.

39. 50 g to mg

40. 2,500 mL to L

41. 10 nL to μL

42. 5.0 mm to nm

43. 35 pg to μg

44. 7.2 mg/mL to mg/dL

45. 48 pg/nL to g/L

46. 595 mg/L to μg/mL

47. 50% to μg/L

48. 15 ng/mL to %

49. 8,000 square nm to square μm

50. 115 cubic mm to cubic cm

APPLICATIONS

Molecular Diagnostics

A reaction requires a particular amount in units of an enzyme. The enzyme is purchased in concentrated form, 5 units per microliter (units/μL). There are 20 samples and controls in the run. The procedure calls for addition of enzyme to a concentration of 0.01 unit/μL to each reaction.

1. If each reaction requires 50 μL, how much reaction mix must be prepared for 20 reactions + 1 extra to accommodate pipetting error?
2. What volume of concentrated enzyme must be added to the total reaction mix?

Clinical Chemistry

1. Acidity is expressed as millimoles acid per liter. If 3.2 mL of 0.1 N NaOH neutralizes 25 mL, what is the acidity?
2. The upper limit of the dynamic range of the instrument used for measurement of lipase levels in serum was exceeded by an undiluted patient specimen. The sample was therefore diluted into pooled serum (50 mg/dL lipase) to bring the specimen concentration into measurement range. One milliliter of sample was mixed with 19 mL of pooled serum for a total of 20 mL. The diluted specimen is measured, and the concentration of the mixture was 65.0 mg/dL. What is the concentration of the original sample? What would be the results if the sample had been tested using a 1:20 ratio of sample to diluent?

CHAPTER 7

LOGARITHMS AND EXPONENTIAL FUNCTIONS

Before the development of electronic calculating instruments, multiplying or dividing very small or very large numbers was tedious and prone to error. The use of exponents simplified these calculations somewhat, but a resulting exponential number, such as 25^2, still had to be converted to a natural number, 625. The derivation and use of logarithms have been greatly facilitated by electronic calculators and computer software. Logarithms are frequently used in laboratory calculations, for expression of hydrogen or hydroxyl ion concentrations and in spectrophotometry.

LOGARITHMS

An exponential expression has two parts, the **base** and the **exponent**. A logarithm is the exponent of an exponential expression (Box 7-1); (Fig. 7-1).

Real or natural numbers are converted to logarithms by first expressing them in exponential form. The number 512 can be expressed as 8^3. In this example, 8 is the base and **3** is the exponent. The number 512 can be expressed logarithmically in the base 8 as **3**. That is:

$$\log_8 512 = 3$$

The $\log_8$ of 512 is then 3. The $\log_8$ of 64, (8^2) is 2. The log is the exponent in the given base (Box 7-2). The same log can indicate a different number in a different base. Compare the $\log_8$ of 64 with the $\log_5$ of 25, (5^2):

$$\log_8 64 = 2$$
$$\log_5 25 = 2$$

The value of 2 represents 25 or 64, depending on the base.

LEARNING OUTCOMES
- Define logarithms.
- Distinguish common and natural logarithms.
- Derive logarithms from natural numbers.
- Define the two parts of the logarithm, characteristic and mantissa.
- List the algebraic properties of logarithms.
- Define antilogarithms.
- Convert logarithms to natural numbers.

Box 7-1 Logarithm History

John Napier, a Scottish mathematician and religious scholar, is credited with the invention of logarithms. His original logarithms, published in 1614, were based on an irrational number *e*, which is approximately equal to 2.7. Napier intended his system to be used by astronomers to save time and prevent errors in calculations. The logarithms facilitated calculations using sines, a term for the relationship between sides of a triangle. In 1617, Napier devised a mechanical multiplication method using metal rods marked with numbers to be used along with his logarithmic system. This device was the basis for modern calculators.

Working together, Napier and the English mathematician Henry Briggs discovered natural logarithms, logarithms to the base *e*, which were variations of Napier's original logarithms. Napier and Briggs also suggested the calculations of logarithms by extracting roots of the base 10. Briggs compiled the first Table of Common Logarithms in 1624. The definition of logarithms as exponents was proposed by John Wallis in 1685 and John Bernoulli in 1694.

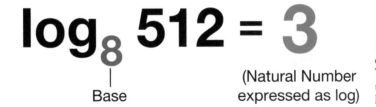

$$8^3 = 512$$

Exponent

Base   (Natural Number)

$$\log_8 512 = 3$$

Base   (Natural Number expressed as log)

Figure 7-1 A logarithm is an exponent of a number (base). The exponent (3) represents the natural number (512) as long as the base (8) is known.

Box 7-2 Logarithmic Expression

Logarithms can be expressed from any base (2^{35}, 100^2, 15^4 are exponential numbers with bases of 2, 100, 15).

Common logarithms are always in the base 10. It is not necessary to indicate the base 10 when writing common logarithms. When the log expression is used without an indication of base, the base 10 is assumed.

The base 10 and the base *e* are used for laboratory applications, and fits well with the decimal system. Logs with the base 10 are called **common** or

Briggsian logs. Common or Briggsian logarithms are abbreviated log (not capitalized and no period). The base *e* is an irrational number (a number that cannot be expressed as a ratio of two natural numbers and that has infinite nonrepeating digits when expressed as a decimal fraction). The base e is approximately 2.7182818284. Logs to the base *e* are called **natural** or **Naperian** (or **Napierian**) logs. Natural logarithms are abbreviated ln or $\log_e$ (not capitalized and no period). Laboratory calculations are mostly in common logarithms; however, some formulae may contain natural logarithmic expressions.

Parts of Logarithms

In common logarithms, the log of 1 is 0 ($10^0 = 1$; log 1 = 0), and the log of 10 is 1 ($10^1 = 10$; log 10 = 1).

10^0 = 1	log 1 = 0
10^1 = 10	log 10 = 1
10^2 = 100	log 100 = 2
10^3 = 1,000	log 1,000 = 3
10^4 = 10,000	log 10,000 = 4
10^5 = 100,000	log 100,000 = 5
10^6 = 1,000,000	log 1,000,000 = 6

The numbers 0 to 6 shown on the right above represent a range of multiples (or powers) of 10 from 1 to 1,000,000. Logs of numbers less than 1 (between 0 and 1) are expressed using a negative sign:

10^{-1} = 0.1	log 0.1 = −1
10^{-2} = 0.01	log 0.01 = −2
10^{-3} = 0.001	log 0.001 = −3
10^{-4} = 0.0001	log 0.0001 = −4
10^{-5} = 0.00001	log 0.00001 = −5
10^{-6} = 0.000001	log 0.000001 = −6

The numbers −1 to −6 shown on the right above represent a range of fractions of 10 from $\frac{1}{10}$ to $\frac{1}{1,000,000}$ (decimal fractions 0.1 to 0.000001; Box 7-3)).

Positive and negative whole numbers are just one part of the logarithm, called the **characteristic** or log characteristic. The characteristic indicates the placement of the decimal point in the number that the logarithm represents.

Box 7-3 | **Negative Exponents**

There are no logarithms of negative numbers. Numbers between 0 and 1, however, have negative exponents.

For whole numbers, the log characteristic is always positive and one less than the number of digits to the left of the decimal point. The number 575 is three places to the left of the decimal, so the log characteristic for this number is **2**. The number 1,780,276 is seven places to the left of the decimal point, so the log characteristic for this number is 6.

For numbers between 0 and 1, the log characteristic is negative and one more than the number of zeroes to the right of the decimal point. The number 0.00575 has 2 zeroes to the right of the decimal point, so its characteristic is –3. The number 0.575 has no zeroes to the right of the decimal point, so its characteristic is –1.

> Because of the way in which logarithm tables were originally written, logarithms of numbers between 0 and 1 are not the same as the actual exponents of 10 for these numbers. This is apparent when using calculators to find logarithms. Calculators find the actual exponents of 10.

Common logarithms express multiples and fractions of 10. How then does one express the logarithm of a number between powers of 10, such as 575? Scientific notation can be used, as discussed in Chapter 2. First determine the power of 10 in the number. The number 575 is a multiple of two powers of 10 or 10^2. Then convert 575 to a number between 1 and 10. The number, 575, expressed in scientific notation in the form:

a x 10^b

would be

5.75 x 10^2

Another part of the log expression is required to express numbers between multiples of the base (10 in common logarithms, *e* in natural logarithms). This is the **mantissa**. The mantissa is always a decimal number. Whereas the characteristic indicates the multiple of 10 (0.1, 10, 1,000), the mantissa estimates the point between the two orders of 10 at which the natural number lies. For the log of a number between log100 and log1,000, (2 and 3), a mantissa of 0.9999, (2.9999) is very close to an exponent of 3, indicating a natural number close to 10^3 10^3 = 1,000. So, $10^{2.9999}$ would be close to 1,000.

Natural numbers:	100...................................1,000
Powers of 10:	10^2.....................$10^{2.9999}$......10^3
Logarithms:	2.........................2.9999.........3

A mantissa of 0.0001 (2.0001) is very close to an exponent of 2 or a natural number of 100.

Natural numbers:	100...................................1,000
Powers of 10:	10^2.....$10^{2.0001}$........................10^3
Logarithms:	2.......2.0001..........................3

Consider the number, **575 = 5.75 x 10²**. The characteristic for 575 is 2, and the mantissa for 575 is 0.7597. (How this mantissa is determined is discussed in the next section.)

Natural numbers: 100.........575....................1,000

Powers of 10: 10^2..........$10^{2.7597}$.................10^3

Logarithms: 2..............2.7597....................3

log 100 = 2.0000

log 1,000 = 3.0000

log 575 = 2.7597

The mantissa is determined either with a table of mantissas or by using a calculator.

THE MANTISSA

The mantissa is an estimation of the distance between the powers of 10 indicated by the characteristic. In the example given earlier, the number 575 is expressed as a logarithm with a four-place mantissa as 2.7597. The mantissa 0.7597 is determined from a table of mantissas or a calculator.

Mantissas are the same for all powers of 10 of a number. The 0.7597 mantissa is the same for 5,750 or 575,000 or 0.00000575. The characteristic accounts for the placement of the decimal point.

log 575 = 2.7597

log 5,750 = 3.7597

log 575,000 = 5.7597

log 0.00000575 = −6.7597

Although logarithmic tables were used extensively before the advent of electronic systems, the medical laboratory professional will likely use calculators, software, or computer applications for this task.

Determining the Mantissa Using a Calculator

Scientific calculators are rapid and relatively simple to use for the conversion of natural numbers to logarithms. Electronic calculators have variable configurations, so refer to the instruction manual supplied with any particular unit. In general, there should be a key designated "log" on the keyboard. Some calculators may have this function noted above or below a key, meaning that a shift key must be pressed to access the log function. In some calculators, the natural number must be entered first and then the log key pressed. In others, press the log key first and then the natural number. The logarithm, characteristic and mantissa, should appear. It may be necessary to press the "=" or "exe" key to reveal the logarithm. The instruction manual will indicate which order is correct.

Using a calculator, determine the logarithms for 575. Enter 575 and then log (or log and then 575). When the "log" or "exe" key is pressed, the resulting number is the complete logarithm, including the characteristic and mantissa 2.7597. The mantissa is carried out to more than four places by the calculator as it is mathematically computing the actual exponent of 10:

> **Result from a log table:** $10^{2.7597} \sim 575$
>
> **Result from a calculator:** $10^{2.759667845} \sim 575$

Entering 5,750 yields a logarithm with the same mantissa and different characteristic: 3.7597 (rounded off).

> **Result from a log table:** $10^{3.7597} \sim 5,750$
>
> **Result from a calculator:** $10^{3.759667845} \sim 5,750$

Using the calculator to find the logarithm of numbers less than 1 (between 0 and 1) will yield a mantissa different from a logarithm found in logarithmic tables. This is because the calculator is finding the exponent of 10 that would yield the natural number expression. Calculations for numbers less than 1 yield a negative mantissa. There are, however, no negative mantissas in table logarithms.

To find the table logarithm for a number between 0 and 1 on a calculator, first determine the mantissa by adding a positive whole number to the negative exponent of 10. The added number should be high enough to produce a positive sum. The mantissa will be the digits to the right of the decimal point. Use this with the characteristic to form the table log.

To find the table log of log 0.00000575, find the log (exponent of 10) on the calculator.

> **log 0.00000575 = −5.2403**

Add 6 (or any whole number larger than 5).

> **−5.2403 + 6 = 0.7597**

This is the mantissa. Inspect the number, to find the characteristic (−6). The table log is −6.7597.

Logarithms are used for a number of laboratory applications including chemistry, spectrophotometry, and molecular biology. As demonstrated in later chapters, the numbers generated on calculators, and not table logarithms, are used in these applications.

Box 7-4   Naperian Logs

Naperian (Napierian) logs or logs to other bases are not frequently used in routine laboratory work. They can be calculated in the same manner described in the text, by substituting the "ln" key on the calculator or software for the "log" key. Naperian logs are more frequently used in business and financial calculations. Business calculators may have only Naperian log capabilities (only the "ln" key and no "log" key).

Determining Logarithms Using Computer Software

With the rapid advances of technology, computers are an integral part of the classroom as well as the laboratory. A variety of software programs will automatically convert natural numbers to logs and vice versa with minimal effort. In the Microsoft Excel Spreadsheet program, the logarithm of a number is determined using the function option (fx) and then selecting log10 (logarithms in the base 10 or common logs). A window will appear into which the natural number is entered. The logarithm (exponent of 10) equivalent to that number will then be calculated. Like calculators, this program yields exponents of 10 and not table logarithms for numbers between 0 and 1.

Dedicated programs are linked to applications in which the log is being used, such as software associated with instruments. In some cases, the use of the logarithm may not be apparent within the calculations. To use these systems, follow the online instructions or manuals provided with the software.

ANTILOGARITHMS

Presented with a logarithm, one may have to determine the natural number represented by that logarithm. The natural number in this case is the **antilogarithm** (antilog).

Antilogs can be found using antilog tables, log tables in reverse, or a calculator or computer.

The method to find an antilog on a calculator depends on the brand and type of calculator, and so refer to the operations manual for detailed instructions. In general, there may be an "antilog" key or a key labeled "10^x" on the calculator. Press the antilog or 10^x key and then the logarithm, including the characteristic. You may have to press the "=" or exe key to obtain the natural number or antilog. Thus, the log of 0.00575 is –2.24033 by calculator, and the antilog of –2.24033 is 0.00575 using the antilog key. Some calculators may require entering the logarithm and then pressing the "antilog" or "10^x" key.

ALGEBRAIC PROPERTIES OF LOGARITHMS

Logarithms have characteristics of exponents. The following equations are for common logs (base 10), but they hold for any base.

1. The log of 1 is always 0.

$$\log 1 = 0$$

Examples:
$$10^0 = 1$$
$$8^0 = 1$$
$$e^0 = 1$$
$$a^0 = 1$$

2. The log of any number to its own base is always 1.

$$\log_b b \ = \ 1$$
$$\log_{10} 10 \ = \ 1$$

Examples:　$10^1 = 10$

$8^1 = 8$

$e^1 = e$

$a^1 = a$

3. The log of the product of two numbers is the sum of the log of each number.

$$\log (xy) = \log x + \log y$$

Example:　$\log (8 \times 3) = \log 8 + \log 3$

$\log 8 + \log 3 = 0.9031 + 0.4771 = 1.3802$

To confirm:　$8 \times 3 = 24$

$\log 24 = 1.3802$

This rule can be used to find the logarithm (exponent of 10) of a number in scientific notation ($a \times 10^{-b}$).

$\log (7.61 \times 10^{-3}) =$

$\log 7.61 + \log (10^{-3}) =$

$0.8814 + (-3) = -2.1186$

4. The log of the quotient of two numbers is the difference of the log of the divisor subtracted from the log of the dividend.

$$\log (x/y) = \log x - \log y$$

Example:　$\log (9/5) = \log 9 - \log 5$

$\log 9 - \log 5 = 0.9542 - 0.6990 = 0.2552$

To confirm:　$9/5 = 1.8$

$\log 1.8 = 0.2553$

5. The log of the reciprocal of a number is the negative log of the number.

$$\log (1/x) = -(\log x)$$

Example:　$\log (1/20) = -(\log 20)$

$\log 1 - \log 20 = 0 - 1.3010 = -1.3010$

$(\log 1/20) = -1.3010$

To confirm:　$1/20 = 0.05$

$\log 0.05 = -1.3010$

6. The log of an exponential number is the exponent times the log of the number.

$$\log x^n = n \times \log x$$

Example:
$$\log 25^2 = 2 \times \log 25$$
$$\log 25 = 1.3979$$
$$2 \times 1.3979 = 2.7959$$

Check:
$$25^2 = 625; \log 625 = 2.7959$$

CALCULATING WITH LOGARITHMS

Electronic calculators and computer software have facilitated all levels of mathematical calculations, including those with very large and very small numbers. Logarithms were originally used for multiplication and division of numbers greater than 0 through their exponential expressions. Calculations using logarithms were estimates of the actual results. Results are now automatically calculated on a computer or calculator. The advantage of logarithmic expressions is the simplification of very large and very small numbers. Scales can be shortened on instruments, and results may be more easily interpreted.

PRACTICE PROBLEMS

1. What is the base of an exponential expression?

2. What is the exponent of an exponential expression?

3. What is the base of natural (Naperian) logarithms?

4. What is the base of common (Briggsian) logarithms?

5. For the number 5^3, what is the base and what is the exponent?

6. For the number 10^3, what is the base and what is the exponent?

7. In expressing the number 10^3 as a common logarithm, what is the characteristic?

8. Without using a calculator, find the characteristics of the following numbers.

   25
   25,000
   377
   2.5×10^9
   0.002
   7
   7.237
   0.27
   1.3×10^{-4}
   1.000003

9. In expressing the number 10^3 as a common logarithm, what is the mantissa?

10. Find four-place mantissas of the following numbers by using a calculator.

   25
   25,000
   377
   2.5×10^9
   0.002
   7
   7.237
   0.27
   1.3×10^{-4}
   1.000003

Continued

11. What are the logarithms of the following numbers?

25
25,000
377
2.5×10^9
0.002
7
7.237
0.27
1.3×10^{-4}
1.000003

12. Find the base 10 exponents of the following numbers by using a calculator. (i.e., $10^x = 25$, what is x?)

25
25,000
377
2.5×10^9
0.002
7
7.237
0.27
1.3×10^{-4}
1.000003

Finish the following equations for logarithms in the base 10.

13. $\log(xy) =$

14. $\log 1 =$

15. $\log x - \log y =$

16. $\log (1/x) =$

17. $\log x^k =$

18. $\log_e x =$

APPLICATIONS

Physiology

Body surface area measurements guide drug dosage and adjustment of physiological assessments. Body surface area is a function of height and weight. A formula used to determine body surface area (A) in square meters is:

$$\log A = (0.425 \times \log W) + (0.725 \times \log H) - 2.144$$

where W is weight in kg and H is height in cm.

Determine the body surface area of a person who is 6 feet tall and weighs 235 pounds.

CHAPTER 8

IONIC
SOLUTIONS

IONS

Matter is composed of atoms, which are combinations of protons, electrons, and other subatomic particles. Electrons are negatively charged, whereas protons carry a positive charge. In an **ion**, the number of protons in an atom is not equal to the number of electrons. If the number of protons exceeds the number of electrons, the ion carries a positive charge and is a **cation.** If the number of electrons exceeds the number of protons, the ion carries a negative charge and is an **anion.**

Many chemical reactions take place with the attraction of cations and anions by electromagnetic forces. Cations and anions form **ionic bonds.** Pure anions combined with pure cations form large repeating structures, or crystals (Fig. 8-1).

LEARNING OUTCOMES

- Define ions.
- Define acids, bases, and salts.
- Describe ionic dissociation.
- Define pH and pOH.
- Calculate pH from ionic concentration.
- Convert pH to molar concentration.
- Describe the preparation of a solution when given the pH.
- Illustrate how a buffer resists pH change.
- Define and describe the preparation of buffered solutions.
- Describe buffering in body fluids.

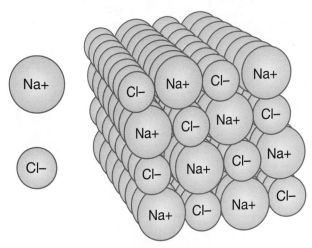

Figure 8-1 Negatively charged anions (Cl⁻) and positively charged cations (Na⁺) form ionic bonds (e.g., making NaCl). When bonded anions and cations form repeating structures called crystals, such as salt crystals, that become large enough to see with an unaided eye.

ACIDS, BASES, AND SALTS

When dissolved in water (in aqueous solution), an **acid** releases hydrogen ions (H^+). H^+ represents a proton. H^+ exists as such for only a very short time before it joins a water molecule (H_2O) to form a positively charged **hydronium ion** (H_3O^+). A **base** in aqueous solution releases hydroxyl ions (OH^-). OH^- can accept or combine with a proton to form a water molecule (Fig. 8-2).

Lowry and Bronsted defined an acid as a substance that donates a proton and a base as a substance that accepts a proton. When an acid loses a proton (H^+), it becomes a **conjugate base**.

Acid	Conjugate base
$H_2PO_4^-$	$\leftrightarrow$ HPO_4^- + H^+
NH_4^+	$\leftrightarrow$ NH_3 + H^+
HCl	$\leftrightarrow$ Cl^- + H^+

As indicated by $\leftrightarrow$, the conjugate base can accept a proton to become a **conjugate acid**. The conjugate acid has one more H^+ (and one less negative charge) than its conjugate base. A conjugate base has one less H^+ (and one more negative charge) than its conjugate acid. Every acid has a conjugate base and every base has a conjugate acid.

A **salt** is a combination of the cation (positive ion) of the base and the anion (negative ion) of the acid. A salt neither donates nor accepts protons, nor does it release H^+ or OH^-. Salts are formed when acids and bases are mixed together:

Acid + Base	$\rightarrow$ Salt
HCl + $NaOH$	$\rightarrow$ $NaCl$ + HOH
H_2SO_4 + 2 KOH	$\rightarrow$ K_2SO_4 + 2 HOH

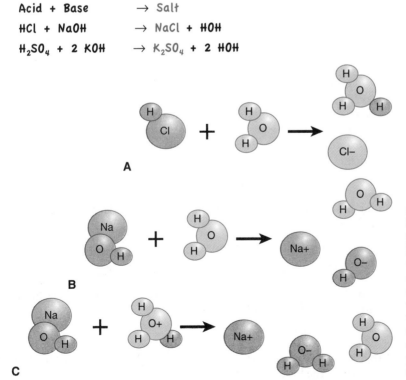

Figure 8-2 (A) Acids, such as hydrochloric acid (HCl), in water release hydrogen ions (H^+, which exist as hydronium ions, H_3O^+). (B) Bases (e.g., sodium hydroxide [NaOH]) in water release hydroxyl ions (OH^-) that can replace OH^- in the water molecules. C, When an acid is present, the OH^- can combine with excess protons and neutralize the solution.

In this reaction, the acid **neutralizes** the base (or the base neutralizes the acid) as the OH^- and H^+ released from the base and acid, respectively, join to form water molecules.

IONIC DISSOCIATION

In aqueous solutions, the H^+ released by acids are attracted by the negative charge on the oxygen atom of H_2O, to form H_3O^+.

HNO_3	$+$	H_2O	$\leftrightarrow$	$NO_3^- +$	H_3O^+
Acid		Conjugate base		Conjugate base	Acid

In this equation, H_2O is the conjugate base of H_3O^+ because it accepts an H^+, and H_3O^+ becomes the acid. Conversely, NO_3^- is the conjugate base of nitric acid (HNO_3). H_3O^+ and H_2O are a **conjugate pair**, as are NO_3^- and HNO_3.

Separation of a compound into ions is called ionic dissociation or **ionization**. The degree to which an acid ionizes varies among acids and is a measure of the strength of that acid. Strong acids are almost 100% ionized in water, thus producing the maximum amount of H^+ in solution. In contrast, weak acids exist mostly in the un-ionized form. They are only partially ionized acids and release fewer H^+ ions in solution.

Ionizable acids are **monoprotic**, meaning that they contain only one ionizable hydrogen atom, or **polyprotic** (diprotic, triprotic), with more than one ionizable hydrogen atom. A polyprotic acid can be both a strong and a weak acid because one hydrogen atom may ionize more readily than the other. Sulfuric acid readily ionizes one of its hydrogen atoms and less readily ionizes the other:

$$H_2SO_4 + H_2O \rightarrow HSO_4^- + H_3O^+$$
$$HSO_4^- \leftrightarrow SO_4^{--} + H_3O^+$$

Thus, H_2SO_4 is a strong acid, whereas HSO_4^- is a weak acid (and a conjugate base to H_2SO_4).

Bases also ionize to different extents in aqueous solution, releasing hydroxyl groups (OH^-). Strong bases ionize completely, whereas weak bases ionize to lesser extents. As with acids, ionizable bases can be **monobasic**, such as sodium hydroxide (NaOH):

$$NaOH \rightarrow Na^+ + OH^-$$

or **polybasic** (dibasic, tribasic). Barium hydroxide ($BaOH_2$) is dibasic and can ionize twice:

$$Ba(OH)_2 \rightarrow BaOH^+ + OH^-$$
$$BaOH^+ \rightarrow Ba^{++} + OH^-$$

If acid is present in the same solution with a base, the OH^- combines with H^+ from the acid to form HOH or H_2O.

$$OH^- + H^+ \rightarrow H_2O$$

This effectively lowers both the OH^- and the H^+ concentrations in the mixture; that is, the base (or acid) is neutralized.

Compounds without hydroxyl groups can also act as bases. A compound containing an amino group, RNH_2 (R represents the rest of the molecule), takes a hydrogen atom from solution forming RNH_3^+ and leaves a hydroxyl ion. The formation of the negative hydroxyl ion is the same as adding an OH^- to solution.

$$RNH_2 + HOH \leftrightarrow OH^- + RNH_3^+$$

Conversely, ammonium ion (NH_4^+) in aqueous solution releases H^+ (H_3O^+) and ammonia (NH_3). This makes a solution more acidic.

$$NH_4^+ + H_2O \rightarrow NH_3 + H_3O^+$$

The Ionization Constant

The degree of ionization of an acid in aqueous solution is described by how extensively it separates from its hydrogen ion. This degree of ionization defines an **ionization constant** (K_a) for the acid. Acetic acid is a weak acid that only ionizes to a small extent as shown in the following formula (H^+ represents H_3O^+ in aqueous solution):

$$H_3CCOOH \leftrightarrow H^+ + H_3CCOO^-$$

Using brackets [ ] to indicate concentration, a formula can be written:

$$[H_3CCOOH] \leftrightarrow [H^+] + [H_3CCOO^-]$$

That is, the concentration of intact acetic acid is more than the sum of the concentrations of its dissociated ions. The ionization constant (K_a) is:

$$K_a = \frac{[H^+] \times [H_3CCOO^-]}{[H_3CCOOH]}$$

Because acetic acid is a weak acid and it ionizes very little, the concentrations of the ions, H^+ and H_3CCOO^-, are very low compared to the concentration of the intact acid H_3CCOOH. This will make the K_a of acetic acid very small (1.8×10^{-5}). K_a is a constant and so it remains the same regardless of the concentration of acid. The ratio of the product of the [H^+] and [H_3CCOO^-] ion concentrations to the intact acid concentration will be 1.8×10^{-5}, regardless of the acetic acid concentration. Low K_a values indicate minor ionization (weak acids). K_a is used only for weak acids. It is not calculated for strong acids because they ionize completely in solution and leave little or no intact acid.

In the following general formula, HA represents any acid, and H^+ represents H_3O^+ in aqueous solution. A^- represents the conjugate base.

$$K_a = \frac{[H^+] \times [A^-]}{[HA]}$$

A similar formula can be used for ionization constants of weak and strong bases (K_b). The general formula can be written for ionization of base in aqueous solution:

$$K_b = \frac{[B^+] \times [OH^-]}{[BOH]}$$

A weak base such as ammonia will not produce OH^- ions on its own, but partially ionize water to generate OH^- ions:

$$NH_3 + H_2O \longleftrightarrow OH^- + NH_4^+$$

The ionization constant for the base is:

$$K_b = \frac{[OH^-] \times [NH_4^+]}{[NH_3]}$$

A strong base such as NaOH completely ionizes into Na^+ and OH^- ions. Like strong acids, the K_b for a strong base is very large.

Acids and bases that ionize more than once have multiple ionization constants. K_a will vary with the ease of ionization of each ion.

$$H_3PO_4 \longleftrightarrow H_2PO_4^- + H^+$$
$$H_2PO_4^- \longleftrightarrow HPO_4^- + H^+$$
$$HPO_4^- \longleftrightarrow PO_4^{--} + H^+$$

In H_3PO_4, ionization becomes weaker with each hydrogen dissociation (i.e., K_a becomes smaller):

$$K_{a1} = \frac{[H_2PO_4^-] \times [H^+]}{[H_3PO_4]} = 7.5 \times 10^{-3}$$

$$K_{a2} = \frac{[HPO_4^-] \times [H^+]}{[H_2PO_4^-]} = 6.8 \times 10^{-8}$$

$$K_{a3} = \frac{[PO_4^-] \times [H^+]}{[HPO_4^-]} = 1.0 \times 10^{-12}$$

Examples of acids and bases and their ionization constants are shown in Table 8-1.

Hydrogen Ion Concentration

The molecular weight of hydrogen is 1 g/mole; in other words, 1 mole of H^+ is equal to 1 g of H^+. Therefore, the concentration of H^+ in grams per liter is is the same as the concentration in moles per liter or equivalents per liter.

$$\frac{(1 \text{ g/L})}{(1 \text{ g/mole})} = 1 \text{ mole/L} = 1 \text{ molar solution}$$

$$\frac{(1 \text{ g/L})}{(1 \text{ g/Eq})} = 1 \text{ Eq/L} = 1 \text{ normal solution}$$

The H^+ concentration in an acid solution depends on the degree of ionization (% ionization) and the concentration of the acid in equivalents per liter (normality of the acid):

$$\text{Normality} \times \% \text{ ionization} = [H^+] \text{ in Eq/L or g/L or moles/L}$$

The % ionization is converted to a decimal number to perform the multiplication (10% ionization = 0.10) before solving the equation. A 0.5 N acid with 10% ionization has an H^+ concentration of:

$$0.5 \times 0.1 = 0.05 \text{ N } H^+ = 0.05 \text{ g/L } H^+ = 0.05 \text{ moles/L } H^+$$

Table 8-1   Strong and Weak Acids and Bases

Classification	Compound	Ionization Constant
Weak Acids	Acetic	1.8×10^{-5}
	Boric	1.8×10^{-5}
	Carbonic, K_{a1}	4.2×10^{-7}
	Carbonic, K_{a2}	4.8×10^{-11}
	Formic	2.1×10^{-4}
	Hydrofluoric	6.9×10^{-4}
	Hydrogen peroxide	2.4×10^{-12}
	Nitrous	4.5×10^{-4}
	Phosphoric, K_{a1}	7.5×10^{-3}
	Phosphoric, K_{a2}	6.8×10^{-8}
	Phosphoric, K_{a3}	1.0×10^{-12}
Weak Bases	Ammonium hydroxide	1.8×10^{-5}
	Calcium hydroxide, K_1	3.74×10^{-3}
	Calcium hydroxide, K_2	4.0×10^{-2}
	Hydrazine	1.7×10^{-6}
	Hydroxylamine	1.07×10^{-8}
	Lead hydroxide	9.6×10^{-4}
	Silver hydroxide	1.1×10^{-4}
	Zinc hydroxide	9.6×10^{-4}
Strong Acids	Hydrochloric	
	Hydrobromic	
	Nitric	
	Perchloric	
	Sulfuric	
Strong Bases	Barium hydroxide	
	Calcium hydroxide	
	Cesium hydroxide	
	Lithium hydroxide	
	Magnesium hydroxide	
	Potassium hydroxide	
	Rubidium hydroxide	
	Sodium hydroxide	
	Strontium hydroxide	

K_a, ionization constant. Subscript numbers denote strength of ionization.

Acetic acid, a weak acid, ionizes 0.6% in solution. The 0.6% ionization is 0.006 in the formula. So, a 0.5 N solution of CH_3COOH has an H^+ concentration of:

$$0.5 \times 0.006 = 0.003 \text{ Eq/L } H^+ = 0.003 \text{ g/L } H^+ = 0.003 \text{ moles/L } H^+$$

A strong acid, such as hydrochloric acid (HCl), completely ionizes in solution. The 100% ionization is 1.00 in the formula, which makes the H^+ concentration the same as that of the acid. A 0.20 N solution of HCl has an H^+ concentration that is the same as the normality (Box 8-1):

$$0.20 \times 1.00 = 0.20 \text{ N } H^+ = 0.20 \text{ g/L } H^+ = 0.20 \text{ moles/L } H^+$$

> **Box 8-1** **Weak and Strong Acids**
>
> The terms *strong acid* and *weak acid* do not refer to the concentration of an acid in solution. Concentration is described as concentrated or dilute.

Hydrogen Ions and Hydroxyl Ion Concentrations

All aqueous solutions contain H^+ and OH^-, and the degree of acidity or basicity of the aqueous solution depends on the relative amount of these ions. A solution with more H^+ than OH^- is acidic, whereas a solution with more OH^- than H^+ is basic.

The relative concentration of H^+ than OH^- ions is determined using a particular property of aqueous solutions:

$$[H^+] \times [OH^-] = 1 \times 10^{-14}$$

Regardless of its acidity, neutrality or basicity, the molar concentration of $[OH^-]$ multiplied by the molar concentration of $[H^+]$ is always 10^{-14}.

Therefore, $[H^+]$ can be calculated from $[OH^-]$ and vice versa, as long as one of the two concentrations is known. If, in a solution the $[H^+]$ was 2.8×10^{-4}, then the $[OH^-]$ concentration would be:

$$2.8 \times 10^{-4} \times [OH^{--}] = 1.0 \times 10^{-14}$$

$$[OH^{--}] = \frac{1.0 \times 10^{-14}}{2.8 \times 10^{-4}} = 0.36 \times 10^{-10} = 3.6 \times 10^{-11} \text{ moles/L}$$

pH AND pOH

pH is defined as the log of the reciprocal of the $[H^+]$:

$$pH = \log(1/[H^+])$$

Another expression of the relationship between pH and the $[H^+]$ is derived by expanding the equation:

$$pH = \log 1 - \log [H^+]$$

$\log 1 = 0$,

$$pH = 0 - \log [H^+]$$

$$pH = -\log [H^+]$$

The advantage of using the pH system is that it converts the large range of $[H^+]$ (1 to 0.00000000000001) to numbers ranging from 0 to14. Furthermore, when $[H^+]$ increases, $[OH^-]$ decreases and vice versa. $[OH^-]$ expressed as pOH, also ranges from 0 to14 (Table 8-2). The property of acid and base concentrations in aqueous solutions, $[H^+] \times [OH^-] = 1 \times 10^{-14}$, then becomes a simpler formula:

$$pH + pOH = 14$$

Table 8-2 Hydrogen and Hydroxyl Ion Concentrations, pH, and pOH

[H$^+$] (Moles/L)	pH	[OH$^-$] (Moles/L)	pOH
1.0	0	0.00000000000001	14
0.1	1	0.0000000000001	13
0.01	2	0.000000000001	12
0.001	3	0.00000000001	11
0.0001	4	0.0000000001	10
0.00001	5	0.000000001	9
0.000001	6	0.00000001	8
0.0000001	7	0.0000001	7
0.00000001	8	0.000001	6
0.000000001	9	0.00001	5
0.0000000001	10	0.0001	4
0.00000000001	11	0.001	3
0.000000000001	12	0.01	2
0.0000000000001	13	0.1	1
0.00000000000001	14	1.0	0

pOH, hydroxyl ion concentration.

CALCULATING pH AND pOH FROM IONIC CONCENTRATION

As pH is the log of 1/[H$^+$], similarly, pOH is the log of 1/[OH$^+$].

$$pH = log\ 1/(H^+) = -log(H^+)$$
$$pOH = log\ 1/(OH^-) = -log(OH^-)$$

Using the relationships shown in Table 8-2, pH and [H$^+$] can be used to determine pOH and [OH$^-$]. Conversion from pH and pOH to molar concentration of acids or bases is frequently used to make solutions of specified acidity or basicity.

Mixes of acid and basic solutions, such as mono- and dibasic sodium phosphate or Tris HCl [Tris(hydroxymethyl)–aminomethane hydrochloride] and Trizma base [2-Amino-2-(hydroxymethyl)-1,3-propanediol] are used in a variety of applications where stable pH is required. To achieve the proper pH, the acid and base components are mixed in a molar ratio that can be calculated from the pH. Mixing tables that provide the g/L or volume of 1 molar of the acid and base components required to produce the desired pH are available from commercial suppliers.

Neutral pH

Pure water has a pH that can be determined from its own low levels of ionization:

$$2H_2O \longleftrightarrow H_3O^+ + OH^-$$

Measurements of electrical conductivity have shown that 1 L of pure water contains 0.0000001 g H⁺. The [H⁺] of pure water is then:

$$0.0000001 \text{ g/L} = 1.0 \times 10^{-7} \text{g/L}$$

This is equivalent to 1.0×10^{-7} moles/L [H⁺]. The pH of pure water is:

$$pH = -log[H^+] = log(1.0 \times 10^{-7}) = -(-7) = 7$$

The [OH⁻] of pure water is:

$$[H^+] \times [OH^-] = 1 \times 10^{-14}$$

$$[OH^-] = \frac{(1 \times 10^{-14})}{[H^+]} = \frac{(1 \times 10^{-14})}{(1 \times 10^{-7})} = (1 \times 10^{-7})$$

And so the pOH of pure water will also be:

$$pOH = -log[OH-] = -log(10^{-7}) = -(-7) = 7$$

Using the relationship between pH and pOH:

$$pH + pOH = 14$$
$$7 + pOH = 14$$
$$pOH = 14 - 7 = 7$$

pH 7 is considered **neutral pH**; that is [H⁺] = [OH⁻].

Converting [H⁺] and [OH⁻] to pH and pOH

Laboratory protocols use pH expressions to describe solutions. If a solution is developed or optimized with changes in component concentrations, then the pH may also be different. In these cases, the pH can be calculated from a known [H⁺].

For [H⁺] (moles/liter) that are exact powers of 10 (0.1, 0.01, 0.001, 0.0001), the pH will be the negative exponent of 10 (Table 8-2):

$$[H^+] = 0.00000001 = 10^{-8}$$
$$pH = -log[H^+] = -log(10^{-8}) = -(-8) = 8$$
$$[OH^-] = 0.001 = 10^{-3}$$
$$pOH = -log[OH-] = -log(10^{-3}) = -(-3) = 3$$

For [H⁺] that are between powers of 10, the pH is calculated using logarithms. With the use of calculators, the simplest conversion of [H⁺] to pH is to use the formula:

$$pH = -log[H^+]$$

Conversion requires finding the log of the fractional number, usually by using a calculator or other computer (see Chapter 7).

If [H⁺] is 0.00032, what is the pH?

$$pH = -log[H^+] = -log(0.00032) = -(-3.5) = 3.5$$

If [OH⁻] is 0.0021, what is the pOH?

$$pOH = -log[OH⁻] = -log(0.0021) = -(-2.7) = 2.7$$

An alternative method to determine the pH is to use [H⁺] expressed in scientific notation:

$$a \times 10^{-b}$$

In this format, an [H⁺] of 0.0003 moles/L would be expressed as:

$$[H⁺] = 3 \times 10^{-4} \text{ moles/L}$$

Substituting $(a \times 10^{-b})$ for [H⁺] in the pH formula:

$$pH = -log [H⁺]$$
$$pH = -log (a \times 10^{-b})$$

Rearranging terms:

$$pH = - [(log\ a) + log\ (10^{-b})]$$
$$pH = - [(log\ a) + (-b)]$$
$$pH = - (log\ a - b)$$
$$pH = -log\ a + b$$
$$pH = b - log\ a$$

This formula is then used to find the pH. For an [H⁺] of 0.0003 moles/L, first express 0.0003 in scientific terms, and then use the formula derived previously:

$$0.0003 = 3 \times 10^{-4} = a \times 10^{-b}$$
$$pH = b - log\ a$$
$$pH = 4 - log\ (3)$$
$$pH = 4 - 0.4771 = 3.5$$

An 0.01 *N* acid solution is 70% ionized. What is the pH?
  First determine the [H⁺] based on the percent ionization of the acid:

$$[H⁺] = 0.01 \times 0.70 = 0.007$$

Then express [H⁺] in scientific notation and use the formula:

$$0.007 = 7 \times 10^{-3} \text{ moles/L}$$
$$pH = b - log\ a$$
$$pH = 3 - log\ (7)$$
$$pH = 3 - 0.8451 = 2.15$$

pOH can be determined in the same way. For an [OH⁻] = 0.00018:

$$0.00018 = 1.8 \times 10^{-4} \text{ moles/L}$$
$$pOH = b - log\ a$$
$$pOH = 4 - log\ (1.8)$$
$$pOH = 4 - 0.2553 = 3.74$$

Converting pH and pOH to [H⁺] and [OH⁻]

A laboratory procedure may require preparation of a solution for which only the components and pH are given. To know how much of each ingredient is required, first determine the [H⁺]. Concentration is immediately apparent if the pH is a whole number. Invert the sign of the pH, and express the number as an exponent of 10. That is the [H⁺]:

pH = 3
[H⁺] = 10⁻³ = 0.001 moles/L

Similarly, for pOH:

pOH = 6
[OH⁻] = 10⁻⁶ = 0.000001 moles/L

When the pH is a fractional number, invert the sign of the pH, and find the antilog of the negative number, most conveniently by using a calculator or computer software.

If pH = 7.9, find the [H⁺]:

pH = −log [H⁺]
7.9 = −log [H⁺]
−7.9 = log [H⁺]
antilog of −7.9 = 0.000000012 moles/L

An alternative method is use the same formula, pH = $b - \log a$. For pH = 7.9:

pH = b − log a
7.9 = b − log a

This equation is problematic in that it has two unknowns, **a** and **b**. To continue with the calculation, either *a* or *b* must be known. The following examples show that because *b* is an exponent and is, along with a, part of the scientific notation of the [H⁺], equation a × 10⁻ᵇ, any number may be used for b. The value of *b* modifies the value of *a* in the equation.

Although any number can be used for *b*, the most convenient number is the next integer greater than the pH. For pH = 7.9, the most convenient number for *b* would be **8**:

pH = b − log a
7.9 = b − log a
7.9 = 8 −log a
log a = 8 − 7.9
log a = 0.10
a = antilog 0.10
a = 1.2
[H⁺] = a × 10⁻ᵇ
[H⁺] = 1.2 × 10⁻⁸ moles/L

To show that any number may be substituted for b, substitute 100 for b:

$$7.9 = b - \log a$$
$$7.9 = 100 - \log a$$
$$\log a = 100 - 7.9$$
$$\log a = 92.1$$
$$a = \text{antilog } 92.1$$
$$a = 1.2 \times 10^{92}$$
$$[H^+] = a \times 10^{-b}$$
$$[H^+] = (1.2 \times 10^{92}) \times 10^{-100}$$
$$[H^+] = 1.2 \times 10^{-8} = 0.000000012 \text{ moles/L}$$

PREPARATION OF SOLUTIONS OF A SPECIFIED pH

Conversions such as those described earlier are helpful for making solutions when only the pH is given.

A protocol may require 300 mL of HCl, pH 2.50. What molarity of HCl should be used? With the molarity and molecular weight, the mass of HCl required can be calculated. The molarity of this strong acid is determined from the pH:

$$pH = b - \log a$$
$$2.50 = b - \log a$$
$$2.50 = 3 - \log a$$

(The most convenient value for b in this case is 3, but any number could have been used.)

$$\log a = 0.50$$
$$a = 3.16$$
$$[H^+] = a \times 10^{-b}$$
$$[H^+] = 3.16 \times 10^{-3} \text{ moles/L}$$

Because HCl is 100% ionized, the $[H^+]$ is the same as the acid concentration. For 300 mL of HCl at a concentration of 3.16×10^{-3} moles/L:

$$0.300 \text{ L} \times (3.16 \times 10^{-3} \text{ moles/L}) = 0.948 \times 10^{-3} \text{ moles}$$

$$9.48 \times 10^{-4} \text{ moles} \times 36.46 \text{ g/mole} = 3.46 \times 10^{-2} \text{ g HCl} = 34.6 \text{ mg HCl}$$

This solution requires 34.6 mg HCl brought to 250 mL with water (Box 8-2).

 CAUTION: Never add water to acid. For the example described in the text, slowly add the acid to about 100 mL of water and then bring the mixture to 250 mL.

> ### Box 8-2   Specific Gravity and Purity
>
> If this solution is being made with a commercial preparation of HCl that has a specific gravity of 1.19 and a purity of 37%, the volume containing 28.8 g must be determined.
>
> $$1.19 \text{ g/mL} \times 0.37 = 0.44 \text{ g HCl/mL preparation}$$
> $$28.8 \text{ g/}(0.44 \text{ g/mL}) = 65.4 \text{ mL}$$
>
> To make 250 mL of HCl, pH 2.5, add 65.4 mL commercial HCl preparation to about 100 mL water, and then bring the final volume to 250 mL.

Similar calculations are used to calculate the amount of base required to make a basic solution of a given pH. A method calls for 500 mL of NaOH, **pH 12.2**. First, determine pOH and the $[OH^-]$:

$$pOH = 14 - pH = 14 - 12.2 = 1.8$$
$$pOH = b - \log a$$
$$1.8 = b - \log a$$

As with pH, the most convenient number to use for b is the next larger integer over the pOH, which is 2:

$$1.8 = 2 - \log a$$
$$\log a = 2 - 1.8$$
$$\log a = 0.2$$
$$a = \text{antilog } 0.2$$
$$a = 1.58$$
$$[OH^-] = a \times 10^{-b}$$
$$[OH^-] = 1.58 \times 10^{-2}$$

Because NaOH is completely ionized, the NaOH concentration is the same as $[OH^-]$, or 1.58×10^{-2}. To make 500 mL of NaOH at a concentration of 1.59×10^{-2} moles/L:

$$0.50 \cancel{L} \times (1.58 \times 10^{-2} \text{ moles/}\cancel{L}) = 0.008 \text{ moles}$$
$$0.008 \cancel{\text{moles}} \times 40 \text{ g/}\cancel{\text{mole}} = 0.32 \text{ g NaOH}$$

Bring 0.32 g NaOH to 500 mL.

BUFFERS

Buffers maintain reaction pH when samples are introduced. A highly acidic or basic sample added to a reaction mix could alter the pH such that enzymes or other components of the reaction will not work efficiently. Buffers are mixtures of a strong acid and a weak base that resist change in pH.

Every acid has a conjugate base that has one fewer H^+ and one more negative charge than the acid. The conjugate base of acetic acid, CH_3COOH, is acetate, CH_3COO^-:

$$CH_3COOH \rightarrow CH_3COO^- + H^+$$

If the base acquires one more H^+, it becomes the conjugate acid:

$$CH_3COO^- + H^+ \rightarrow CH_3COOH$$

Acetic acid (a weak acid) and sodium acetate (a strong base) mixed together comprise a buffer. This buffer reduces or eliminates unwanted changes in pH through the **common ion effect**. Two substances that dissociate to the same ion (common ion, such as the acetate ion), dissociate less than if either were present alone. When sodium acetate is mixed with acetic acid, both will yield acetate anion, most of which will come from the completely ionized salt (sodium acetate).

Acetic acid: $CH_3COOH \leftrightarrow CH_3HCOO^- + H^+$

Sodium acetate: $CH_3COONa \rightarrow CH_3COO^- + Na^+$

The low $[H^+]$ ionized from the acetic acid is even lower in the presence of the salt because of the common ion effect, in which excess acetate ions, CH_3COO^-, collect H^+ released by the acid. If a strong acid is added to this solution, the extra H^+ from the added acid will combine with the excess acetate ions and form acetic acid. If a strong base is added to the buffer, the OH^- from the base will react with the available H^+ to form water, thus forcing more of the acetic acid to ionize and replace the H^+ ions. In both cases, the $[H^+]$ remains unchanged.

Buffering ability (the ability to resist pH change) depends on the degree of ionization of the weak acid (i.e., the degree to which it ionizes into H^+ and the conjugate base). Because the ionization constant of a compound does not change, the relative proportion of ionized and un-ionized components remains the same.

In an acetate buffer, the pH is controlled by the degree of ionization of acetic acid:

$$CH_3COOH \leftrightarrow CH_3COO^- + H^+$$

or, in more general terms:

$$HA \leftrightarrow A^- + H^+$$

and because the ionization of acetic acid is a constant, K_a,

$$\frac{[A^-][H^+]}{[HA]} = K_a$$

Rearranging this equation,

$$[H^+] = K_a \times \frac{[HA]}{[A^-]}$$

Take the log of both sides of the equation:

$$\log[H^+] = \log K_a + \log \frac{([HA]}{[A^-])}$$

Multiplying both sides of the equation by −1 will yield the terms for pH (−log [H⁺]) and a similar term, pKₐ, for −log Kₐ:

$$-\log[H^+] = -\log K_a - \log \frac{([HA]}{[A^-])}$$

$$pH = pK_a - \log \frac{([HA]}{[A^-])}$$

In logarithms, $-\log (x/y) = +\log (y/x)$

$$pH = pK_a + \log \frac{([A^-]}{(HA])}$$

The foregoing formula is a version of the **Henderson-Hasselbalch equation:**

$$pH = pK + \log \frac{[base]}{[acid]}$$

The Henderson-Hasselbalch equation is used to determine the pH of a buffer system. Here pK (= pKₐ) is the −log of the ionization constant (Kₐ) of the weak acid, HA, into H⁺ and its conjugate base anion, A⁻. Using the Henderson-Hasselbalch equation, the pH of a buffer can be determined if the concentration of the acid and its conjugate base are known. The pK (pKₐ) of the acid is listed in resource tables. An example of pK values is shown in Table 8-3.

Table 8-3	Acid pK Values
Compound	pK$_a$
Acetic acid	4.76
Boric acid	9.27
Citric acid	3.2
Formic acid	3.75
Urea	0.10
Lactic acid	3.08
Creatine, K$_{a1}$	2.63
Creatine, K$_{a2}$	14.3
Ascorbic acid, K$_{a1}$	4.10
Ascorbic acid, K$_{a2}$	11.79
Phosphoric, K$_{a1}$	2.16
Phosphoric, K$_{a2}$	7.21
Phosphoric, K$_{a3}$	12.32

K$_a$, ionization constant; pK and pK$_a$, negative log of the ionization constant. Subscript numbers denote strength of ionization.

Example: Determine the pH of a buffer composed of 0.05 molar acetic acid and 0.10 molar sodium acetate. The pK of acetic acid is 4.76. Use the Henderson-Hasselbalch equation:

$$pH = pK + \log \frac{[base]}{[acid]}$$

$$pH = 4.76 + \log \frac{0.10 \text{ molar}}{0.05 \text{ molar}}$$

$$\frac{0.10 \text{ molar}}{0.05 \text{ molar}} = 2$$

$$pH = 4.76 + \log 2$$

$$pH = 4.76 + 0.301$$

$$pH = 5.06$$

The Henderson-Hasselbalch equation predicts that an increase in [base] will increase the pH. Compared with the previous solution, if the [base] was 0.15 molar, the pH would be:

$$pH = 4.76 + \log \frac{0.15 \text{ molar}}{0.05 \text{ molar}}$$

$$\frac{0.15 \text{ molar}}{0.05 \text{ molar}} = 3.0$$

$$pH = 4.76 + \log 3.0$$

$$pH = 4.76 + 0.48$$

$$pH = 5.24$$

Conversely, an increase in [acid] will lower the pH. Compared with the previous solution, if the [acid] was 0.07 molar, the pH would be:

$$pH = 4.76 + \log \frac{0.10 \text{ molar}}{0.07 \text{ molar}}$$

$$\frac{0.10 \text{ molar}}{0.07 \text{ molar}} = 1.43$$

$$pH = 4.76 + \log 1.43$$

$$pH = 4.76 + 0.16$$

$$pH = 4.92$$

Buffer systems prevent changes in pH as long as they are not overwhelmed with acidic or basic ions. The Henderson-Hasselbalch equation makes buffers for selected [H^+] or pH. The relative concentration of acid and salt required to make a solution, when given the pH can be determined by rearranging the equation:

$$pH = pK + \log \frac{[base]}{[acid]}$$

$$-\log \frac{[base]}{[acid]} = pK - pH$$

$$\log \frac{[base]}{[acid]} = pH - pK$$

Prepare 100 mL of 0.20 molar sodium borate buffer, pH 10.0. The pK of boric acid is 9.27.

$$\log \frac{[\text{base}]}{[\text{acid}]} = pH - pK$$

$$\log \frac{[\text{base}]}{[\text{acid}]} = 10.0 - 9.27$$

$$\log \frac{[\text{base}]}{[\text{acid}]} = 0.73$$

$$\frac{[\text{base}]}{[\text{acid}]} = \text{antilog } 0.73$$

$$\frac{[\text{base}]}{[\text{acid}]} = 5.37$$

$$\frac{\text{molar borate}}{\text{molar boric acid}} = 5.37$$

The *ratio* of borate to boric acid should be 5.37, that is, for 1 part boric acid, there are 5.37 parts sodium borate salt. The total parts of boric acid and borate salt are **1 + 5.37 = 6.37**. Knowing that the sum of the *concentrations* of the salt and acid is **0.20 molar** and that there are 6.37 total *parts*, ratio and proportion are used to determine the molar concentrations in a total of 0.20 moles for 1 L.

$$\frac{\text{Total moles borate + boric acid}}{\text{moles boric acid}} = \frac{0.2 \text{ M}}{x \text{ M boric acid}}$$

$$\frac{6.37}{1.0} = \frac{0.2 \text{ M}}{x \text{ moles boric acid}}$$

$$\frac{6.37 \text{ x}}{} = \frac{0.2 \text{ moles}}{}$$

$$x = \frac{0.2}{6.37} = 0.03 \text{ molar boric acid}$$

If the boric acid and borate salt total concentration is 0.20 molar, then the molarity of the borate salt will be:

$$\text{Total molarity} - \text{Acid molarity} = \text{Salt molarity}$$

$$0.20 \text{ molar} - 0.03 \text{ molar} = 0.17 \text{ molar}$$

The 0.20-molar buffer will contain 0.03 molar boric acid and 0.17 molar borate salt. To make the buffer, determine the amount of each component using their molecular weights (boric acid, 61.83 g/mole; sodium borate, 381.37 g/mole):

$$0.03 \text{ moles/L} \times 61.83 \text{ g/mole} = 1.85 \text{ g/L boric acid}$$

$$0.17 \text{ moles/L} \times 381.37 \text{ g/mole} = 64.8 \text{ g/L sodium borate}$$

For the final solution of 100 mL,

$$1.85 \text{ g/1,000 mL} = x \text{ g/100 mL}$$

$$x = 0.185 \text{ g boric acid}$$

$$64.8 \text{ g/1,000 mL} = x \text{ g/100 mL}$$

$$x = 6.48 \text{ g sodium borate}$$

To make the buffer, bring 0.185 g boric acid + 6.48 g sodium borate to 100 mL.

Buffers are made according to the range of pH and the component ions appropriate for their use, such as work with deoxyribonucleic acid which requires buffers with a pH of 8.0. Compounds have the strongest buffering capacity (resistance to pH change) at their own pK. A mixture of Tris-HCl ($pK_a = 8.06$) and Trizma base ($NH_2C(CH_2OH)_3$) is an effective buffer in this pH range. Antigen-antibody binding studies may require a more acid environment. A buffer that could be used for this lower pH range (pH 3 to 6) is citrate buffer consisting of citric acid ($H_3C_6H_5O_7$, $pK_{a1} = 3.2$) and sodium citrate. The concentrations and relative amounts of weak acid and conjugate base can be adjusted to accommodate higher or lower concentrations of added acids and bases. Ideally, pH is measured at room temperature (22°C to 25°C). The pH reading will be slightly different when the solution temperature is higher or lower than this (Box 8-3).

Enzyme-catalyzed reactions, product detection, and stability of reaction components are all affected by pH in aqueous solutions. Laboratory methods specify the type and concentration of buffer solutions required for optimal test performance. The type of buffer to use is determined in the development of the test procedure because buffer components can also affect reactions. Using buffers avoids changes in pH that may occur on addition of sample to a reaction mix. Changes in pH affect enzyme activity, signal production, or instrument function. Buffers that resist these changes allow addition of acidic or basic specimens without changing the accuracy of the testing method.

pH IN BODY FLUIDS

Acid-base balance in cells and body fluids is maintained by a complex array of buffering reactions. The normal pH of blood is 7.35 to 7.45. This pH is maintained by a buffer system of carbonic acid (H_2CO_3) formed from carbon dioxide (CO_2) and water (H_2O).

$$CO_2 + H_2O \longleftrightarrow H_2CO_3$$

The H_2CO_3 ionizes to its conjugate base, HCO_3^- and H^+ at a constant rate:

$$H_2CO_3 \longleftrightarrow H^+ + HCO_3^-$$

Box 8-3 Temperature and pH

Temperature affects pH in two ways. The actual pH of a solution changes with temperature. For this reason, pH of a solution is reported with temperature, for example, pH 7.8 at 23°C. The other way that pH is affected by temperature has to do with the effect of temperature on the instrument used to measure pH (pH meter). The electrode, which senses pH in millivolts (mV), is affected by temperature such that the mV output increases with increasing temperature. Some pH meters automatically adjust for the temperature of the solution. For others, the solution temperature is manually entered before measuring the pH.

In other words, the concentrations of $[H^+]$ and the conjugate base, $[HCO_3^-]$ relative to the acid, $[H_2CO_3]$ remain constant and is represented as K':

$$\frac{[H^+][HCO_3^-]}{[H_2CO_3]} = K'$$

In body fluids, the concentration of CO_2 is 1,000 times the concentration of H_2CO_3:

$$[CO_2] = [H_2CO_3] \times 1,000$$

Multiplying both sides of the K' equation by $\frac{1}{1,000}$:

$$\frac{[H^+][HCO_3^-]}{[H_2CO_3] \times 1,000} = \frac{K'}{1,000}$$

Substituting $[CO_2]$ for $[H_2CO_3] \times 1,000$:

$$\frac{[H^+][HCO_3^-]}{[CO_2]} = \frac{K'}{1,000}$$

The term $(K'/1,000)$ can be expressed as K:

$$\frac{K'}{1,000} = K$$

Then:

$$\frac{[H^+][HCO_3^-]}{[CO_2]} = K$$

To calculate $[H^+]$, rearrange this formula:

$$[H^+] = \frac{K[CO_2]}{[HCO_3^-]}$$

$$[H^+] = K \times \frac{[CO_2]}{[HCO_3^-]}$$

The $[H^+]$ can be converted to pH using logs. Take the log of both sides of the equation:

$$\log[H^+] = \log K + \log\frac{[CO_2]}{[HCO_3^-]}$$

Multiply both sides of the equation by -1, which yields the term for pH on the left side of the equation:

$$-\log[H^+] = -\log K - \log\frac{[CO_2]}{[HCO_3^-]}$$

By the rules of logarithms, $-\log x/y = +\log y/x$. Then:

$$-\log[H^+] = -\log K + \log\frac{[HCO_3^-]}{[CO_2]}$$

Because $-\log[H^+]$ is pH, $-\log K$ can be called pK:

$$pH = pK + \log\frac{[HCO_3^-]}{[CO_2]}$$

The previous formula is a version of the Henderson-Hasselbalch equation. Thus the Henderson-Hasselbalch equation is used to calculate the pH of blood, or concentration of carbonate.

The equation can also be used to determine the cause of abnormal blood pH less than 7.35 (acidosis) or more than 7.45 (alkalosis). Increased carbonate base or decreased CO_2 raises pH, whereas decreased carbonate base or increased CO_2 lowers pH. Normal carbonate concentrations range from 20 to 29 mM. Normal CO_2 concentrations are expressed as dissolved CO_2 (dCO_2), which is calculated from the **partial pressure** of CO_2 (PCO_2). Blood PCO_2 levels normally range from 35 to 45 mm Hg. (Pressure is measured in millimeters of mercury [mm Hg].)

Although pH can be measured directly, carbonate and dCO_2 levels cannot. The PCO_2 measurement is used to determine dCO_2.

PCO_2

CO_2 exists in the body in the form of gas and in solution (dCO_2). PCO_2 is the contribution of CO_2 to the total gas pressure in a body space. CO_2 concentration in solution is proportional to the partial pressure of gaseous CO_2 (PCO_2) times a proportionality constant, a, which for this reaction is 0.0306 mM (= 0.07 mL%). If the pH is known, carbonate concentration, which cannot be directly measured, is determined using blood gas CO_2 in solution converted to millimolar concentration with the proportionality constant, a (carbonic acid pK = 6.10):

$$pH = pK + \log \frac{[HCO_3^-]}{[a \times Pco_2]}$$

The causes of acid-base imbalance can be determined from measuring pH and PCO_2, and calculating $[HCO_3^-]$. These levels are important even when pH is normal because the body compensates for acidic or alkaline conditions by retaining or excreting carbonate and CO_2.

A blood pH is measured at 7.40 and dCO_2 at 40 mm Hg. What is the carbonate ion concentration?

$$pH = pK + \log \frac{[HCO_3^-]}{[a \times Pco_2]}$$

$$7.40 = 6.10 + \log \frac{[HCO_3^-]}{(0.0306 \times 40)}$$

$$1.3 = \log \frac{[HCO_3^-]}{1.224)}$$

$$antilog\ 1.3 = \frac{[HCO_3^-]}{1.224}$$

$$19.9 = \frac{[HCO_3^-]}{1.224)}$$

$$19.9 \times 1.224 = [HCO_3^-]$$

$$24 = [HCO_3^-]$$

In this example, pH, P_{CO_2} and carbonate ion are within normal range. A normal pH level may not always reflect normal P_{CO_2} and carbonate ion, for instance, high P_{CO_2} (lowering pH) can compensate for alkaline conditions resulting from high $[HCO_3^-]$ levels. Knowledge of these levels will direct appropriate medical treatment.

CAUTION: Normal ranges of analytes vary among laboratories, depending on the methods and instruments used to measure them. Most instruments flag abnormal levels as high or low, depending on the acceptable ranges of the laboratory's validated protocols.

PRACTICE PROBLEMS

1. Cations have a _____ charge.

2. Anions have a _____ charge.

3. Cations have more _____ than _____ .

4. Anions have more _____ than _____ .

5. Cations are attracted to ions with a net _____ charge.

6. Cations and anions form _____ bonds.

7. _____ are substances that release hydrogen ions, whereas _____ are substances that release hydroxyl ions.

8. A strong acid will/will not almost completely ionize.

9. Loss of a proton from an acid leaves its _____.

10. What are the conjugate bases of the following acids?

Carbonic acid (H_2CO_3)
Hydrofluoric acid (HF)
Formic acid ($HCHO_2$)
Acetic acid ($HC_2H_3O_2$)
Oxalic acid ($H_2C_2O_4$)

11. What is the hydrogen ion concentration in moles per liter if the concentration of $[H^+]$ is 0.01 g/L?

Calculate the hydrogen ion concentration in grams per liter of the following solutions.

12. 0.20 *N* acetic acid, 10% ionized

13. 0.10 *M* acetic acid, 1.0% ionized

14. 0.25 *M* hydrochloric acid, 100% ionized

15. 0.015 *M* boric acid, 0.10% ionized

16. What is the pH or pOH corresponding to the following ion concentrations?

$[H^+] = 1.0 \times 10^{-7}$ moles/L
$[H^+] = 1.0 \times 10^{-10}$ moles/L
$[H^+] = 2.5 \times 10^{-2}$ moles/L
$[OH^-] = 5.0 \times 10^{-4}$ moles/L
$[OH^-] = 2.0 \times 10^{-8}$ moles/L

17. What is the hydrogen ion concentration of water?

18. An acid solution has a pH of 2.14. What is its hydrogen ion concentration?

19. An acid solution has a pH of 1.88. What is its hydrogen ion concentration?

20. A basic solution has a pH of 10.2. What is its hydrogen ion concentration?

21. What is the hydroxyl ion concentration of the solution in question 20?

Continued

PRACTICE PROBLEMS *cont.*

Convert the following ion concentrations to pH and pOH.

22. $[H^+] = 1.0 \times 10^{-3}$ moles/L

23. $[H^+] = 5.0 \times 10^{-6}$ moles/L

24. $[H^+] = 9.8 \times 10^{-12}$ moles/L

25. $[H^+] = 6.4 \times 10^{-2}$ moles/L

26. $[H^+] = 15.8 \times 10^{-9}$ moles/L

27. $[OH^-] = 1.0 \times 10^{-14}$ moles/L

28. $[OH^-] = 5.0 \times 10^{-5}$ moles/L

29. $[OH^-] = 3.5 \times 10^{-10}$ moles/L

30. $[OH^-] = 2.1 \times 10^{-7}$ moles/L

Convert the following ionic concentrations to cH.

31. $[H^+] = 6.4 \times 10^{-2}$ moles/L

32. $[H^+] = 7.3 \times 10^{-8}$ moles/L

33. $[H^+] = 3.4 \times 10^{-5}$ moles/L

34. $[OH^-] = 6.8 \times 10^{-9}$ moles/L

35. $[OH^-] = 1.0 \times 10^{-10}$ moles/L

36. $[OH^-] = 7.8 \times 10^{-2}$ moles/L

Convert the following pH and pOH to cH.

37. pH = 7.3

38. pH = 3.5

39. pOH = 7.3

40. pOH = 12

41. pOH = 2.0

Describe how to prepare a solution with the following pH or pOH.

42. One liter HCl, pH = 2.0 from commercial HCl (1.18 g/mL, 36% pure)

43. 500 mL H_2SO_4, pH = 1.5 from commercial H_2SO_4 (1.84 g/mL, 85% pure)

44. 700 mL NaOH, pOH = 4.2

45. 2 L NaOH, pOH = 6.0

Use the Henderson-Hasselbalch equation to determine the base:acid ratio in the following buffers.

46. Acetate buffer, pH = 6.00; pK of acetic acid = 4.76

47. Phosphoric acid buffer, pH = 4.20; pK of H_3PO_4 = 2.15

Find the molarity of the acid and base necessary to make 1 mole/L solutions of the buffers in questions 46 and 47.

48. Acetate buffer, pH = 6.00; pK of acetic acid = 4.76; [base]/[acid] = 17.4

Phosphoric acid buffer, pH = 4.20; pK of H_3PO_4 = 2.15; [base]/[acid] = 112

49. Calculate the volume of commercial acetic acid necessary to make the 1-*M* solution of the buffer in question 46. Acetate buffer, pH = 6.00; pK of acetic acid = 4.76; [base]/[acid] = 17.4; 0.06 *M* acetic acid

50. Calculate the volume of commercial phosphoric acid necessary to make the 1-*M* solution of the buffer in question 47. Phosphate buffer, pH = 6.00; pK of phosphoric acid = 2.15; [base]/[acid] = 112; 0.009 M phosphoric acid

APPLICATIONS

Clinical Chemistry

Acid-base balance in cells and body fluids is maintained by a complex array of buffering reactions. The main buffer system in humans is the formation of carbonic acid from carbon dioxide and water.

$$pH = pK + \log \frac{[HCO_3^-]}{[a \times P_{CO_2}]}$$

A patient's pH level was measured at 7.60, with a P_{CO_2} of 39. What is the carbonate concentration? What would be the dCO_2 level if the pH were normal (7.40) with the same carbonate concentration?

Microbiology

Human pathogens (bacteria) grow best at or near neutral pH. Acid-base balance is naturally maintained in body fluids, even with bacterial infection. Growing bacteria from patients' samples (isolates) in the laboratory requires acid-base conditions similar to those maintained in body fluids. In the laboratory, isolates are introduced to specialized solutions of nutrients, energy sources, and other factors required by the bacterial cells. As the bacteria grow, they release metabolites that can affect the pH of the medium. A buffering system is included to avoid changes in pH that would ultimately kill the culture. A common buffer used for this purpose is composed of dipotassium phosphate (K_2HPO_4, a strong base) and monopotassium phosphate (KH_2PO_4, a weak acid, pK = 7.2).

What would be the relative concentrations of these components in a culture that must be maintained at pH 7.5? If the final buffer concentration is 0.15 molar, how much of each of the buffer components would be required to make 1 L of buffered culture?

CHAPTER **9**

SPECTROPHOTOMETRY

Electromagnetic energy exists in repeating waves (Fig. 9-1). The distance from the crest of one wave to the next is called the **wavelength (λ)**. "Light" is that part of the electromagnetic spectrum with wavelengths ranging from 200 to 900 nm (Table 9-1). Measurement of light absorbance and transmittance is a useful method to determine the presence, state, or concentration of substances. Laboratory instruments detect light at specified wavelengths. Laboratory tests may involve light measurement from any wavelength in the ultraviolet (UV)–visible-infrared (IR) range (200 to 900 nm). Substances absorb or transmit light at different wavelengths, thus making it possible to use light for the detection and measurement of specific compounds by spectrophotometry. Examples are protein, which most efficiently absorbs light at a wavelength of 280 nm, and benzene, which most efficiently absorbs light at 180 nm. The degree to which light at 280 nm is absorbed by a solution indicates the amount of protein present. The amount of light absorbed at 180 nm indicates the amount of benzene present. Substances that do not absorb light can be measured by using a reagent, or chromophore, that produces color (absorbs light) in the presence of the test material. Automated instruments make use of natural or induced absorbance to measure substance concentrations in the chemistry laboratory, such as cholesterol levels measured by enzymatic production of a quinone chromophore that absorbs light at 500 nm.

Unknown substances are identified or characterized by the wavelength at which they most efficiently absorb light. A series of wavelengths is called a **spectrum**. Spectral analysis is testing the absorbance of light at a series of wavelengths to find the wavelength at which peak absorbance occurs (Fig. 9-2). Light-detecting instruments such as capillary electrophoresis systems and quantitative polymerase chain reaction thermal cyclers may require a spectral calibration with wavelength standards to ensure that they are identifying targets at the intended wavelengths (Box 9-1).

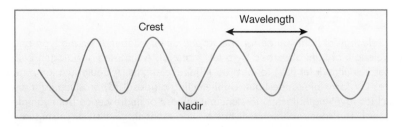

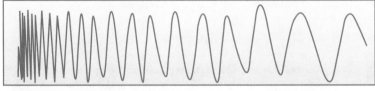

Ultraviolet (100–400 nm)   Visible (400–700 nm)   Infrared (700–900 nm)

Figure 9-1 Light travels in waves (*top*). A wave is measured in wavelengths, the distance in nanometers from the highest point (crest) of one wave to the crest of the next wave. The lowest point of a wave is the nadir. Light is a part of the electromagnetic spectrum. Ultraviolet light includes wavelengths from less than 200 to 400 nm. Visible light includes wavelengths from 400 to 700 nm. Infrared light wavelengths measure from 700 to 900 nm. Substances absorb light at characteristic wavelengths. Spectrophotometers measure the absorbance or transmittance of light at set wavelengths.

Table 9-1 Light in the Electromagnetic Spectrum	
Region	Wavelength (nm)
Ultraviolet (UV)	200–400
Visible (vis)	400–700
Infrared (IR)	700–900

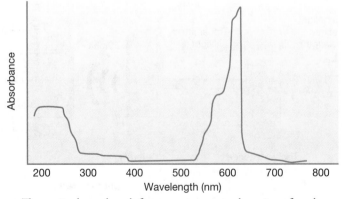

Figure 9-2 The optimal wavelength for measurement or detection of a substance is determined by scanning across a spectrum of wavelengths to find the wavelength at which the greatest amount of light is absorbed. In the example shown, the substance shows peak absorbance at 600 nm. A procedure to measure or detect this substance by spectrophotometry would include setting the wavelength and reading at 600 nm.

> **Box 9-1**   Spectrophotometer Light Sources
>
> The selection of light source for spectrophotometry depends on the type and wavelength of light absorbed by a test material. A tungsten or halogen bulb generates ultraviolet (UV) to infrared (IR) wavelengths. A deuterium lamp generates UV to visible-range light. Light-emitting diodes (LED) produce light at a specific wavelength (lasers) to stimulate release of fluorescence from sample material. The spectrophotometer has a filter, monochromator, or prism that further separates light from the light source by limiting the wavelengths of the beam of light that passes through the test substance.

! CAUTION: Laboratory tests require measurement of light throughout the UV-visible-IR range. Visible light is not harmful under normal use; however, UV and IR light can be hazardous. UV light is dangerous to skin and eyes. It can result in burn-like damage to skin and damage to the retina. Do not expose your unprotected eyes or skin to these high-energy waves. Full face shields to protect face and eyes should be available in the laboratory. Many laboratories have incorporated closed systems in which UV light is contained within a hood or detector so that direct exposure is avoided. IR light is less frequently encountered for measuring concentration in the laboratory. It is the source of energy for some detection, remote control, or heating devices. Although not as dangerous to skin as UV light, IR light can also damage eyes. Avoid looking directly into any light.

A **spectrophotometer** directs light through a substance contained in a **cuvette** and measures the amount of that light that is absorbed or transmitted by that substance (Fig. 9-3). A simple spectrophotometer is a combination of a spectrometer that produces incident light (L_o) and a photometer that

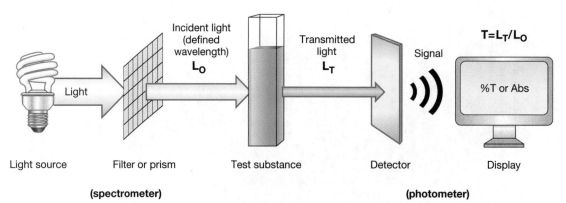

Figure 9-3 A spectrophotometer consists of a light source and a light detector. Various light sources produce light at the desired ranges of wavelength. Filters, prisms, or other light separation devices direct light of a more precisely defined wavelength into the test substance (L_o). The transmitted light, L_T, (that is not absorbed by the substance) is detected, and readout is calculated as absorbance or percent (%) transmittance.

detects transmitted light (L_T). The photometer sends an electrical signal to a processor and display device. A **fluorometer** measures light emitted from a substance after excitation of substances that re-emit light after being energized by outside light (fluorophores). Capillary gel electrophoresis systems used for applications such as bone marrow engraftment monitoring and DNA fingerprinting are fluorometers. A **luminometer** measures light emitted from a substance as a result of a chemical reaction or chemiluminescence. Examples of luminometers are plate readers for enzyme-linked immunoassays (ELISA) and pyrosequencers that detect genetic mutations.

Filtered light from the light source is directed to the test solution held in a **cuvette**. The cuvette must be transparent (i.e., not absorb light on its own). The cuvette should not interfere with the access or penetration of light. Cuvettes of different materials are transparent at certain wavelengths. Quartz cuvettes are recommended for UV light measurements because some plastics absorb UV light even though they are transparent to visible light. Specialized spectrophotometers do not require cuvettes because they measure light absorbance directly through the test material in a permanent flow-through cuvette or are held in place by surface tension.

Based on the amount of light applied to a substance (**incident light**, I_o or L_o), the spectrophotometer measures the light that penetrates the substance (**transmitted light**, I or L_T) and determines the amount of light absorbed by the substance (**absorbance, A**; Box 9-2).

The amount of light transmitted through the test solution depends on the concentration of substance (c) and how far the incident light has to travel through the substance, also called the **path length**, b. The path length differs with the size of the cuvette containing the test substance. Although it is constant for methods using the same cuvette size, the path length may vary from one instrument or method to another.

Transmittance (T) is the ratio of light that is detected after passage through the test solution (L_T) relative to the incident light, L_o, that can pass through a blank sample containing no test substance (Box 9-3).

$$T = L_T/L_o$$

This number is expressed as percent.

$$\%T = L_T/L_o \times 100$$

The range of values for transmittance is, therefore, 0%, at which none of the incident light is transmitted ($L_T = 0$), to 100%, at which all the incident light is transmitted ($L_T = L_o$; Fig. 9-4).

Box 9-2   Transmittance and Absorbance

The intensity of the light that is transmitted through the substance is inversely proportional to the concentration of molecules in the solution (c) that can absorb light. These molecules absorb light as it passes through the substance.

> **Box 9-3** Relation of Light Absorbance to Transmission
>
> The logarithmic relationship of absorbance of light to transmission is derived from the formula:
>
> $$T = 10^{-abc}$$
>
> where T is the transmittance, b is the path length, c is the substance concentration, and a is a measure of the extent to which light is absorbed (molar absorptivity), which is a constant for each substance.
>
> $$\% \, T = 10^{-abc} \times 10^2$$
> $$\% \, T = 10^{-abc \, +2}$$
> $$\log \% \, T = -abc + 2$$
> $$-2 + \log \% \, T = -abc$$
>
> or,
>
> $$2 - \log \% \, T = abc$$
>
> For a path length of 1 cm ($b = 1$), abc becomes absorptivity (absorbance of a 1-molar concentration of the test substance) times the concentration in moles/L:
>
> $$abc = a/1 \; \text{(mole/liter)} \times 1 \times c \; \text{moles/liter} = A$$
>
> or,
>
> $$A = abc$$
>
> and
>
> $$2 - \log \% \, T = A$$

Percent transmittance

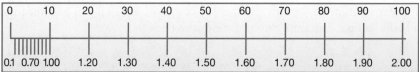

Absorbance

Figure 9-4 Percent transmittance will range from 0%, at which all incident light is absorbed and 0% is transmitted, to 100%, at which no incident light is absorbed and 100% is transmitted. Absorbance is logarithmically related to percent transmittance and ranges from more than 0 to 2.00.

BEER'S LAW

Beer's Law or the Beer-Lambert Law relates the concentration of a substance to the amount of light absorbed (rather than transmitted) by that solution. The more concentrated a solution is, the more light it absorbs and the less it transmits (Fig. 9-5).

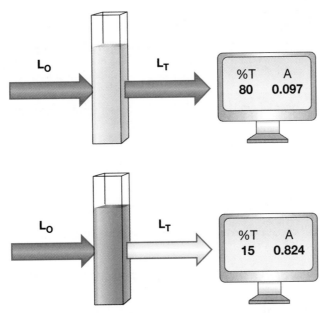

Figure 9-5 Absorbance and percent transmittance are inversely related: as percent transmittance (%T) goes up (low concentration), absorbance (A) goes down. As percent transmittance goes down (high concentration), absorbance goes up. The relationship between percent transmittance and absorbance is expressed by the formula $A = 2 - \log \%T$. L_o, incidence light; L_T, transmitted light (T).

Absorbance (A) and transmittance (T) are related by the following formula:

$$A = -\log T$$

The formula showing the relationship of concentration, absorbance, and transmittance is:

$$T = 10^{-abc}$$

where b is the path length through the test substance, c is the test substance concentration, and a is a constant.

Starting with the formula for the absorbance and transmittance,

$$A = -\log T$$

and substituting 10^{-abc} for transmittance,

$$T = 10^{-abc}$$
$$A = -\log T$$
$$A = -\log (10^{-abc})$$
$$A = -(-abc) = abc$$

That is, the absorbance of a compound is the product of the path length (b), the substance concentration (c), and the constant (a), which is the **molar extinction coefficient** or **molar absorptivity**. Pure substances have a specific molar extinction coefficient defined as the amount of light absorbed by a 1-molar concentration of the substance with a 1-cm path length. The molar extinction coefficient is a characteristic of each substance at a given wavelength of light (Box 9-4).

> **Box 9-4**   **Optical Density**
>
> When $b = 1$ cm, A is also called the **optical density** or OD. The letter A is most often used for absorbance. It does not imply a specific path length.

Beer's Law is presented with varying terms representing the molar absorptivity (ε, a), and path length (b, d), as shown in the following examples:

$$A = adc$$
$$A = abc$$
$$A = \varepsilon bc$$
$$A = \varepsilon dc$$

All these expressions represent the same formula for Beer's Law. **A = abc** is used here (Box 9-5).

CONVERSION OF SPECTRAL READINGS TO CONCENTRATION

Determining Concentration Relative to a Standard

An unknown concentration (c_u) can be determined without using the molar extinction coefficient by making the calculation relative to a standard solution of the same substance (c_s). The formula for the absorbance of the standard (A_s) is:

$$A_s = a_s b_s c_s$$

The formula for the absorbance of the unknown (A_u) is:

$$A_u = a_u b_u c_u$$

There are two ways to approach the calculation of concentration of the unknown (c_u). Colorimetric instruments may use either of these methods.

Direct Colorimetry

In **direct colorimetry**, test and reference materials are measured so that the path length is the same for the unknown, u, and the standard, s, ($b_u = b_s$). The absorbance of the test substance relative to the standard is used to determine concentration:

$$A = abc$$
$$A_u = a_u b_u c_u \qquad\qquad A_s = a_s b_s c_s$$
$$b_u = A_u/(a_u c_u) \qquad\qquad b_s = A_s/(a_s c_s)$$
$$b_u = b_s$$
$$A_u/(a_u c_u) = A_s/(a_s c_s)$$

The molar absorptivity term (a) can be dropped because the standard and unknown are the same substance and $a_u = a_s$:

$$A_u/(\cancel{a_u} c_u) = A_s / (\cancel{a_s} c_s)$$
$$A_u/(c_u) = A_s / (c_s)$$

> **Box 9-5**   Concentration, Transmittance and Absorbance
>
> The equation $A = abc$ demonstrates that the relationship between concentration and absorbance is linear. Because the relationship between absorbance and transmittance is logarithmic ($A = -\log T$), the relationship between concentration and transmittance is also logarithmic.

Solving for c_u:

$$c_u = (A_u/A_s) \times c_s$$

Direct colorimetry is also called **photometric colorimetry** because the absorbance of the unknown, A_u, is directly related to the concentration of the unknown (i.e., as the concentration increases, so does the absorbance). High concentrations have high absorbance, and low concentrations have low absorbance relative to the standard.

The direct colorimetry formula is conveniently used to determine concentration from absorbance readings of the unknown and standard, as long as the substance obeys Beer's Law.

A standard has a concentration of 24.0 g/dL and an absorbance reading of 0.420, and an unknown test sample has an absorbance reading of 0.210. The unknown concentration is:

$$c_u = (A_u/A_s) \times c_s$$
$$c_u = (0.210/0.420) \times 24.0 \text{ g/dL}$$
$$c_u = 0.50 \times 24.0 \text{ g/dL} = 12.0 \text{ g/dL}$$

Not all substances obey Beer's Law. If absorbance does not double when concentration doubles, or absorbance does not triple as concentration triples the direct colorimetry formula cannot be used. For those substances, reading of a standard curve determines concentration. The standard curve will show whether a substance obeys Beer's Law. If so, subsequent absorbance measurements can be converted to concentration by the direct colorimetry formula.

Inverse Colorimetry

Concentrations determined by inverse colorimetry are based on path length, b, rather than absorbance. The path length of the unknown is adjusted until its absorbance is equal to that of the standard substance. In inverse colorimetry, the absorbance is therefore the same for the unknown, u, and for the standard, s, ($A_u = A_s$). The path length of the unknown substance relative to the standard is used to determine concentration:

$$A_u = a_u b_u c_u \qquad A_s = a_s b_s c_s$$

The constant $a_u = a_s$ because the unknown and the standard are the same substance. These terms can be dropped from both sides of the equation.

$$A_u = b_u c_u \qquad A_s = b_s c_s$$

The absorbances, A_u and A_s, are the same because of the adjustment of the path length.

$$A_u = A_s$$
$$b_u \, c_u = b_s \, c_s$$
$$c_u = (b_s \, c_s)/b_u$$

The path length is inversely proportional to the concentration, so higher concentrations have shorter path lengths and lower concentrations have longer path lengths.

To find the concentration of a substance with a path length of 1.80 cm compared with the standard (250 mg/dL) with a path length of 1.00 cm:

$$c_u = (b_s \, c_s)/b_u$$
$$c_u = (1.00 \times 250)/1.80$$
$$c_u = 139 \text{ mg/dL}$$

Concentration From Transmittance

Spectrophotometric readings are expressed as absorbance or transmittance. **Transmittance** (L_T) is determined from **transmission** of light through a substance relative to the incident light (L_o) for test substance and blank.

$$\text{Transmission of test} = L_T/L_o$$
$$\text{Transmission of blank} = B/L_o$$
$$\text{Transmittance of test} = \frac{(L_T/L_o)}{(B/L_o)} = \frac{L_T}{B}$$

Because the blank contains none of the test substance, its transmission (B) is high. Only any incidental loss of transmission from the solvent or diluent is present. Therefore, the value of L_T/B is less than 1.

Spectrophotometers convert the test transmittance as a fraction of L_T divided by the blank to percent of the blank transmission, or %T.

$$\%T = T \times 100$$
$$T = \%T/100$$

%T can be converted to absorbance. The formula for conversion of %T to absorbance is derived from the formula for conversion of T to absorbance:

$$A = -\log T$$
$$A = -\log (\%T/100)$$
$$A = -(\log \%T - \log 100)$$
$$A = -\log \%T + 2$$
$$A = 2 - \log \%T$$

This formula is then used to convert $\%T$ to absorbance.

If a 100 mg/mL standard read 45% transmittance and the reading for the unknown was 75%, then:

$$A = 2 - \log \%T$$

The absorbance of the standard is:

$$A_s = 2 - \log 45 = 2 - 1.653 = 0.347$$

The absorbance of the unknown is:

$$A_u = 2 - \log 75 = 2 - 1.875 = 0.125$$

$$c_u = (A_u/A_s) \times c_s$$

$$c_u = (0.125/0.347) \times 100 \text{ mg/mL}$$

$$c_u = 0.360 \times 100 \text{ mg/mL} = 36.0 \text{ mg/mL}$$

Absorvance can be calculated directly from transmittance according to the formula, $A = -\log T$ In this case, the result is displayed directly on the calculator. For the previous example:

$$A_s = -\log 0.45 = -(-0.347) = 0.347$$

$$A_u = -\log 0.75 = -(-0.125) = 0.125$$

Either formula may be used to convert transmittance to absorbance. Using $A = 2 - \log \%T$ avoids the use of negative exponents; however, using a calculator, $A = -\log T$ may be faster. Press log and then the value of T (not $\%T$), and change the sign of the negative answer to positive, which will be the absorbance. On some calculators, calculating the log is reversed; that is, enter T (not $\%T$) and then log, and change the sign of the answer.

Conversion of Absorbance Readings to Concentration Using Molar Absorptivity

Under defined conditions of temperature, pH, and solvent, pure substances absorb light to a characteristic extent at a specific wavelength. This molar absorptivity is expressed in absorbance units as the molar extinction coefficient, a. It is defined as the absorbance of 1-molar solution of a pure substance.

The molar absorptivity changes depending on the wavelength at which absorbance is read. Concentration is evaluated from absorbance at the wavelength of peak absorbance for a compound. In common practice, this wavelength has already been established and provided. It is found by reading absorbance of a compound over a range of wavelengths (**spectrum;** see Fig. 9-2) and choosing the wavelength where the absorbance is greatest. Other wavelengths can be used as long as the corresponding molar absorptivity is included in the calculation.

Reduced nicotinamide-adenine dinucleotide (NADH) is a coenzyme that incorporates niacin. NADH has the following molar extinction coefficients at wavelengths of 366 nm (a_{366nm}), 340 nm (a_{340nm}), and 334 nm (a_{334nm}):

$$a_{366nm} = 3,300$$

$$a_{340nm} = 6,220$$

$$a_{334nm} = 6,000$$

Absorbance readings of NADH at these three wavelengths are different because the ability of NADH to absorb light varies with wavelength.

To find molar concentration, rearrange **A = abc** solving for concentration (*c*):

$$c = A/(ab)$$

An absorbance of 0.2 with a path length of 1 cm from a substance with a molar absorptivity of 60,700, the concentration is:

$$c = A/(ab)$$

$$c = 0.2/(60,700 \times 1)$$

$$c = 3.3 \times 10^{-6} \text{ moles/L or } 3.3 \text{ } \mu M$$

For substances used at low concentrations such as nucleotides used in molecular diagnostics, it is more convenient to use the millimolar absorptivity (*E*) (Box 9-6):

$$E = b/1,000$$

When millimolar absorptivity, *E*, is substituted for molar absorptivity, *a*, the concentration, *c*, is in millimoles per liter rather than moles per liter. In the previous example, if the molar absorptivity is 60,700, the millimolar absorptivity, **E = 60.7**:

$$c = A/(Eb)$$

$$c = 0.2/(60.7 \times 1)$$

$$c = 3.3 \times 10^{-3} \text{ mmoles/L or } 3.3 \text{ } \mu M$$

SUBSTANCE PURITY

Calculating molar absorptivity from the absorbance of known concentrations of a substance reveals the purity of a substance preparation because the pure substance has a predictable molar absorptivity value. The purity is assessed by how close the calculated molar extinction coefficient comes to the actual molar extinction coefficient of the pure substance.

Box 9-6	Millimolar Extinction Coefficient

For compounds measured in the millimolar range, the millimolar absorptivity expressed in absorbance units as the millimolar extinction coefficient, *E*, is used.

The molar absorptivity of a pure substance is known to be 30,000 to 30,200 (30,100 $\pm$ 100). A 5.00-μM (5.00 $\times$ 10^{-6} molar) solution reads 0.150 absorbance units with a 1-cm path length. Is this substance pure (within the acceptable range of molar absorptivity)?

$$a = A/cb$$

$$a = \frac{0.150}{(5.00 \times 10^{-6}) \times 1}$$

$$a = 3.00 \times 10^4 = 30,000$$

This result is within the acceptable range of 30,100 $\pm$ 100 and indicates that the substance preparation is sufficiently pure.

FINDING A DILUTION FACTOR USING MOLAR ABSORPTIVITY

Spectrophotometers read most accurately in their linear range of detection, for instance, between 0.2 and 0.8 absorbance units. The molar extinction coefficient can be used to find an appropriate dilution factor that will bring solutions of high concentration to more dilute concentrations within the linear range of the spectrophotometer.

A substance has a known molar extinction coefficient of 79,800 $\pm$ 200. How would one dilute a 1.00 molar test solution to determine its purity? A target reading of 0.5 is chosen because it is in the center of the desirable range, although other target readings within the range are also acceptable. Calculate a dilution factor (x) so that a reading of 79,800 (1.00 molar) is diluted to a reading of 0.5 absorbance units:

$$79,800 \times \frac{1}{x} = 0.5$$

$$x = \frac{79,800}{0.5} = 159,600$$

The 1.00 molar test substance should then be diluted 1/159,600 before reading absorbance.

If a solution of the test substance was read at this dilution and the absorbance was 0.399 with a 1.2-cm path length, then:

$$C = A/abc$$

$$C = \frac{0.399}{79,800 \times 1.2} = 4.17 \times 10^{-6}$$

$$C = (4.17 \times 10^{-6}) \times 159,600 = 0.665 \text{ molar}$$

The calculated concentration of the solution is 0.66 molar.

PRACTICE PROBLEMS

1. Derive Beer's Law from the formula, $I = I_o \times 10^{-abc}$, given $T = I/I_o$ and $A = -\log T$.

Convert the following spectral readings to molar concentration.

2. Absorbance = 0.280 with a path length of 1.0 cm. The molar absorptivity is 55,000.

3. Absorbance = 0.500 with a path length of 1.0 cm. The molar absorptivity is 55,000.

4. Absorbance of a $\frac{1}{50}$ dilution = 0.150 with a path length of 1.0 cm. The molar absorptivity is 55,000.

5. Absorbance of 0.750 with a path length of 1.50 cm. The molar absorptivity is 125,000.

6. Absorbance of 0.750 with a path length of 1.00 cm. The millimolar absorptivity (E) is 125.

7. Absorbance of a $\frac{1}{100}$ dilution = 0.420 with a path length of 1.50 cm. The millimolar absorptivity is 75.

Convert the following spectral readings to molar concentration by inverse colorimetry.

8. Absorbance = 0.280 with a path length of 1.5 cm. The 100 mg/mL standard reads 0.280 with a path length of 1.0 cm.

9. Absorbance = 0.280 with a path length of 0.8 cm. The 100 mg/mL standard reads 0.280 with a path length of 1.00 cm.

10. Absorbance = 0.280 with a path length of 1.9 cm. The 100 mg/mL standard reads 0.280 with a path length of 1.00 cm.

11. Absorbance of a $\frac{1}{20}$ dilution = 0.180 with a path length of 2.00 cm. The 100 mg/mL standard reads 0.180 with a path length of 1.00 cm.

12. Absorbance of a $\frac{1}{10}$ dilution = 0.080 with a path length of 1.5 cm. The 50 mg/mL standard reads 0.080 with a path length of 1.00 cm.

Convert the following spectral readings to molar concentration by direct colorimetry.

13. Absorbance = 0.280 with a path length of 1.00 cm. The 100 mg/mL standard reads 0.250 with a path length of 1.00 cm.

14. Absorbance = 0.125 with a path length of 1.00 cm. The 100 mg/mL standard reads 0.250 with a path length of 1.00 cm.

15. Absorbance = 0.380 with a path length of 1.00 cm. The 200 µg/mL standard reads 0.500 with a path length of 1.00 cm.

16. Absorbance of a $\frac{1}{5}$ dilution = 0.290 with a path length of 1.50 cm. The 200 mg/mL standard reads 0.500 with a path length of 1.50 cm.

17. Absorbance of a $\frac{1}{20}$ dilution = 0.045 with a path length of 1.50 cm. The 100 mg/mL standard reads 0.250 with a path length of 1.50 cm.

18. Derive the formula for conversion of transmittance to absorbance from percent transmittance, starting with $A = -\log T$.

Continued

PRACTICE PROBLEMS *cont.*

Convert the following percent transmittance values to absorbance.

19. 80%

20. 20%

21. 50%

22. 100%

23. 10%

Convert the following absorbance values to transmittance using the formula, A = −log T.

24. 0.80

25. 0.15

26. 0.55

27. 0.400

28. 0.60

Convert the following absorbance values to percent transmittance.

29. 0.459

30. 0.255

31. 0.100

32. 0.999

33. 0.080

34. 0.859

35. 0.300

36. 0.057

37. 0.950

38. 0.125

Determine the following molar extinction coefficients.

39. A_{330} of a 1.00-μM solution is 0.020 (1.00 cm path length).

40. A_{330} of a 1.00 molar solution diluted $\frac{1}{10,000}$ is 0.320 (1.00-cm path length).

41. A_{330} of a 1.00 molar solution diluted $\frac{1}{10,000}$ is 0.300 (1.50-cm path length).

42. A_{330} of a 0.50 molar solution diluted $\frac{1}{10,000}$ is 0.100 (1.00-cm path length).

43. A_{330} of a 1.50 molar solution diluted $\frac{1}{1,000}$ is 0.350 (1.90-cm path length).

44. A_{330} of a 0.20 molar solution diluted $\frac{1}{100}$ is 0.100 (0.80-cm path length).

PRACTICE PROBLEMS *cont.*

Use molar extinction coefficients to determine concentrations.

45. A_{330} of a solution is 0.147; $a_{330} = 55,000$ (1.00-cm path length).

46. A_{310} of a solution is 0.850; $a_{310} = 45,000$ (1.00-cm path length).

47. A_{250} of a solution diluted $\frac{1}{100}$ is 0.351; $a_{250} = 65,000$ (1.00-cm path length).

48. A_{350} of a solution diluted $\frac{1}{1,000}$ is 0.782; $a_{350} = 25,000$ (1.00-cm path length).

49. A_{250} of a solution diluted $\frac{1}{100}$ is 0.282; $a_{250} = 5,000$ (1.50-cm path length).

50. A_{300} of a solution diluted $\frac{1}{100}$ is 0.282; $E_{300} = 5.00$ (1.50-cm path length).

APPLICATIONS

Molecular Diagnostics

Nucleic acids are used as reagents as well as analytical targets in the medical laboratory. Short chains of DNA oligonucleotides composed of guanine (G), cytosine (C), adenine (A), and thymine (T) monomers are used in reaction mixes for analyses. The millimolar extinction coefficient (E) at 260 nm (A_{260}) is related to the concentration of oligonucleotides by the formula:

$$c = (A_{260})/b\ E$$

where E is the millimolar extinction coefficient and b is the path length. The E of an oligonucleotide (E_{oligo}) is the sum of the E of its component deoxyribonucleotides:

$$E_{oligo} = (n_A \times E_A) + (n_C \times E_C) + (n_G \times E_G) + (n_T \times E_T)$$

where E_A, E_C, E_G, E_T, and n_A, n_C, n_G, n_T are the mM extinction coefficients and the number of each deoxyribonucleotide (A, C, G, T), respectively.

An oligonucleotide is required for a reaction at a concentration of 2 µM. The oligonucleotide is supplied in solution of unknown concentration. The order of deoxyribonucleotides in the oligonucleotide is G-G-T-A-A-C-G-T. When read on the spectrophotometer, the A_{260} reading of the oligonucleotide solution is 0.286 (1-cm path length). Calculate E_{oligo} for this molecule. Then use the following table to calculate the millimolar concentration of the oligonucleotide using E_{oligo}, and ascertain what volume should be used to provide 100 µL of a 2.00-µM solution.

Deoxyribonucleotide	E (mM^{-1}cm^{-1})
A	15.1
C	7.4
G	11.7
T	8.7

Enzymology

Enzymes are molecules that catalyze chemical reactions. Enzyme activity is measured in international units, defined as the amount of enzyme that catalyzes production of 1 µmol of substrate in 1 minute under defined conditions. The change in substrate concentration indicates the enzyme concentration, which are expressed as international units or units per milliliter (International units/mL or units/mL).

Oxidation or reduction of nicotinamide-adenine dinucleotide (NAD) measures enzyme activity on substrates. This is possible because reduced NAD (NADH) absorbs light at 340 nm, whereas the oxidized form (NAD) does not. Depending on the enzyme activity, the absorbance (A) of NADH changes over time. This change can be expressed as difference in A (delta A or ΔA). Delta A of NADH at 340 nm with a 1-cm path length, indicates the enzyme activity on the substrate. If the reaction results in oxidation of NADH, converting it to NAD, the absorbance will decrease. If the reaction results in the reduction of NAD, converting it to NADH, the absorbance will increase.

Continued

APPLICATIONS   cont.

The millimolar absorptivity of NADH is 6.22 at 340 nm with a 1-cm path length. A change in absorbance of 6.22×10^{-3}, therefore indicates a 1-μmol change in substrate concentration. Because international unit concentrations are measured per milliliter, a ΔA of 6.22×10^{-3} (a change of 1 μmol/L) is equivalent to a ΔA of 1 nmol/mL.

The absorbance of a reaction is measured at 340 nm before and after a 1-minute time period. The difference in absorbance (ΔA) is determined by subtracting the lesser from the greater absorbance. A formula for the number of enzyme units per milliliter based on concentration change in substrate can be expressed:

$$\textbf{International units/mL} = \frac{(\Delta A \times V_t)}{(6.22 \times V_s)}$$

Where V_t is the total reaction volume and V_s is volume of test substance (serum) in the reaction.

The absorbance at 340 n*M* of a 5-mL total reaction volume (V_t) containing 1 mL serum (V_s) was 0.288. After a 1-minute incubation, the absorbance was 0.291. What is the enzyme activity in international units per milliliter in this serum sample?

CHAPTER 10

GRAPHS AND STANDARD CURVES

TYPES OF STANDARDS

Standards are solutions of known concentration used for quality control in the laboratory. There are several types of standards, depending on how the solutions are prepared and used. **Reference standards** are used to design and/or validate methods, and **calibrators** are used to calibrate instruments. Organizations such as the U.S. Pharmacopeia (USP) and the National Institute of Standards and Technology (NIST) supply reference standards of known concentration for calibration of laboratory equipment.

Working standards establish instrument response to solute concentration. Working standards are prepared in the laboratory or purchased as a set of solutions of different concentrations. Working standards, used to prepare standard curves, are often made from concentrated stock solutions or stock standards. As an alternative to separate preparations of working standards, a single working standard is used in different volumes, and the resulting concentrations are determined by calculation.

Controls or control standards differ from reference standards in that they are run, usually at one or two concentrations along with each test run. Control results are monitored to ensure that the procedure reagents and equipment are operating properly (see Chapter 11).

> **!** **CAUTION:** It is not recommended to use reference standards as controls. Ideally, controls should be as similar to the test samples as possible. Reference standards may consist of synthetic highly purified compounds, whereas the compound found in a test solution may be mixed with protein or other molecules that could affect its measurement.

LEARNING OUTCOMES

- Compare and contrast types of standards.
- Graph Cartesian coordinates.
- Plot a curve that describes the relationship between variables.
- Define terms used in graphing: origin, axis, abscissa, ordinate, slope, intercept, and extrapolation.
- Compare and contrast reagent blanks and specialized blanks.

GRAPHS AND GRAPHING

The objectives of tests performed in medical laboratory science are to detect, analyze, or otherwise quantify substances in physiological fluids. Quantitative studies are performed using instruments that produce readings associated with substance concentrations, such as tests of blood component concentrations determined by photometry in chemistry analyzers. To interpret instrument data, the relationship between the actual concentrations and the instrument readings must be established. When this relationship is shown to follow certain laws, formulae, such as Beer's Law ($A = abc$), can be used to translate instrument data, such as absorbance readings (A), to concentration (c).

Measurements made in the medical laboratory often use spectrophotometry because many compounds absorb light at specific wavelengths and concentrations can be automatically measured in dedicated instruments. Spectrophotometry depends on the relationship of absorbance (or transmittance) and the substance concentration. If the relationship follows Beer's Law, concentration may be determined mathematically using formulae described in Chapter 9. If a substance does not follow Beer's Law, or if the relationship between concentration and absorbance or other instrument output is unknown, a graph or diagram of the relationship must be prepared.

René Descartes, a French philosopher and mathematician, designed a method that connected algebra to geometry. He developed the Cartesian coordinate system to diagram mathematical equations. Descartes' diagrams revealed the mathematical relationships between pairs of numbers, one of each pair dependent on the value of the other such as instrument readings and concentration.

Cartesian Graphing

An algebraic equation defines a value for an unknown. To use an instrument reading to determine concentration, the reading has to be related to concentration. This relationship is established by testing standards of known concentration on the instrument and making a diagram or graph of the instrument reading for each standard concentration.

To make the graph, the instrument readings can be expressed as y and the standard concentrations as x. Because y depends on x, y is the **dependent variable,** and x is the **independent variable.** Each concentration has a corresponding instrument reading. Any of a range of concentrations can be used as x (it is independent), but the value of y depends on the concentration (it is dependent). By convention, the terms x and y are used to indicate these two variables; however, other designations (a and b, m and n) may also be used. A relationship exists between x and y such that there is a specific corresponding value of y for every value of x. Each value of x with its corresponding value of y is a **Cartesian pair**, designated (x,y).

In Cartesian graphing, pairs of data (x,y) are plotted on a **graph** to show the relationship (or lack of a relationship) between them. A graph is a grid of lines centered on a horizontal line (*x*-axis) and a vertical line (*y*-axis; Fig. 10-1). The point at which the two axes cross is the **origin**. In a simple graph, the **origin** is the point where both the value of *x* and the value of *y* are 0. The horizontal and vertical axes divide the graph into four **quadrants**. The upper right quadrant of the graph is most frequently used because it is the quadrant that represents positive numbers for both *x* and *y*. Graphs are drawn showing only the quadrant containing data. Three dimensional graphs have a third axis (*z*) for plotting three related coordinates (*x,y,z*).

To plot the data, that is, to locate the (*x,y*) points, the axes are marked in units corresponding to those expressed in the *x* and *y* values, such as concentration and absorbance units, respectively. Each axis then has its own **scale** marked in units of increasing (or decreasing) values along the axis line. The units are indicated by short lines or ticks representing major or minor units, such as major marks or ticks every 10 units and minor ticks every 5 units. These marks may extend across the quadrants to form a grid (Fig. 10-2A).

Scales of graphs are either linear, logarithmic, or marked in other mathematical functions. Mostly linear and logarithmic scales are used for laboratory work. Graphs can have linear or logarithmic scales on both the horizontal and the vertical axes, or they may have a linear scale on one axis and a logarithmic scale on the other. A graph with one axis in log scale and the other axis in linear scale is a **semi-log graph** (Fig. 10-2B). A graph with both axes in log scale is a **log-log graph** (Fig. 10-2C). Log_{10} scales have **cycles**, corresponding to multiples of 10 (Box 10-1). The number of cycles depends on the range of data being plotted. For instance, a graph of values ranging from 1 to 1,000 units on a linear scale would be either large or difficult to read because the units would be very close to one another. A log scale with three cycles (1 to 10, 10 to 100, and 100 to 1,000) covers this wide range, and there are relative placements of units in each cycle (Fig. 10-2D).

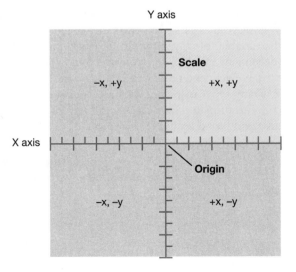

Figure 10-1 A graph comprises horizontal and vertical lines divided into units or scales. Where the lines meet is the origin. The graph is used to diagram the relationship between two sets of numbers. The numbers are paired such that for each number from one set, *x*, there is a coordinate number in the other set, *y*. These pairs of numbers (*x,y*) determine points on the graph.

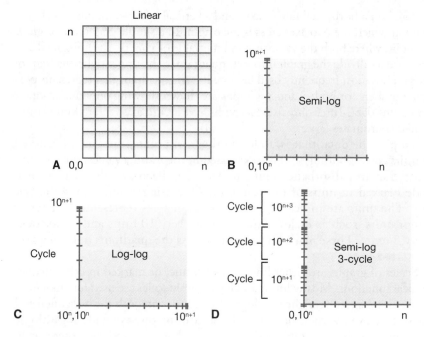

Figure 10-2 Graph scales are linear or logarithmic, or both. Each cycle of a logarithmic scale represents a multiple of 10. In a linear graph (A), both axes are linear; in a semi-log graph, one axis is logarithmic (B and D); and in a log-log graph (C), both axes are logarithmic. Log graphs have varying numbers of cycles representing multiples of 10 (D).

Box 10-1 **Origin in Log Scale**

Because log scales use powers of 10, there is no 0 on log scales. The number at the origin on the log scale is a multiple of 10.

The relationship between Cartesian pairs is diagramed on a graph by placing a point where the value of x on the horizontal axis intersects with the value of y on the vertical axis. The distance from the origin to the x value on the horizontal axis is the **abscissa**. The distance from the origin corresponding to the value of y on the vertical axis is the **ordinate** (see Fig. 10-1). For reading concentrations, the variables of concentration (independent variable) and instrument reading (dependent variable) are represented in table form (Table 10-1). Each pair on the table defines a point or location on the graph (Fig. 10-3).

Many types of paired data are encountered in the laboratory. Substance concentration and instrument reading, work load and reagent cost, and drug dose and blood levels are examples.

Table 10-1 **Examples of Cartesian Coordinates**

Concentration in mg/dL (x)	Instrument Reading (y)
40	0.090
60	0.130
150	0.310
190	0.390

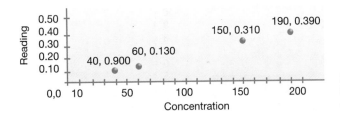

Figure 10-3 At least three (x,y) points are required to define a curve.

The Graph

After point placements, a line is drawn that best connects points for at least three pairs of data values of x and y (x,y). The line is a representation of the relationship between each x and y. The line may be straight (Fig. 10-4A and B) or curved (Fig. 10-4C), or, if there is no apparent connection between x and y, no straight or curved line can be drawn (Fig. 10-4D). The straight line represents a **linear** relationship, whereas a curved line represents a more complex relationship, such as when x or y is a logarithmic expression. The curved line of a logarithmic relationship can be transformed to a straight line by scaling one or both axes in logarithmic numbers of log scale as shown in Figure 10-4E.

A plot of three pairs of values for x and y is shown in Figure 10-5A: (2,1), (6,3), and (8,4). Because a straight line connects these three points (Fig. 10-5B), the relationship between x and y is linear (within the range of values measured). Other relationships would produce a curved line on a graph with linear scales.

The association between variables can also be described mathematically. In a linear relationship (straight line on the graph that goes through the origin), for each change in x (Δx), a corresponding change in y (Δy) occurs

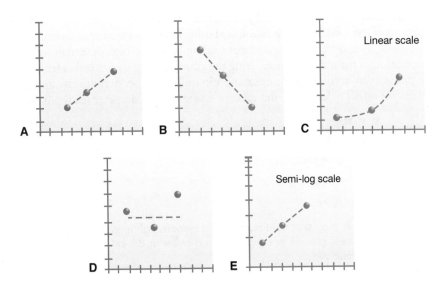

Figure 10-4 A curve may be a straight line (A and B), a curved line (C), or no relationship (D). Curved lines may indicate that the relationship between x and y is not linear. If the relationship is logarithmic, using a semi-log (E) or a log-log graph will yield a straight line with the same data points. If no relationship exists between x and y, then the points will not define a continuous line.

Figure 10-5 (A and B) The distance traveled along the x-axis to reach a point (Δx) is the abscissa. The distance traveled along the y-axis to reach a coordinate point (Δy) is the ordinate. The quotient of (Δy)/(Δx) is the slope, m. The slope for the data shown, m, is equal to 0.5.

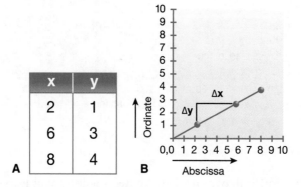

(see Fig. 10-5B). The ratio of Δy to Δx is the **slope** of the curve or m. The value of y, in this case, is x times the slope.

$$y = (\Delta y/\Delta x)\ x$$

$$y = mx$$

In the example in Figure, Δy =2 and Δx = 4; that is when x changes by 4 units, y changes by 2 units. The slope, m, then is:

$$m = \Delta y/\Delta x = 2/4 = 0.5$$

To determine any value of y along this curve from a known value of x,

$$y = mx$$

$$y = 0.5x$$

From the graph, if x = 4.8, then y is 2.4:

$$y = 0.5\ x$$

$$y = 0.5 \times 4.8$$

$$y = 2.4$$

An association between x and y such as an instrument response (y) to concentrations of test substance (x) is established using known concentrations of standard solutions. In this case, the instrument reading is used to find the unknown concentration of the test substance. Using the example slope shown earlier (m = 0.5), suppose y was in colorimetric units and x in milligrams per deciliter (assuming no background). To determine the value of x when the colorimeter reads 3.0 units,

$$y = mx$$

$$3.0 = 0.5x$$

$$x = 6.0\ \textbf{mg/dL}$$

Box 10-2 *y* Intercept

The intercept, b, may represent background response of an instrument when no target substance is present or a signal from a buffer or diluent in which a test substance is dissolved.

All linear relationships do not go through the origin (i.e., when $x = 0$, $y \neq 0$). The value of y when $x = 0$ is the y **intercept**, designated b (Fig. 10-6; Box 10-2). The formula for determining the dependent variable, y, from the independent variable, x, then becomes

y = mx + b

when the graph is a straight line. When possible, instruments are calibrated so that graphs that are used in routine laboratory work go through the origin (i.e., when concentration = 0, the instrument is set at 0). When the graph goes through the origin as in Figure 10-5, b = 0. If background signal readings are unavoidable, the graph will not go through the origin (0,0) when the concentration is 0 as in Figure 10-6 (b ≠ 0). To accommodate the background signal, the instrument may not detect low concentrations. Here, the graph would have a value for x other than 0 when y = 0. In this case, the test method may be adjusted (by eliminating components that produce background) to bring the line back to the origin. Otherwise, it will be necessary to factor in the background and acknowledge the limit on sensitivity.

When establishing a relationship between concentration or other variable and instrument readings, standards (values of x) used must encompass the range of values expected from the unknowns in a test. Readings beyond the curve established by the measured standards (**extrapolation**) are not accurate because the relationships may be linear with a certain range of concentrations, but not above or below this range (see Fig. 10-6B). Some substances obey Beer's Law within a range of concentrations, but not above or below this range.

The slope and intercept are characteristics of the relationship between x and y. When working with reference standards, these values are used to **calibrate** instruments. The reference standards are read on the instrument, a curve is produced, and the instrument readings are adjusted to match the expected slope and intercept.

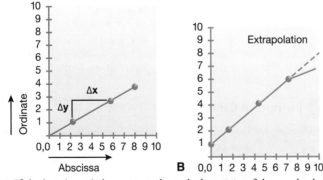

Figure 10-6 If the line (curve) does not go through the origin of the graph, the point where it crosses the y-axis when $x = 0$ is the y intercept or b (A). A curve may not always go through the origin of the graph $(x,y) = (0,0)$ (B). In this case, there will be some value of y other than 0 when x is 0. This value of y (when x is 0) is the **intercept**, or b (A). The intercept is included in the calculation of y or x. Extending a curve beyond the highest (or lowest) coordinate pair point is called extrapolation. Extrapolation may introduce error if the curve becomes nonlinear (B).

INSTRUMENT CALIBRATION

Regular calibration is important for accuracy and reproducibility of results. To calibrate an instrument, a set of calibrators of varying concentrations is run or read on the instrument to be calibrated. There is an expected output or response from the instrument because the calibrator concentrations are known. These numbers are graphed (Fig. 10-7, *dotted line*). To calibrate the instrument, the readings are adjusted to the expected values based on the known concentrations. Alternatively, the absorbance of each concentration is used with a formula, such as Beer's Law, to determine a calibration factor. When samples are run, adjustment by the calibration factor is included in the calculation converting instrument output to concentration (Box 10-3). Laboratory instruments are calibrated on a regular schedule to maintain consistency in test results.

GRAPHING PATIENT MONITORS

Graphs are made to monitor patient states in numerous clinical applications. These include concentrations of natural components or drugs in body fluids. In the microbiology laboratory, viral load over time may be monitored by detection of viral nucleic acid. Patients who have been treated with chemotherapy for leukemia may be monitored for the number of tumor cells/unit volume of

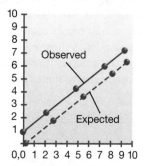

Figure 10-7 Instruments are calibrated with reference standards of known concentration. If the observed instrument readings are higher or lower than the expected readings, the instrument is adjusted to reflect the true concentrations of the reference standards.

Box 10-3 | **Instrument Calibration**

When calibrating an instrument, it is not recommended to try to adjust a graph to pass through (0,0) if other points fall off the curve that goes through the origin of the graph. The actual value of the intercept, b, depends on how many decimals are being used to define the data. It is also helpful to use more than one measurement at each of multiple concentrations of standard when establishing the curve. Reading each concentration only once may produce a curve that does not reflect the true relationship between x and y, especially if the data are "noisy" (i.e.,, the data vary because of influences other than the actual concentration).

---

blood to assess the activity of the therapeutic agent. In this case, the independent variable (x) is time, and the dependent variable is the number of tumor cells determined by the presence of tumor-specfic nucleic acid or other product (y). Ideally, the number of tumor cells should decrease with time, as shown in Figure 10-4B. A similar graph may be made to monitor viral particles or genomes per milliliter of plasma during treatment with antiviral agents.

STOCK STANDARDS

The routine use of a standard requires frequent handling, which may affect its stability or purity. Stock standards are less frequently handled than are working standards. To make working standards, the stock standards are diluted to levels in the range of the concentrations expected from the test specimens.

If a stock standard has a concentration of 10.0 mg/mL, and the working standard is to be 0.2 mg/mL, the working standard is prepared using a dilution factor. The dilution factor is determined from the two concentrations by ratio and proportion:

$$\frac{(\text{Stock standard concentration})}{\text{Dilution factor}} = \frac{(\text{Working standard concentration})}{1}$$

$$\frac{10.0 \text{ mg/mL (stock standard)} \times 1/x}{x} = 0.2 \text{ mg/mL (working standard)}$$

$$x = 50$$

Dilute the 10.0 mg/mL stock standard $\frac{1}{50}$ to prepare the working standard. In continuing the example, if the procedure calls for 100 mL of working standard, use ratio and proportion to determine how much stock standard is required to make 100 mL of the final working standard.

$$\frac{1}{50} = \frac{x \text{ mL}}{100 \text{ mL}}$$

$$x = 2 \text{ mL}$$

Make the working standard by bringing 2 mL stock standard to 100 mL with water or other appropriate dilutent.

STANDARD CURVE

To convert instrument readings to concentration, the relationship between instrument output and actual concentration must be established. Formulae, such as Beer's Law, may be used to calculate concentration; however, not all substances obey Beer's Law or other formulae. In these cases, a custom graph is generated to convert readings to concentration. **Standard curves** (graphs of known values) may also be used to see whether a substance obeys a particular formula. Once this is determined, the formula may be used instead of the graph. If not, the graph is used. Consider the readings in Table 10-2.

A graph of these values reveals that these readings do not obey Beer's Law because when x doubles, y does not, and when x triples, y does not (Fig. 10-8).

Table 10-2	Readings From a Standard Curve
x (Concentration in μg/mL)	y (Instrument Reading)
0	0.000
1	0.167
5	0.833
10	1.667
15	2.500
25	4.167

In this case, a single standard method $[C_u = (A_u/A_s) \times C_s]$ cannot be used to convert readings (A_u) to concentration (C_u). The graph is used instead.

Graphs depict measurements other than concentration. For instance, graphs are used to measure the size of particles in electrophoresis compared with the speed of migration. Particle sizes are calculated in molecular diagnostics by gel electrophoresis, in which the distance migrated in centimeters is graphed versus the size of the particle (Fig. 10-8).

BLANKS: MODIFICATION OF WORKING STANDARD BY PROCEDURE

The high end of a standard curve is the highest standard concentration achievable with the working standard. The low end is a concentration of 0, or a **blank** sample. Blanks are reaction mixes minus the substance being tested. Reading blanks reveal instrument output in the absence of the target substance. This output is generated by background signals in the instrument itself (from stray light or other source of signal in the absence of target) or signals from other components in the reaction mix.

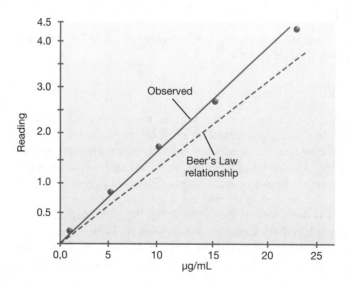

Figure 10-8 A standard curve reveals the relationship between concentration and instrument response. In this example, the substance concentrations being measured do not obey Beer's Law (*dotted line*).

Blanks representing the absence of the analyte may be used in different ways. In one approach (**reagent blank**), the measuring instrument is set at 0 on the blank, and then the readings are taken and transformed to concentration using a standard curve.

Suppose a solution of analyte is to be read on a spectrophotometer. The reagent blank is read first, and the absorbance reading is set at 0.000. The sample is then read, giving an absorbance of 0.500. The corresponding percent transmittance readings are 100% for the blank and 31.6% for the sample. The sample readings are then converted to concentration using a standard curve, which shows the relationship between the readings from the spectrophotometer and actual concentrations (or Beer's Law if the substance obeys Beer's Law).

Alternatively, a **specialized blank** is considered when one of the reagents or a potential contaminant produces a background instrument response. Some buffers absorb light at the same wavelength as the test analyte. For the specialized blanks, the instrument is set at 0 on a sample of water or with an empty cuvette. The blank is then read, and the test sample readings are adjusted according to the specialized blank reading. To make these adjustments, there has to be a linear relationship between the instrument readings and concentration. This means that absorbance can be adjusted, but not transmittance. This is because absorbance and concentration are directly related, whereas logarithmic relationship exists between percent transmittance and concentration.

Suppose a 200 mg/dL solution is read on a spectrophotometer along with a specialized blank. The blank absorbance reading is 0.100. The sample absorbance reading is 0.600. The corresponding percent transmittance readings are 79.5% for the blank and 25.2% for the sample. The sample readings include the absorbance or transmittance from the blank. To determine the correct sample concentration, the sample readings are adjusted to omit that part of the readings resulting from the background signal in the blank so that the readings reflect the correct concentration. There are two ways of doing this: either subtract readings or subtract concentrations.

In one approach, the absorbance reading of the specialized blank is subtracted from the test sample reading. For the absorbance outputs,

> **0.600 (sample) − 0.100 (blank) = 0.500**

Based on the standard curve, 0.500 corresponds to the correct 200 mg/dL. For percent transmittance, however, when the sample percent transmittance is subtracted from the blank percent transmittance

> **79.5% (blank) − 25.2% (sample) = 54.3%**

the resulting 54.3% percent transmittance corresponds to 106 mg/dL, which is incorrect. Adjusting by subtraction of reading can be done only with absorbance readings.

Alternatively, the concentrations are determined from the direct readings for the test samples and the blanks. The resulting "concentrations" (there should be no test substance in the blank) from the blank readings are subtracted from the sample readings. In the previous example, blank readings for both absorbance (0.100) and transmittance (79.5%) correspond to a concentration of 40 mg/dL. Both sample readings without correction for the blank readings correspond to 240 mg/dL. In both cases, absorbance and transmittance, the concentration is determined by subtracting 40 mg/dL from 240 mg/dL, thus yielding 200 mg/dL. This is summarized in Table 10-3.

PLOTTING A STANDARD CURVE

Consider the following rules when preparing a concentration curve from aqueous standards.

1. At least three points (concentrations) are required to establish the curve.

2. The standard concentrations tested must cover the range of expected unknown concentrations.

3. The working standard has to be of sufficient concentration to achieve the highest standard concentration expected.

4. The standard concentrations should be in the units used for reporting of the unknown (g/L, mg/dL, mg/L).

5. Use the appropriate graphing system (linear, log, semi-log) to establish the relationship between concentration and instrument output.

To plot a standard curve, first determine the appropriate working standard by using the calculations shown in the previous section. The working standard concentration should be high enough to reach the upper limit of the concentration range for the procedure, but not so high that there are large gaps between the lower concentrations or stock standard is unnecessarily wasted.

Read the standard concentrations on the detection device, such as absorbance at the appropriate wavelength on a spectrophotometer. Use the blank as a specialized or reagent blank according to the protocol. To do this when measuring transmittance and specialized blanks, calculate concentrations first, and then subtract background in the specialized blank from the concentrations in the test or, in this case, the control samples. A set of example data is shown in Table 10-4. For reagent blanks, adjust the instrument to 0 mg/mL on the blank before reading the standards.

Table 10-3 Adjusting Concentration Measurements Using Specialized Blanks

Method	Adjusted Absorbance Reading	Concentration From Absorbance	Adjusted Percent Transmittance	Concentration From Percent Transmittance
Subtract readings	0.600 – 0.100 = 0.500	200 mg/dL	79.5 – 25.2 = 54.3	106 mg/dL
Subtract concentrations	0.600	240 mg/dL – 40 mg/dL = 200 mg/dL	25.2	240 mg/dL – 40 mg/dL = 200 mg/dL

Table 10-4	Spectrophotometric Readings for a Standard Curve		
Standard	Adjusted C_s (mg/dL)	Absorbance	Percent Transmittance (%)
Blank	0	0.000	100
1	100	0.145	71.6
2	200	0.303	49.8
3	300	0.448	35.6
4	400	0.598	25.2
5	500	0.747	17.9

Figure 10-9 shows a plot of standards in milligrams per deciliter and absorbance readings. A spreadsheet computer program or graphing calculator can be used for this purpose. These electronic sources will also establish a mathematical formula describing the curve that allows automatic calculation of the unknown concentrations from the test readings. Enter the standard concentrations as x and readings as y or as two columns in a spreadsheet. Follow the instructions provided with the calculator or spreadsheet software to determine an unknown x (concentration) from y (absorbance or transmittance reading). Alternatively, the points can be plotted and the graph drawn by hand.

As seen in Figure 10-9, the relationship between concentration and absorbance is linear, producing a straight line on a linear scale. Transmittance, however, is logarithmically associated with absorbance so that the line would be curved using a linear scale (Fig. 10-10A). There are alternative options when collecting transmittance readings. The readings can be converted to absorbance and then graphed. This produces a straight line, but it requires conversion of

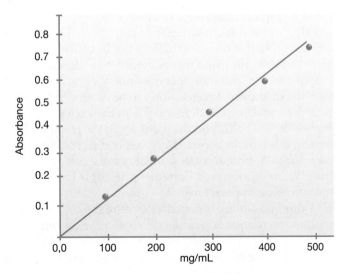

Figure 10-9 A set of standard concentrations and absorbance values plotted on a linear graph. Absorbance is directly related to concentration for this substance.

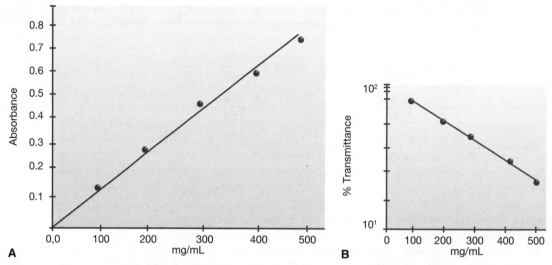

Figure 10-10 Transmittance data for the standard concentrations in Figure 10-9 plotted on a linear graph (A) and a semi-log graph (B). Transmittance is logarithmically associated with concentration. This logarithmic relationship yields a straight line on the semi-log graph.

analyte readings to absorbance before using the graph. Another option is to use a semi-log graph, as shown in Figure 10-10B. This produces a straight line with the transmittance readings but requires conversion of the transmittance readings to logarithms. A third alternative is to use electronic sources to establish a mathematical relationship and calculate the concentrations of the unknown test samples by entering the instrument readings. Many detection systems convert readings to concentration automatically.

DETERMINING CONCENTRATIONS FROM A GRAPH

Once a graph is assembled, it shows one of three options. The graph may reveal an already established relationship between instrument output and concentration. In this case, the readings can be converted using a single standard and a formula. The graph may demonstrate a relationship between instrument output and concentration that does not obey an established formula. In this case, the unknown concentration can be determined directly from the graph. Suppose a specimen reading was 2.5 in the example shown in Figure 10-11. Follow the level of 2.5 on the *y*-axis across the graph to the curve. Then move straight down to the *x*-axis. The corresponding concentration is approximately 14 μg/mL. A more accurate estimate can be achieved using a formula established from the observed Cartesian pairs. This formula may be complex and may involve computer analysis.

A third possibility is that after reading the collection of standard concentrations, no relationship is found between the concentrations and the instrument readings. This could occur if a substance is measured at the wrong wavelength, the method was not operating correctly, the standards were not

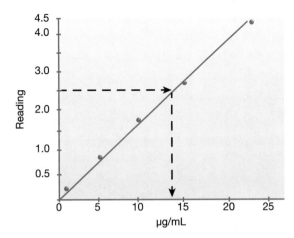

Figure 10-11 To find a concentration using a graph of instrument reading versus concentration, follow the reading level to the curve and then find the corresponding position on the *x*-axis (*dotted lines*).

diluted properly, or there just may be no relationship between the chemical reaction or instrument output used and the substance to be measured. After ruling out any errors in the standard dilutions or method, a new protocol or different measurement device may be required. For more complex relationships, such as logarithmic ones, computer software or instrument-related software systems may be preferred for the determination of the relationship and calculation of concentration.

PRACTICE PROBLEMS

Write the y coordinates for the following relationships:

1. $x = y$, when $x = 0.5$, $x = 2$, $x=19$

2. $y = x + 3.0$, when $x = 0.5$, $x = 2$, $x=19$

3. $y = x - 3.0$, when $x = 0.5$, $x = 2$, $x=19$

4. $2.0y = x$, when $x = 0.5$, $x = 2$, $x=19$

5. $3.0y + 2.0x = 10$, when $x = 0.5$, $x = 2$, $x=19$

Plot a curve that describes the following relationships, using x = 0.0, x = 5.0, and x = 10.

6. $y = x + 2.0$

7. $y = x - 2$

8. $2y = x$

9. $y = - (\frac{10x}{5})$

10. $y = -3x + 10$

11. Match the following terms

Abscissa	Perpendicular line
Origin	$x = 0$
y-axis	Outside plotted coordinates
Slope	Dependent variable
Ordinate	(0,0)
Extrapolation	Independent variable
y intercept	$m = \frac{(\Delta y)}{\Delta x}$

12. How much glucose is required to make 50 mL of a stock standard of 10 mg/mL?

13. Calculate how to make a working standard of 2 mg/mL from a 40 mg/mL stock standard.

14. Calculate how to make a working standard of 25 mg/mL from a 50 g/L stock standard.

15. How much of the 10 mg/mL stock standard is required to make 100 mL of a working standard of 50 μg/mL?

16. Which type of blank (reagent or specialized) is used for an analyte in a diluent such as water that does not absorb light at the test wavelength?

17. Which type of blank (reagent or specialized) is used for an analyte diluted in a buffer mix that contains a component that absorbs light at the same wavelength as the analyte?

18. If a specialized blank reads 0.010 absorbance and the test solution containing analyte reads 0.325 absorbance, what is the corrected absorbance reading of the test solution?

19. If a reagent blank is used to set the 0 concentration at 0 absorbance and the test solution containing analyte reads 0.325 absorbance, what is the absorbance reading of the test solution?

Continued

PRACTICE PROBLEMS   *cont.*

20. If a specialized blank reads 0.050 absorbance and the test solution containing analyte reads 0.158 absorbance, what is the corrected absorbance reading of the test solution?

21. If a specialized blank reads 0.000 absorbance and the test solution containing analyte reads 0.097 absorbance, what is the corrected absorbance reading of the test solution?

22. If a specialized blank reads 90.0% transmittance and the test solution containing analyte reads 35.8% transmittance, what is the corrected absorbance reading of the test solution?

23. Use the graph in Figure 10-9 to estimate concentrations with the following readings:

0.055

0.150

0.200

0.700

0.900

24. Consider the following satisfying the equation for absorbance (y) versus concentration in milligrams per deciliter (x):

$y = 0.0015x$

Find the concentrations of the following unknowns with the following absorbances.

0.088

0.500

0.345

0.125

0.199

25. Consider the following equation for % transmittance (y) versus concentration in milligrams per deciliter (x):
$\log y = 0.0015x$

Find the concentrations of the following unknowns with the following % transmittances.

70%

45%

60%

25%

15%

APPLICATIONS

Pharmacology

Drugs are administered at levels intended to provide the most effective systemic concentrations in the patient. This concentration depends on several factors, including the amount of drug administered and the half-life of the drug in an individual patient. Drug levels were measured over time in a patient, and the results are shown in the following graph (dose-response curve) for three different dosages of drug.

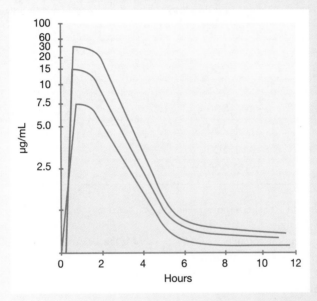

1. Use the graph to approximate the drug concentrations after 2, 3, and 4 hours for the highest dosage (*top line*).
2. What is the half-life of the drug based on these numbers?
3. Estimate the drug concentrations for the two lower dosages. Is the half-life of the drug dependent on the dosage amount?

Molecular Diagnostics

A standard curve was prepared using a commercial reference material of DNA molecules. The reference concentration was 25 nM. The molecular weight of the DNA molecule was 24,532 g/mole. The standard curve of 10-fold dilutions covered eight orders of magnitude in a 20-µL reaction volume. The seventh dilution when tested generated a positive signal, whereas the eighth dilution produced no signal.

1. What was the lowest detectable molar concentration in this assay?
2. What is the lowest absolute number of molecules detected in this assay?

Continued

APPLICATIONS cont.

General Laboratory

After repair and part replacement of a laboratory instrument, calibration was necessary. A reagent blank and a set of reference standards were read on the instrument. The relationship between concentration and instrument output is linear within a limited range. The following data were collected:

C_s (mg/dL)	Expected Reading	Observed Reading
0	0	20
50	125	137
100	250	272
250	625	641
400	1,000	1,025
500	1,250	1,271
600	1,500	1,520
800	2,000	2,019

1. Draw a graph of both readings (y-axis) compared with the standard concentration, C_s (x-axis).
2. Which is the independent variable?
3. Using the expected readings and the formula $y = mx + b$, what is the slope of the curve if $b = 0$?
4. Is the relationship between C_s and light units linear?
5. How should the calibrator be used to adjust the sample concentrations?
   a. Adjust concentrations downward.
   b. Adjust concentrations upward.
   c. No adjustment is necessary.

Molecular Diagnostics

The length of a DNA molecule in base pairs (bp) is determined from its migration speed through a matrix or gel under the force of an electric current (gel electrophoresis). Short molecules of DNA move more quickly than longer ones. The distance of migration through the gel is visualized using a fluorescent dye that binds specifically to nucleic acid and fluoresces under ultraviolet (UV) light. The nucleic acid appears as a band of fluorescence within the gel.

APPLICATIONS cont.

The distance migrated by a double-stranded fragment of DNA in gel electrophoresis is inversely proportional to the log of its length in bp. If a standard collection of DNA fragments of known size in bp (molecular weight marker or DNA ladder) is included on the same gel, one can make a semi-log plot of migration distance versus size of the known fragments to determine the size of an unknown fragment. This graph is generated from a gel image by measuring the distance between the fragment and a reference point on the gel, such as the bottom of the well in the gel into which the sample was loaded. A plot of such distance in centimeters against the known size for each fragment follows (gel image is not to scale):

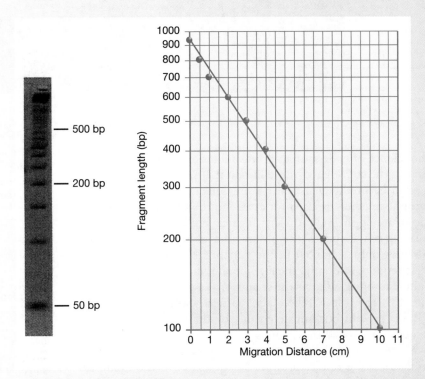

The size of an unknown fragment is estimated by finding the point on the curve that is equivalent to the migration distance of the unknown fragment on the *x*-axis and then finding the corresponding point on the *y*-axis.

1. Is a fragment that migrates 9 cm larger or smaller than a fragment that migrates 3 cm?
2. If a fragment of DNA migrates 6 cm, what is its size in bp?

CHAPTER 11

STATISTICS AND QUALITY CONTROL

STATISTICS

Statistics is the science of collection and interpretation of data. The data are analyzed to test the confidence or likelihood that results accurately reflect reality or can be predicted based on previous observations. In the clinical laboratory, statistics are used for assessing the accuracy of test results and for determining their clinical significance. For example, a positive test result for sickle cell anemia is the observation of a particular type of hemoglobin (hemoglobin S [HbS]) in the patient's blood specimen. To interpret the test result confidently, the likelihood that the test is incorrect must be taken into account. What is the chance that a molecule other than HbS is identified by the test as HbS (false-positive result)? What is the chance that HbS is present but not detectable by the test (false-negative result)? These questions are addressed by statistics. In this way, the technical accuracy of the test is established. A test with high technical accuracy provides confidence in the results produced by the test, in the example, confidence that HbS will be detected and what the test detects is always HbS. Another aspect of testing is the predictive value of a test analyte. The predictive value is the association of the test result with the disease state. Do all patients carrying HbS have sickle cell anemia? Are there cases of sickle cell anemia that do not have HbS?

Like technical accuracy, predictive value is established using statistics. Once an association between the test's result and disease is known, the test method can be put into practice. The reagents and instruments used must be shown to produce the expected result for samples known to contain the test analyte (positive controls) and samples known not to contain the test analyte (negative controls). Even if a test has a high accuracy, its predictive value may not be 100%, conversely erroneous results from technical failure or error can compromise its association with a disease and poses potential harm to patients.

Observations

Observations are detectable or recognizable characteristics. Two types of observations are made in the laboratory. One type of observation is non-numerical or **qualitative**, such as the texture, odor, or color of a sample. Microscopic observation of a particular bacterial morphology that stains with a special stain in a sputum sample is likely *Mycoplasma tuberculosis* which is associated with tuberculosis. The other type of observation is **quantitative**, meaning countable, such as number of red blood cells per microliter, or milligrams of glucose per deciliter. High red blood cell counts in excess of 15 million cells/µL are associated with diseases such as polycythemia vera, heart disease, or dehydration. Low red blood cell counts are found in patients with anemia. High or low glucose levels are associated with diabetes or hypoglycemia, respectively.

A series of related observations is referred to as **data,** such as log of blood glucose quantities over a period of hours. Each single observation is a datum or data point. Statistics makes use of data to characterize the nature of the groups to assess confidence in conclusions made from the data.

In statistics, qualitative observations are categorized; that is, each observation is put into one category or another. So cloudy fluid specimens may be put in one category, whereas clear specimens of the same fluid may be put in a different category.

Qualitative observations are classified in defined categories such as yes/no or positive/negative for reporting and for statistical analysis. **Cutpoints** or cutoff levels are used to convert quantitative results to qualitative data. An example would be measured levels of a human immunodeficiency virus ranging from 10 to more than 5,000 viruses/mL. If a cutpoint is set at 50 viruses/mL, then any result less than 50 viruses/mL is considered negative (reported as less than 50 viral particle/mL), and any result of 50 viruses/mL or greater is considered positive. The selection of cutpoint levels for quantitative data depends on the detection capacity of the test method and the predictive value of the analyte. Quantitative values assigned to categories (positive/negative, high/low) are **dichotomized.**

Quantitative observations that are not dichotomized are statistically treated as either **discrete** or **continuous**. Discrete observations are separated by specific increments, such as the numbers of tests ordered or the numbers of blood cells in a microscopic field (Box 11-1). The information or data will be in the form of whole numbers. There would be no order for one half of a test nor a fraction of a cell. In contrast, continuous data consist of any number within a range, such as diameters of cells or amounts of uric acid excreted in a day.

Box 11-1 Discrete Observations

There are two types of discrete observations. One is nominal, in which the observations have no order, such as blood type or Rh factor. In the other type of discrete observation, ordinal, observations have an order to them, such as stages of cancer, or days on medication.

Laboratory tests are intended to provide information about patients' state of health or disease. Ideally, to describe a tissue or body fluid from a patient effectively, one would have to test all the tissue or the entire volume of fluid, which is not possible. One could not count every red blood cell in a patient to determine the number of red blood cells in that patient. To obtain a close estimate of this information, a **sample** is collected (Box 11-2). Data are calculated from testing the sample and are used to estimate the true characteristics or **parameters** of the whole population. Statistics are used to interpret the sample data.

Variability

The observations being evaluated statistically are called **variables**. The word, variable implies that data have variability; that is, all data points collected, even in identical circumstances, are not necessarily the same. This is **test variability**. So, if serum amylase was measured at 75.2 mg/dL in a sample, reading the same sample again may give a result of 75.4 or 75.1 mg/dL. Taking a sample from a population also introduces variability between the sample and the whole population, or **sample variability**. An example would be measurement of glucose concentration in a sample specimen. Interpretation of the data of concentration, say, 125 mg/dL, of blood glucose must account for the sample variability. Pre-analytical treatments such as the time of day the sample was taken or whether a patient has been fasting or has just eaten a meal contribute to sample variability (Box 11-3). Sample variability has to be considered when interpreting test results and making conclusions from the collected data. Thus, a test result of 125 mg/dL must allow for the test variability, that is, if multiple samples were taken from the same sample, how each measurement would be expected to vary from 125 mg/dL (Box 11-4).

Samples are considered to be representative of a larger population of data, so a few milliliters of blood are a sample of all blood in the circulatory system, or relatively small numbers of people are a sample of a defined

---

Box 11-2   Sample Size

The size of the sample is very important statistically as well as biologically. In both cases, the sample must be large enough to be representative of the overall population. A tiny sample, such as a microliter of blood, may not be representative, especially if rare cells or infectious viruses are of interest. Conversely, drawing a liter of blood would not be practical either, because it would harm the patient and would be difficult to handle in the laboratory. The size of the sample depends on several factors, including the expected frequency of testing, levels of the target cells or molecules being tested and the methodology used. Laboratory procedures are designed to use the appropriate sample size through validation procedures. Validation procedures test known sample targets and define the capabilities and limitations of the test method.

> **Box 11-3   Sample Collection**
>
> Sample collection may generate an additional source of variability. An example would be a measurement of glucose concentration in a sample specimen. Interpretation of the data of concentration, say, 125 mg/dL, must account for the sample variability. Testing protocols include sample collection requirements (e.g., fasting glucose) and their effect on final results. Sampling procedures are designed to limit this source of variability.

> **Box 11-4   Implied Variability**
>
> Variability is implied in how many significant figures are reported. A result of 75.2 mg/dL implies that the actual value is between 75.15 and 75.25 mg/dL. A more correct expression would be 75 mg/dL, thus implying that the actual value is between 74.5 and 75.5 mg/dL. See Chapter 1 for additional discussion of significant figures. Variability depends on the precision of the analyzer and the number of significant figures given for the standard.

population. Samples must be taken at random, that is, without bias to any particular part or characteristic of the population. For discrete variables, for instance, when choosing individuals from a community to test for the presence of an infectious agent, a computer system should be used to determine which individuals will make up the sample to describe the frequency of infection of the entire community. Using a computerized or mechanical sampling would avoid any inherent and unintended human bias in the selection process.

STATISTICAL CALCULATIONS

Central Tendency

A group of values that cover a range from the smallest to the largest value with the values clustered in the middle of this range is called a **normal (or Gaussian) distribution**. This means that if the data were plotted on a graph with values on the *x*-axis and number of data points with those values on the *y*-axis, the curve would be bell-shaped peaking at the center value (Fig. 11-1). The symmetry of the curve depicts the **central tendency**, which means that most of the values are in the center, with fewer and fewer values much greater than or less than the central value. The central value in a normal distribution is the **average** or **mean** value. Values more than the average or less than the average are less and less frequent. The width of the curve showing the range of the values can be very wide or very narrow (Fig. 11-2). Normally distributed data peak at the center of the curve, regardless of the range of values. Data that do not peak at the center are considered skewed or biased (Fig. 11-3).

The central tendency is a very important characteristic of a group of data. It defines the general nature of the group and can be used to compare one set of values with another, such as the glucose levels of a group of people with insulin deficiency compared with the glucose levels of a similar group with normal insulin function. The three ways to consider central tendency are mean, median, and mode.

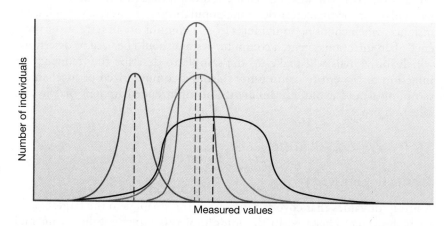

Figure 11-1 Normally distributed data center on the average or mean value of the population of data. Values become less and less frequent as they approach levels much more than or much less than the mean.

Figure 11-2 Data can be normally distributed around the mean (*dotted lines*) with greater or lesser range, the difference between the largest and smallest value. The mean is determined by the number and range of values.

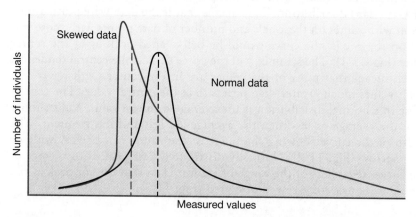

Figure 11-3 Data that center on the mean are said to have central tendency (*dotted line*). Data that are not normally distributed (skewed data) are not centered around the mean (*solid blue line*).

Mean

The **mean** value, often also called the average value, of a set of numbers is calculated by adding all the numbers in the set and dividing that sum by the number of values in the set. The formula for the mean of a set of sample values is:

$$\bar{x} = \sum x_i / n$$

The sample mean is indicated by $\bar{x}$. Each number in the sample group is indicated by x_i where the subscript i represents any number in the group. The sigma symbol, $\sum$, denotes the sum of all the numbers in the sample group. This formula describes the mean of a sample, the sample representing a larger population. Statistically, different notations are used to describe an entire population (Box 11-5).

Consider a set of data: The enzyme serum glutamic oxaloacetic transaminase (SGOT) is found in the liver and muscles. This enzyme is elevated when there is tissue damage and is decreased in vitamin B deficiency. Use the formula to find the mean of the following set of 11 liver enzyme levels in international units per microliter (optimal level, 21 international units/μL):

15, 20, 18, 22, 27, 22, 23, 27, 18, 16, 22

The mean is:

$$\bar{x} = \sum x_i / n$$
$$\bar{x} = (15 + 20 + 18 + 22 + 27 + 22 + 23 + 27 + 18 + 16 + 22)/11$$
$$= 230/11 = 20.9$$

Many calculators determine the mean of a set of numbers. A calculator with this capability has an "$\bar{x}$" (mean) key and another key, "DT," with which to enter data. You may have to go to a STAT mode using a mode key. Before beginning the calculations, clear the statistical memory by entering shift, CLR, SCL or as directed for your calculator. Enter each number followed by DT. The calculator may give a readout of n (number of data points) after each entry. After all the numbers are entered, press shift (if necessary) and the "mean" key. Additional entries may be required, depending on the calculator. Not all calculators have the capacity to find the mean. You may have to use the shift key to access these functions. Consult the instructions for your specific calculator.

Median

Another description of central tendency is the **median.** The median is the center value of the range of data. For the previous example, the median is found by first putting the numbers in order of increasing value:

15, 16, 18, 18, 20, 22, 22, 22, 23, 27, 27

> **Box 11-5** **Population Mean**
>
> The calculations shown are for a sample of values from a larger population. The mean of these numbers is the sample mean. Whereas the sample mean is indicated by $\bar{x}$, the mean of the entire population from which that sample is taken is indicated by m. A different version of this formula is used to indicate the mean of the entire population.
>
> $$m = \sum \bar{x}_i / N$$
>
> A designation of N is used to indicate the number of values in the entire population, and n is used for the number of values in the sample.

The median is the central number in this group, or 22. Five values are greater than the median, and five values are less than the median.

15, 16, 18, 18, 20, 22, 22, 22, 23, 27, 27

Median numbers are another indicator of central tendency. Median measurements are reported for effects of treatment on a disease state or disease recurrence.

The previous example has an odd number of values, thus making the median easy to determine as the center number. For data with an even number of values, the median is halfway between the two center numbers. Suppose there was an extra reading of 20 in the group:

15, 16, 18, 18, 20, 20, 22, 22, 22, 23, 27, 27

With an even number of values, the two center values determine the median:

15, 16, 18, 18, 20, 20, 22, 22, 22, 23, 27, 27

Five values are greater than the two center values, and five values are less than the two center values. The median here would be halfway between 20 and 22. To find this number, add the two central values and divide by 2:

$$\frac{(20 + 20)}{2} = 21$$

The median for this set of values is 21.

Mode

The **mode** is the number that occurs most frequently occurring number in the sample population. It is another way to assess central tendency. Continuing with the previous example, the mode is 22 because it appears three times in the data set, more than any other number. In another example, observe the following blood urea nitrogen (BUN) values in milligrams per deciliter:

12, 15, 10, 15, 7, 20, 23, 8, 19, 15, 16, 20, 17, 15, 10, 8

The mode is 15 mg/dL because there are more of this value than any of the others:

12, **15,** 10, **15,** 7, 20, 23, 8, 19, **15,** 16, 20, 17, **15,** 10, 8

A set of data may have more than one mode, as in the following data:

15, **18,** 17, **13,** 17, **12,** 15, 15, **19,** 17, 17, 15, 17, **16,** 20, 15

There are five values of 15 and five values of 17. This set of data has two modes, 15 and 17; it is bimodal. A set of data where each value is unique or appears with equal frequency as all other values will have no mode, as in the following numbers:

12, **18,** 10, **15,** 7, 20, 23, 8, 19, **14,** 16, 20, 17, 13

This set of values has no mode.

The central tendency of a set of data can be assessed by comparing the mean, median, and mode. For normally distributed data, the mean, median, and mode approach the same value. If the data do not have central tendency, the mean, median, and mode will differ.

Range

Another description of a group of numbers is the **range**, which is the distance from the smallest to the largest value. To determine the range, subtract the smallest value from the largest value:

Largest value – Smallest value = Range

Cholesterol is a lipid substance synthesized in the liver and is also absorbed from the diet. Elevated cholesterol levels have been observed in cases of diabetes and pregnancy. Malnutrition, liver insufficiency, anemia, and infection may result in low cholesterol levels. Exact measurements may differ among laboratories, instruments, and methods, but cholesterol levels of 120 to 240 mg/dL are frequently observed. The range in this case would be:

Largest value – Smallest value = Range
240 – 120 = 120

Two types of cholesterol are high-density lipoprotein (HDL) and low-density lipoprotein (LDL). HDL is a good blood component, in contrast to LDL, high levels of which are associated with arterial blockage. For HDL levels of 40 to 60 mg/dL, the range is:

60 – 40 = 20

For LDL levels of 60 to 130 mg/dL, the range is:

130 – 60 = 70

The range shows how far the data in a set of observations vary from the mean.

Standard Deviation and Error

The purpose of measurements or counts of items is to find the number that describes the population from which the sample is taken. This number may be represented by the mean, the average, of many measurements. Individual values in the population should fall closely to the real number or average.

Serum thyroxine is an indicator of thyroid function. If the average serum thyroxine level for a patient is 7.9 µg/dL, results of repeat tests for thyroxine in this patient may not be exactly 7.9 µg/dL, but they should be close to this value. The distance or deviation from the average is **error**.

Standard Deviation

Error is measured in terms of how many values fall within a defined distance from the mean. This distance is called **standard deviation** whose symbol is s. The standard deviation is an indication of how closely a set of values is clustered around the mean. It is mathematically calculated from the mean and the range of values in a normal distribution.

$$s = \sqrt{\frac{\sum (x_i - \bar{x})^2}{n - 1}}$$

That is, subtract the mean value from each value and square the difference. After doing this for all values ($i = 1 \ldots n$), sum the squared differences and divide by $n - 1$. Finally, find the square root of that number (Box 11-6).

This formula is not practical for manual calculations. Calculators or, more often, spreadsheets or statistical software programs automatically find the standard deviation of a group of entered numbers. Instrument-dedicated software may also calculate s as part of a test procedure.

Calculators with the capacity to find the mean may also have the capacity to determine standard deviations. Enter individual values using the DT function in the STAT mode, as described previously for the mean. Determining standard deviation is similar to the method described for finding the mean, by substituting $x_{\sigma n-1}$ (the standard deviation key) for the mean key and then pressing the exe or equal key. Calculators have different designations for the standard deviation or average deviation key. Consult your calculator instructions.

Graphically, the standard deviation is represented as shown in Figure 11-4. The mean plus or minus 1 standard deviation covers 68.3% of the values in a normal distribution. The mean plus or minus 2 standard deviations covers 95.4% of the values, and the mean plus or minus 3 standard deviations covers 99.7% of the values. The precision, or reproducibility, of a series of measurements is assessed by the closeness of the data points to the mean (Box 11-7). The standard deviation shows how close these values are to the mean. Measurements are expressed as being within 1 to 3 or more

---

Box 11-6 Population Standard Deviation

The standard deviation formula for an entire population uses slightly different symbols representing the same terms:

$$\sigma = \sqrt{\frac{\sum (x_i - \mu)^2}{N}}$$

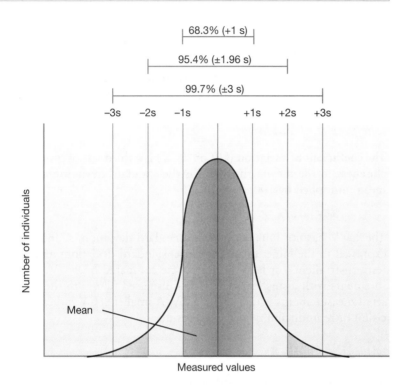

Figure 11-4 The spread of data is defined by the standard deviation. For all normally distributed data, 68.3% of values will fall within 1 standard deviation of the mean (*shaded area*). The mean ± 2 standard deviations include 95.4% of values.

Box 11-7 Calculation of Standard Deviation

For purposes of laboratory application, standard deviation is calculated electronically. Because there are other ways of computing the standard deviation using *n* instead of (*n* – 1) in the equation, it is important to make sure that the correct processes are being entered. In spreadsheets, choose Standard Deviation result, using the "unbiased," or "*n* – 1," method code for the cell where the calculated standard deviation is to be placed.

---

standard deviations from the mean. The standard deviation in these cases defines the allowable error.

Variance

Variance is another expression of error or spread of data from the mean. Variance, designated s^2, or σ^2, is the square of the standard deviation. The standard deviation is also defined as the square root of the variance. For a sample of a population, the variance is

$$s^2 = \frac{\sum (x_i - \bar{x})^2}{n}$$

Like standard deviation, variance is a measurement of the likelihood of values falling on or around the mean. In data that are normally distributed, that probability becomes smaller as the distance from the mean increases. The variance is a characteristic or parameter of a population calculated from a sample without observing the entire population. For laboratory tests, a method is designed to determine a real value in a patient from a sample, such as the concentration of a substance in a body fluid. The distance from the mean of the obtained result is a measure of whether the value is "normal."

Coefficient of Variation

The **coefficient of variation** (CV or %CV) is a third test of spread of data and closeness to the mean. The %CV is the standard deviation divided by the mean multiplied by 100:

$$\%CV = s/\bar{x} \times 100$$

The %CV has no units because the standard deviation, s, and mean, $\bar{x}$, are expressed in the same units. Therefore, standard deviations among different tests, instruments, or laboratories can be compared by %CV. A set of measurements with a smaller %CV is less dispersed (closer to the mean) than a set of measurements with a larger %CV. A smaller %CV indicates better **precision** or reproducibility of the test results.

QUALITY CONTROL

Measurements of deviation from the average are not only very useful in the interpretation of laboratory test results but also in the monitoring of laboratory performance. The latter process is called **quality control**. The **Clinical Laboratory Improvement Amendments (CLIA)** were passed by the U.S. Congress in 1988 to establish quality testing standards to ensure consistent patient test results in the clinical laboratory. CLIA specifies standards for quality control and quality assurance for laboratories.

Test Performance

Development and use of methods in the clinical laboratory require validation of the performance of methods and reagents (Box 11-8).

Test performance is determined by the ability of the technology to distinguish the presence or absence of the target molecule (**analytical sensitivity**) and only the target molecule without producing a false-positive result based on a cross reaction with an unrelated molecule (**analytical specificity**). To determine analytically true positive and true negative, a reference standard is used.

> **Box 11-8** **Test Performance and Clinical Accuracy**
>
> Although test performance is assessed by the accuracy of the test for the presence or amount of the target molecule in the specimen, clinical accuracy is determined by the association of a positive test result with the presence of disease (clinical sensitivity or positive predictive value) and the absence of disease when the test result is negative (clinical specificity or negative predictive value).

Qualitative Results

Analytical sensitivity and specificity are calculated by comparison of results to those of a reference or "gold standard" method with established accuracy. **True-positive** results are those where the positive reference tests positively and **true-negative** results are those where the negative reference tests negatively. A test without perfect accuracy produces **false-positive** results (the negative reference tests positively) and **false-negative** results (the positive reference tests negatively).

The sensitivity of a test is:

$$\frac{TP}{(TP + FN)} \times 100$$

and specificity of a test is:

$$\frac{TN}{(TN + FP)} \times 100$$

where TN = true negative, TP = true positive, FN = false negative, and FP = false positive.

The accuracy of a test is the sum of all true measurements divided by the total number of measurements (true and false) $\times$ 100:

$$\frac{(TN + TP)}{(TN + TP + FN + FP)} \times 100$$

Suppose a new test is developed to detect cytomegalovirus (CMV) in tissue samples. Even though the currently established method used in the laboratory is 100% accurate, the new test is more rapid and cost-effective than the current method. One hundred samples previously tested by the established procedure (current method) are retested using the new test. The results obtained are shown in Table 11-1.

Table 11-1 **Positive and Negative Results of a Retest**

New Test Method	Current Method	
	Positive	Negative
Positive results	10 (true-positive)	2 (false-positive)
Negative results	0 (false-negative)	88 (true-negative)

The sensitivity of the new test is:

$$\frac{TP}{(TP + FN)} \times 100$$

$$\frac{10}{(10 + 0)} \times 100 = 100\%$$

The specificity of the new test is:

$$\frac{TN}{(TN + FP)} \times 100$$

$$\frac{88}{(88 + 2)} \times 100 = 97.8\%$$

The accuracy of the new assay then equals:

$$\frac{(88 + 10)}{(88 + 10 + 0 + 2)} \times 100 = 98.0\%$$

The new test is 100% sensitive; that is, it detected the presence of CMV in all of the positive test samples. This sensitivity may be at the cost of specificity, however, because the new test produced false-positive results in two specimens in which CMV was not present. Overall, the accuracy of the test is 98% compared with the established method.

Quantitative Results

In addition to being accurate, quantitative results must be reproducible; that is, repeated testing of the same reference should yield the same result (Box 11-9). This reproducibility of results is referred to as the precision of the assay. Precision is especially monitored in quantitative tests in which the reproducibility of results is monitored. Precision does not necessarily indicate accuracy (Fig. 11-5A). Loss of precision as a result of inaccuracy is random error. Loss of accuracy consistently to a reproducible value different from the mean is systemic error (Fig. 11-5B).

Technical accuracy depends on design of the method specifically to detect the intended target molecules, such as the presence of a human papillomavirus (HPV) or a particular strain of HPV that causes cervical cancer. The method must also have the capacity to detect small numbers of virus particles (Box 11-10).

Analytical sensitivity can further be defined by the **detection limit** or lower limit of detection. The detection limit is the lowest number or concentration of molecules that is detectable by the assay. Some results are reported as positive with any detection of the target molecule, not matter how low. Alternatively,

---

Box 11-9 Control Samples

Control samples are included each time a test is run to monitor the test performance. Controls are known positive and negative samples that should yield the same results with every run. For quantitative results, the mean test results for the positive control should be very close to the actual value. The results will likely not be exactly the same for each repeat, and the error or standard deviation around the mean is established to define acceptable results.

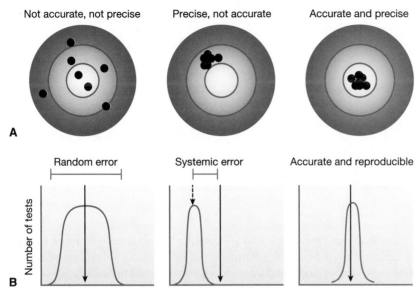

Figure 11-5 Laboratory data are intended to represent true measurements of values. (A) Random error causes most of the measurements to fall close to but not exactly on the expected value. A significant amount of random error results in a wide range of measured values centered around the expected measurement. More precise measurements fall close to the mean, which should also be the intended value. Precision does not guarantee accuracy, as shown in the center diagrams. (B) Values that consistently fall to one side of the mean define a systemic error. Both random and systemic errors require adjustment of the method to measure the target substance more accurately.

Box 11-10   Clinical Sensitivity and Analytical Sensitivity

Clinical sensitivity is different from analytical sensitivity. Analytical sensitivity is defined as the ability of the assay to detect the presence of the target molecule, whereas clinical sensitivity refers to the association of the target molecule, once detected, with actual disease state.

---

a cutpoint quantity is established above which is considered positive and below which is negative.

Quantitative methods also have an **analytical** or **dynamic range**, that is, test values between the lowest and highest levels at which the test result is accurate (Fig. 11-6). Instruments are designed to measure accurately, but they can do so only within a finite range. Instruments become inaccurate with very concentrated or very dilute solutions. Quantitative test performance is monitored in each run by inclusion of high, low (sensitivity), and negative controls in each run. Routine laboratory assays may also have normal and abnormal controls. An abnormal control is outside of the normal range of the analyte, whereas a normal control would be within that range. For an analyte that normally measures between 3.5 and 8.5 mg/dL, a normal control would have a concentration within this range. An abnormal control would have a concentration greater than 8.5 or less than 3.5 mg/dL. The normal and abnormal controls should be within the analytical range of the measuring instrument.

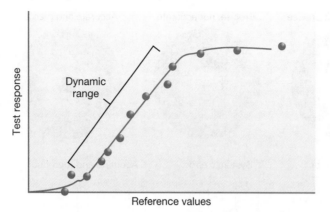

Figure 11-6 Instrument response should increase with increased concentration of test substance. Test response is measured using a set of samples with known values. Reference standards are used to define the dynamic range or the range of values where the test is most accurate.

The analytical range of an assay is established by measuring dilutions of known concentrations of a reference standard and establishing a direct correlation between test output and standard concentrations (standard curve). The raw data should be consistent with the known concentrations of the standard. If a viral load is interpreted as negative, the raw measurement should be below the cutoff value established for the test. Calculations and comparisons with standards used to verify test results are described in the laboratory test validation documents.

Quality Assurance

Quality control in the laboratory is used to ensure accuracy and precision of a measuring system within a series of measurements. These measurements are taken as part of test runs containing patients' samples and controls. Periodic review and documentation of test results are required for all clinical testing. Test performance is measured by comparison of the numbers of positive and negative results with expected numbers from independent sources, such as published results, over time, or assessment of the degree of variation of quantitative results.

A reliable test procedure would have no errors other than random inherent imprecision resulting from variability in specimens or specimen handling. If errors occur, the variation from the mean or intended value is recorded. The numbers of consecutive errors in subsequent runs are also noted, if they occur. Successive runs with errors can reveal the presence of systemic error caused by reagent or instrument deterioration or other factors. The frequency and duration of errors are considered in method design and selection of control samples used to monitor runs.

Levey-Jennings Charts

Levey-Jennings charts monitor error in terms of trends or shifts in control results in quantitative assays (Box 11-11). These plots are based on the mean and standard deviation of results from repeated measurement of control samples. The acceptable range of values to expect from controls on each run is based on the standard deviation.

Box 11-11	**Control Charts**

In the 1930s, Walter A. Shewhart first described control charts to be used in industry. Twenty years later, Levey and Jennings introduced similar control charts for clinical laboratories. These charts were based on the mean and range of results from control samples. Henry and Segalove simplified the method to include plotting of individual control results on a single chart.

To make a Levey-Jennings plot, first calculate the mean and standard deviation of results from control samples in multiple runs over a period of time. The number of values required depends on the frequency the test is to be done, such as 20 days for a test that is run once a day.

Figure 11-7 shows a graph with the run number or test day on the *x*-axis and the observed results for the control measurement on the *y*-axis. Horizontal lines mark the mean and **control limits** based on the standard deviation of the result values. Control limits are upper and lower values that define a range of acceptable results. A run is considered in control when the control values fall within these limits and out of control when control values fall outside of this range. When values repeatedly fall outside of the acceptable range, action must be taken, perhaps by repeating the run or checking the control integrity. The limits are chosen in the development and validation of the assay based on the expected inherent variability (error) of the data.

Table 11-2 shows an example of control measurements over 10 days, with two runs performed per day, one in the morning (a.m.) and one in the afternoon (p.m.). The actual concentration of the control is 50 mg/dL.

To draw a Levey-Jennings chart for this data, first determine the mean for all the runs by adding all the values together (Σx) and dividing by the number of runs, *n*:

$$\bar{x} = (\Sigma x)/n = 1{,}002/20 = 50.1$$

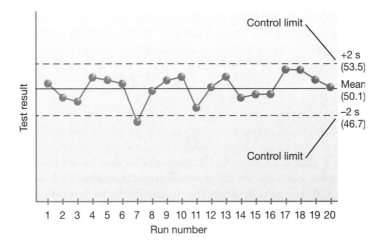

Figure 11-7 In a Levey-Jennings plot of in-control data, control values fall within defined limits (here, mean ±2 standard deviations) and on either side of the mean.

Table 11-2	Control Measurements Over 10 Days		
Run	a.m. Control (mg/dL)	Run	p.m. Control (mg/dL)
1	51	2	49
3	48	4	52
5	52	6	51
7	45	8	49
9	51	10	53
11	47	12	50
13	51	14	48
15	49	16	50
17	53	18	52
19	51	20	50

The standard deviation is:

$$s = \sqrt{\frac{\sum (x_i - \bar{x})^2}{n - 1}}$$

$$= \sqrt{\frac{\sum (x_i - 50.1)^2}{19}} = 2.05$$

Using the mean and standard deviation, the chart is drawn showing the limits of acceptable error. The standard deviation predicts the range of values to be expected from future runs (precision). Limits are set at ±1 or more standard deviations from the mean. The mean represents the closeness to the actual value of the control (accuracy).

A Levey-Jennings plot of the data is shown in Figure 11-7. The solid line is the mean of the data (50.1). The acceptable range for this particular set of data is defined as the mean ±2 standard deviations (±2s). The 2s value is determined by multiplying the calculated standard (2.05) deviation by 2. In this example, the control range is **(50.1 - 4.1) = 46.0 to (50.1 + 4.1) = 54.2.** Most commonly, a method is considered in control if the control values fall in a range of mean ± the selected number of standard deviations, usually, ±2 or 3s, that is, the mean ±2s or mean ±3s. If the data are normally distributed, an acceptable test result range is mean ±2s, then 95.4% of control results should fall within this range. (A control range may be stated to be the mean ±3s. A range of mean ±3s includes 99.7% of the control values; a range of mean ±1s includes 68.3% of the control values.) Figure 11-7 demonstrates a method that is in control. The chart shows that values fall above and below the mean, but close to the mean. Variation beyond 2s is depicted as points outside of the area between the dotted lines. All but one of the 20 control measurements (run 7) fall within the acceptable range. Because 95.4% of the values will fall within 2s in a normal distribution, **100% - 95.4% = 4.6%** of the data is expected to fall outside of this range. One point in 20 runs that does so is not considered an indication that the method is out of control. Depending on the laboratory protocol, repeating the control analysis for run 7 may be required. Many instruments are programmed to do this. When re-run, the control value should fall back into the ±2s range.

Examples of data that are out of control as a result of inaccurate measurement are shown in Figure 11-8. Figure 11-8A shows data with unacceptable random error. More than 5% (one in twenty) of the measurements fall outside of the ±2s control limits. This pattern is evidence of reagent or instrument instability or operator inconsistency. Figure 11-8B shows a shift in control values. There is a sudden change in control values between runs 3 and 4. Controls for runs 4 to 10 fall above the control limit. This sudden change is an essential characteristic of a shift. A shift can be upward as shown or downward, but the error is in the same direction; that is, the data fall to one side of the mean, higher or lower. If a mean were calculated from data in runs 4 to 10, it would be greater than the actual mean represented by the solid line. Patients' test results from these runs are likely to be inaccurate, probably higher than their true measurement. A change in reagent lot or instrument setting may cause this kind of error.

Figure 11-8C shows a trend pattern. Here there is a gradual change away from the mean in one direction. Controls of consecutive runs are higher than the previous run. A more obvious trend pattern is seen in runs 17 to 20 on this plot, where data trended out of control. Trends can be upward or downward. Fading lamps or other detection devices, improperly stored reagents, or incomplete instrument maintenance can cause trends in control data. The pattern shown in Figure 11-8D represents data from an assay done twice a day, once in the morning (1a, 2a, 3a, ...) and once in the evening (1p, 2p, 3p, ...). The assay shows accuracy in the morning runs, but a shift downward and out of control in the evening runs. The performance of the assay in the morning runs indicates that the reagents and instrument are functioning properly. In this case the evening runs are being affected by some aspect of testing at that time in the laboratory. This may occur if reagents are freshly prepared for the morning run and are reused later in the day, when they may have deteriorated. Alternatively, the instrument may have been left on between runs or turned off and not properly restarted, thus causing less than peak operating conditions by the evening run.

As demonstrated, some control results fall outside of a defined acceptable range (e.g., ±2s) simply because of random error. Rules have been established in monitoring the control measurements from run to run to define limits of acceptability for a test procedure (Westgard Rules). These rules are expressed in the form, A_L, where A is the number of control measurements outside of the acceptable range and $_L$ is the statistic, such as ±3 standard deviations, used to define the acceptable range. If a control limit is set such that no more than one measurement falls outside of 3 standard deviations, the designation would be 1_{3s}. If a control limit is set such that no more than three consecutive measurements fall outside of 2 standard deviations, the designation would be 3_{2s}. Control limits can also be defined by the range of the control data (R, the difference between the consecutive control values; a type of random error), the number of measurements consecutively falling on one side of the mean (N_x; a type of systemic error), or the number of measurements in an upward or downward trend (N_T; a type of systemic error). Table 11-3 shows examples of control limits and their definitions. These limits are applied to measurements made directly from controls (individual-value control charts).

A run containing a control that exceeds the defined limit is rejected, unless the limit has been set as a warning value. A warning demands careful inspection of the control data using additional rules. An error of 1_{2_s} is an example of a warning. If, however, the control measurement also violates another limit such as R_{4s}, then the run should be rejected.

Cumulative Sum Plots

Further statistics may be performed on individual values with establishment of additional control limits. Data from a Levey-Jennings plot can be used to make a **cumulative sum (cusum)** plot. Here, the difference between a measurement

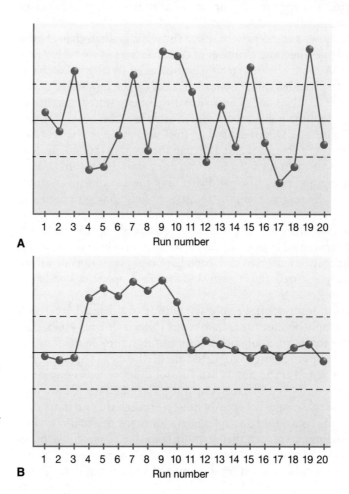

Figure 11-8 Out-of-control data are of different types. In random error, control values fall outside of the defined limits, on either side of the mean (A). In a systemic error (B), values from consecutive runs fall inside or outside of the control limit, to one side of the mean. A trend

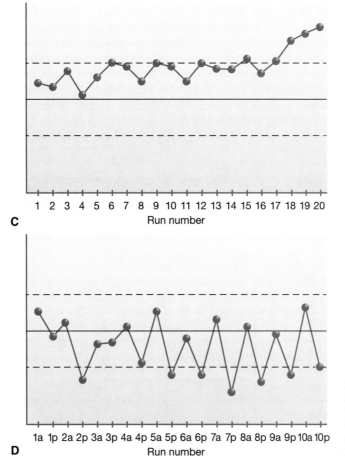

C

Figure 11-8—cont'd (C) results when a systemic error increases gradually with each test run. In D, a systemic error is frequently occurring in evening runs (p), but not in morning runs (a).

D

Table 11-3	**Examples of Control Limits**
Rule Abbreviation	Definition
1_{2s}	One control measurement falls outside of ±2 standard deviations
2_{2s}	Two consecutive control measurements fall outside of ±2 standard deviations
3_{2s}	Three consecutive control measurements fall outside of ±2 standard deviations
3_{1s}	Three consecutive control measurements fall outside of ±1 standard deviation
4_{2s}	Four consecutive control measurements fall outside of ±2 standard deviations
R_{3s}	The difference between consecutive control measurements exceeds 3 standard deviations
5_x	Five consecutive control measurements fall to one side of the mean
10_T	Ten consecutive control measurements show an upward or downward trend

and a target value (mean) is added to that difference from the previous measurement (Table 11-4). A trend or systemic error results in a steep slope on the cusum plot. The sum of differences from a mean (rounded to 50) for a set of data is shown in Figure 11-9A. Because the control values randomly fall above and below the mean value, the points fall close to the zero line.

The cusum plot of data from Table 11-5 reveals a systemic error in the data where control values start to fall continuously to one side of the mean (runs 4 to 11; Fig. 11-9B). The slope of the cusum plot may be positive for systemic error above the mean or negative for systemic error below the mean. The error

Table 11-4	Cumulative Sum of Differences From the Mean for Runs 1 to 20				
Run	Difference	Cumulative Sum	Run	Difference	Cumulative Sum
1	1	1	2	−1	0
3	−2	−2	4	2	0
5	2	2	6	1	3
7	−5	−2	8	−1	−3
9	1	−2	10	3	1
11	−3	−2	12	0	−2
13	1	−1	14	−2	−3
15	−1	−4	16	0	−4
17	3	−1	18	2	1
19	1	2	20	0	2

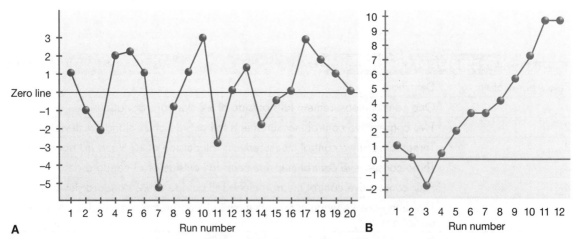

A   Run number

B   Run number

Figure 11-9 A cusum plot measures cumulative error from run to run. Random error results in a cusum plot that goes back and forth across the zero line (A). Systemic error produces a line sloping away from the center line (runs 4 to 11; B). Whether the error is enough to reject or adjust the test method depends on limits set by the laboratory.

Table 11-5	Cumulative Sum of Differences From the Mean	
Run	Difference	Cumulative Sum
1	1	1
2	−1	0
3	−2	−2
4	2	0
5	2	2
6	1	3
7	0	3
8	1	4
9	1	5
10	2	7
11	2	10
12	0	10

is judged by the steepness of the slope of the cusum plot. A control cusum limit may be set based on this slope.

Control charts allow close monitoring of test performance and accuracy. In this way, medically important errors are detected before release of results that may affect patient care. Various modifications of quality control charts and statistics are designed for specific tests and control types. Levey-Jennings plots offer the advantage of plotting individual control readings. Other approaches, such as the cusum plot, require incorporation of prior data and calculations.

Quality control statistics measure but do not prevent error. Laboratory procedure defines the acceptable levels of error and the rules for collecting control data. The overall goal is consistent, accurate, and timely production of laboratory results.

PRACTICE PROBLEMS

1. Find the mean, median, and mode of the following data:

   26, 52, 37, 22, 24, 45, 58, 28, 39, 60, 25, 47, 23, 56, 28

2. Do the data in question 1 demonstrate central tendency (normal distribution)?

3. Find the mean, median, and mode of the following data:

   126, 125, 130, 122, 124, 125, 125, 128, 129, 130, 125, 124, 123, 126, 125

4. Do the data in question 3 demonstrate central tendency (normal distribution)?

5. Find the mean, median, and mode of the following data:

   0.38, 0.52, 0.55, 0.32, 0.37, 0.38, 0.38, 0.35, 0.29, 0.38, 0.28, 0.39, 0.40, 0.38, 0.38, 0.38

6. Do the data in question 5 demonstrate central tendency (normal distribution)?

7. What is n for the number sets in questions 1, 3, and 5?

8. If the standard deviation of is 8.90 and the mean is 127, what is the coefficient of variation (%CV)?

9. Given the following standard deviations for questions 1, 3, and 5, what is the %CV for the data in questions 1, 3, and 5?

   a. s = 14.0 (question 1)
   b. s = 2.43 (question 3)
   c. s = 0.07 (question 5)

10. What are the values for the mean −2s and mean +2s for question 1?

11. What are the values for the mean +1s and mean −1s for question 3?

12. What are the values for the mean +3s and mean −3s for question 5?

13. Find the mean, median, and mode of the following data:

   0.76, 1.89, 0.88, 1.12, 0.07, 1.62, 0.11, 0.02, 0.13, 0.01

14. Do the data in question 13 demonstrate central tendency (normal distribution)?

15. Find the mean, median, and mode of the following data:

   9, 8, 9, 10, 9, 9, 10, 8, 9, 8, 10, 9

16. Do the data in question 15 demonstrate central tendency (normal distribution)?

17. If the standard deviation of the values in question 13 is 0.70, what is the variance?

18. If the standard deviation of the values in question 15 is 0.74, what is the variance?

19. What is the %CV for the data in question 13?

20. What is the %CV for the data in question 15?

21. Compare the %CV in questions 19 and 20. Which data set has the highest variability?

Continued

PRACTICE PROBLEMS *cont.*

22. Which would describe data with the greatest precision?

   a. Large standard deviation, low mean
   b. Low standard deviation, large mean
   c. High standard deviation, high mean
   d. High standard deviation with the same mean

Hematocrit is a measure of the percent (%) of blood volume that consists of red blood cells. Hematocrit readings in % for 20 males and 20 females are shown in the following table:

Males (%)	Females (%)
41	35
44	40
52	39
35	36
49	36
40	38
45	39
43	35
41	40
49	41
52	38
37	42
40	33
42	37
41	38
45	38
50	39
44	41
43	38
45	40

23. What are the mean % values for males and females?

24. What are the median % values for males and females?

25. What are the mode values for males and females?

26. If the standard deviations are 4.6 for males and 2.3 for females, what would be the range that would include 95.4% of values based on the numbers given?

27. What is the %CV for the test for males and females?

PRACTICE PROBLEMS   *cont.*

28. If s = 2.5 and the mean is 20, what is the mean ±2s?

29. If s = 3.0 and the mean is 20, what is the mean ±1s?

30. If s = 17 and the mean is 298, what is the mean ±3s?

Observe the Levey-Jennings plot of the following data showing the mean with ±1s control limits (53.6 ±2.8).

Run Number	Positive Control Result
1	56
2	56
3	55
4	57
5	56
6	54
7	51
8	51
9	50
10	50

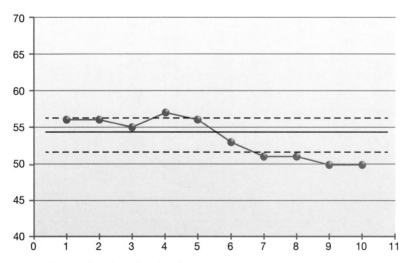

31. If ±1s is the control limit, what does the plot show?

　　a. The runs are within the control limits.
　　b. There is random error.
　　c. There is a systemic error.

Continued

PRACTICE PROBLEMS *cont.*

32. Which of the following rules is violated in question 31?

a. 4_{2s}
b. 6_x
c. 10_T
d. 2_{1s}

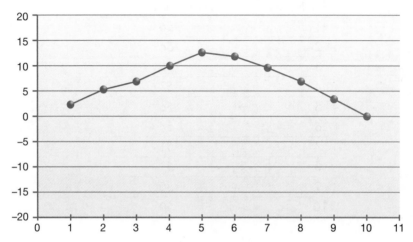

33. Consider the cusum plot shown here. What characteristic of the cusum plot suggests error in values for runs 1 to 5?

34. What does the cusum plot suggest for runs 6 to 10 in question 33?

The following plot was drawn for controls in a test for concentration of triglycerides in blood. The mean value of the previous 15 runs was 103 mg/dL, and the standard deviation was 2.4. The control limits are 103 ±2s (98 to 108 mg/dL).

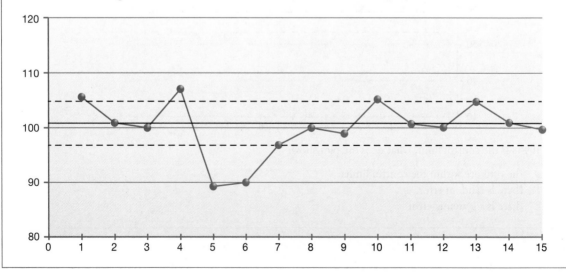

35. Which of the following rules is violated over the course of the 15 runs in question 34? (More than one answer may be correct.)

   a. 3_{2s}
   b. 4_{2s}
   c. R_{4s}
   d. 6_T

The following cusum plot was drawn for another triglyceride test:

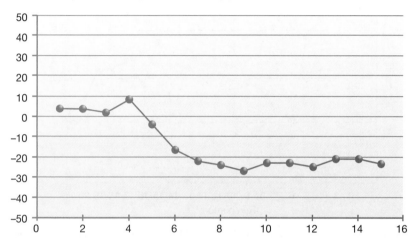

36. What does this cusum plot suggest for runs 4 to 7?

37. Which rule is violated over the course of 15 runs?

   a. Five consecutive run control results have fallen below the mean.
   b. Five consecutive run control results have fallen above the mean.
   c. Runs 1 to 4 control results are unacceptably high.
   d. Runs 9 to 15 control results are unacceptably low.

Continued

PRACTICE PROBLEMS *cont.*

38. Which type of error is apparent?

    a. Acceptable random error
    b. Unacceptable random error
    c. No error
    d. Systemic error

Observe the following plot:

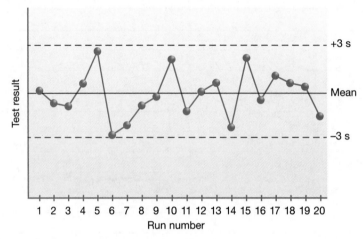

39. Which rule(s) is/are violated over the course of 20 runs? (More than one answers may be correct.)

    a. 4_{3s}
    b. 6_T
    c. R_{4s}
    d. 2_{4s}

40. Which type of error is apparent?

    a. Acceptable random error
    b. Unacceptable random error
    c. Acceptable systemic error
    d. Unacceptable systemic error

Observe the following plot:

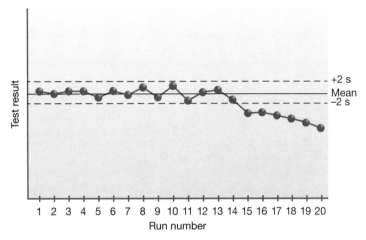

41. Which rule(s) is/are violated over the course of 20 runs? (More than one answers may be correct)

    a. 2_{2s}
    b. 5_T
    c. 3_{2s}
    d. R_{2s}

42. Which type of error is apparent?

    a. Acceptable random error
    b. Unacceptable random error
    c. Acceptable systemic error
    d. Unacceptable systemic error

Continued

PRACTICE PROBLEMS *cont.*

43. If each of two technologists performed every other run, what could be the cause of the observed results?

   a. Technologist error
   b. Reagent preparation
   c. Sample collection
   d. Instrument failure

A new reagent lot was incorporated in run 13. The control results are shown in the following plot:

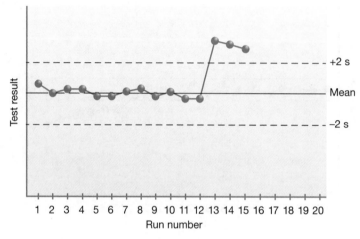

44. Which rule(s) is/are violated over the course of 20 runs? (More than one answers may be correct)

   a. 2_{2s}
   b. 5_T
   c. 3_{2s}
   d. R_{2s}

45. Which type of error is apparent?

   a. Acceptable random error
   b. Unacceptable random error
   c. Acceptable systemic error
   d. Unacceptable systemic error

46. Based on the information given, which of the following could be the cause of the results observed in question 44?

    a. Technologist error
    b. The new reagent lot
    c. Sample collection
    d. Instrument failure

After 13 runs, a new lot of test reagent was implemented. The cusum plot is shown as follows:

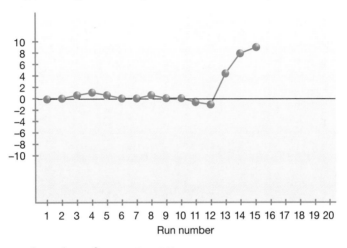

47. What does the cusum plot indicate for runs 1 to 12?

48. Which type of error is apparent from a cusum plot for runs 13 to 15 in question 47?

    a. Acceptable random error
    b. Unacceptable random error
    c. Acceptable systemic error
    d. Unacceptable systemic error

49. Which of the following changed in runs 13 to 15 with the new reagent lot in question 47?

    a. Accuracy of control results
    b. Precision of control results
    c. Acceptability of control results
    d. Unacceptable systemic error

50. What would be the predicted error in the measurement of the patient specimens in runs 13 to 15 in question 47, based on the effect of the new reagent lot on the controls?

    a. Results will be inaccurate and low.
    b. Specimen results will not be affected.
    c. Results will be inaccurate and high.
    d. Only specimens with low-level readings will be affected.

APPLICATIONS

General Laboratory

A reference laboratory performs a test for concentration of an analyte (target molecule). The laboratory operates on three shifts daily. Runs for the first 5 days of the month are shown below. A positive control of 100.0 mg/dL is included with each run, and the mean for the control results for the first 5 days is 101.8 mg/dL, with a standard deviation of 2.36. Differences from the mean $(x_i - x)$ and the cumulative sum of these differences $S(x_i - x)$ are also shown.

Day	Shift	Run	Control mg/dL	$x_i - x$	Cumulative Sum
1	1	1	105.5	3.7	3.7
	2	2	101.2	–0.6	3.1
	3	3	100.1	–1.7	1.4
2	1	4	103.4	1.6	3.0
	2	5	99.9	–1.9	1.1
	3	6	100.2	–1.6	–0.5
3	1	7	105.1	3.3	2.8
	2	8	100.0	–1.8	1.0
	3	9	99.0	–2.8	–1.8
4	1	10	105.4	3.6	1.8
	2	11	100.8	–1.0	0.8
	3	12	100.1	–1.7	–0.9
5	1	13	104.8	3.0	2.1
	2	14	101.1	–0.7	1.4
	3	15	99.8	–2.0	–0.6

Continued

APPLICATIONS cont.

A Levey-Jennings chart for the 15 runs was made. The control limits were mean ±2s.

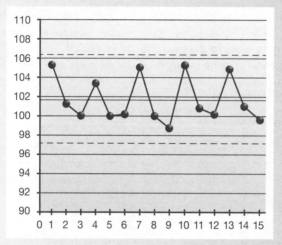

A cusum plot was also made.

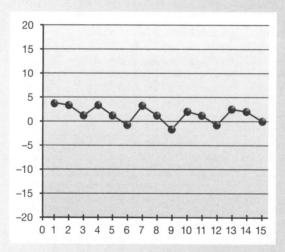

1. Is this method in control?
2. Compare the results on each shift. Is there systemic or random error within shifts? If so, what could explain the observation?

ANSWERS TO PRACTICE PROBLEMS AND APPLICATIONS

CHAPTER 1

PRACTICE PROBLEM ANSWERS

Fundamental Concepts

1. A test result is reported in increasing units of color with the degree of pigment in the sample. A darkly pigmented sample yields a result value lower than that of a lightly pigmented sample. Is this expected? **No, the darkly pigmented sample should have more units of color because it has more pigment than the lightly pigmented sample.**

2. If a handwritten test result has a value of 1 crossed out with a value of 2 written below it, what is the result? **The correct result is 2.**

3. A sample is diluted 1/10. The test reading of the diluted sample is 10 times less than the original undiluted substance. Is this correct? **Yes. A diluted substance will produce a reading less than the original substance. In this example, the reading should be 10 times less because the diluted sample contains 10 times less of the substance.**

4. Test results for substance A are reported in percent format (40%, 10%, 60%). Is a result of "50" correctly reported? **No. The result must be reported in the proper format, 50%.**

5. Scientist A makes a quick mental calculation on how much reagent is required for a test. Because the amount calculated is conveniently the same amount of reagent available, the scientist proceeds with the test. Is this correct? **No. Calculations should be documented and verified before proceeding with the test.**

6. A smaller mass weighs more than a larger mass of the same substance. Is this acceptable without reviewing the process? **No. The larger mass should weigh more than the smaller one. The process and instrumentation should be reviewed before proceeding.**

7. Your calculator gives an unexpected value. Is this necessarily correct, because you used your calculator? No. A number may have been miskeyed into the calculator. The instrument will perform the mathematical operations correctly, but only on the numbers entered.

8. True or False: When handwritten values for a repetitive protocol are illegible, the values most frequently observed in previous tests should be assumed. False. Even if results from a protocol are repeatedly similar, values may differ occasionally.

9. Your automatic pipet is intended to pick up a volume twice as large as a volume previously pipetted; however, the amount in the pipet tip looks smaller than the amount previously pipetted (see Fig. 1-5). Which pipetted amount is likely incorrect, the previous amount (1) or the current amount (2), or both? Both the previous and the current amount are likely incorrect. The pipet is not drawing up accurate amounts and should be repaired or recalibrated to work properly.

10. If a calculation calls for division of a whole number into a dividend, should the answer be greater or smaller than the dividend? Whenever a number is divided by a whole number, the result (quotient) will be smaller than the original number.

Numerals

Perform the following mathematical exercises.

11. $\frac{1}{2} + \frac{3}{4} = (\frac{2}{4} + \frac{3}{4}) = \frac{5}{4} = 1\frac{1}{4}$

12. $5\frac{1}{2} + 3\frac{1}{4} = (\frac{11}{2} + \frac{13}{4}) = \frac{22}{4} + \frac{13}{4} = \frac{35}{4} = 8\frac{3}{4}$

13. $\frac{2}{3} - \frac{1}{2} = (\frac{4}{6} - \frac{3}{6}) = \frac{1}{6}$

14. $\frac{7}{8} + \frac{1}{9} - \frac{2}{3} = (\frac{63}{72} + \frac{8}{72}) - \frac{48}{72} = \frac{23}{72}$

15. $\frac{3}{7} \times \frac{2}{3} = \frac{6}{21} = \frac{2}{7}$

16. $6\frac{1}{4} \times 2\frac{1}{3} = (\frac{25}{4} \times \frac{7}{3}) = \frac{175}{12} = 14\frac{7}{12}$

17. $7 \times (3\frac{1}{2} + \frac{3}{7}) = 7 \times (\frac{7}{2} + \frac{3}{7}) = 7 \times (\frac{49}{14} + \frac{6}{14}) = 7 \times \frac{55}{14} = \frac{385}{14} = 27\frac{7}{14} = 27\frac{1}{2}$

18. $(\frac{6}{4})/(\frac{1}{2}) = (\frac{6}{4} \times \frac{2}{1}) = \frac{12}{4} = 3$

19. $(5\frac{2}{3}) / (7\frac{1}{3}) = [(\frac{17}{3})/(\frac{22}{3})] = (\frac{17}{3} \times \frac{3}{22}) = \frac{51}{66} = \frac{17}{22}$

20. $\{[(\frac{4}{5}) / (\frac{2}{3})] \times \frac{1}{4}\} + 100 = \{[\frac{4}{5} \times \frac{3}{2}] \times \frac{1}{4}\} + 100 = \{\frac{12}{10} \times \frac{1}{4}\} + 100 = \frac{12}{40} +$

$100 = 100\frac{12}{40} = 100\frac{3}{10}$

Express the following numbers in decimal fractions and percentages. (Round to the nearest whole percent.)

21. $\frac{7}{10} = 0.7 = 70\%$

22. $\frac{3}{6} = 0.5 = 50\%$

23. $\frac{1}{3} = 0.33... = 33\%$

24. $\frac{1}{5} = 0.2 = 20\%$

25. $2\frac{2}{3} = 2.66... = 267\%$

26. $\frac{5}{100} = 0.05 = 5\%$

27. $1\frac{7}{9} = 1.77... = 178\%$

28. $\frac{24}{52} \approx 0.46 = 46\%$

29. $\frac{505}{100} = 5.05 = 505\%$

30. $\frac{466}{1000} = 0.466 = 47\%$

Write the reciprocal of the following numbers.

31. 98 $\frac{1}{98}$

32. $\frac{1}{7}$ 7

33. $\frac{6}{10}$ $\frac{10}{6}$

34. x $\frac{1}{x}$

35. $\frac{a}{b}$ $\frac{b}{a}$

Use common and decimal fractions to solve the following problems.

36. How many units comprise $\frac{1}{2}$ of 50 units?

    50 units $\times \frac{1}{2} = \frac{50}{2}$ units = 25 units

37. If you make five aliquots out of a 3-ounce sample, how many ounces would be in each aliquot?

    3 oz $\times \frac{1}{5} = \frac{3}{5}$ oz = 0.6 oz

38. One tenth of the sum of 4 parts plus 2 times 3 parts is how many parts?

    $\frac{(4 + 3 \times 2)}{10} = \frac{[4 + (3 \times 2)]}{10} = \frac{[4 + 6]}{10} = \frac{10}{10} = 1$ parts

39. What is 0.5 of 0.25?

   0.25 x 0.5 = 0.125

40. How many parts are in ¼ of a ⅓ aliquot of 30 parts?

   $\frac{1}{3}$ x 30 = 10 parts

   $\frac{1}{4}$ x 10 = 2.5 parts

Round off the following values and express in three significant figures.

41.	1.754	1.75
42.	0.86237	0.862
43.	0.001747	0.00175
44.	100.96	101
45.	1,531.2	1,530
46.	0.0115	0.0115
47.	0.0125	0.0125
48.	124.7	125
49.	1,111,111	1,110,000
50.	0.000999	0.000999

APPLICATION ANSWERS

Laboratory Inventory

Each run consists of a total of 25 samples, 22 for specimens plus two controls and one blank. The number of units required for each run would be:

$$10 \text{ units/} \sout{sample} \times 25 \text{ } \sout{samples} = 250 \text{ units}$$

If the test is performed twice a week, the number of units per week would be:

$$250 \text{ units/} \sout{run} \times 2 \text{ } \sout{runs}/\text{week} = 500 \text{ units/week}$$

A package containing 1,000 units would last 2 weeks:

$$\frac{1,000 \sout{units}}{(500 \text{ } \sout{units}/\text{week})} = 2 \text{ weeks}$$

The number of packages to order per month would be:

$$\frac{4 \text{ } \sout{weeks}}{(2 \text{ } \sout{weeks}/\text{package})} = 2 \text{ packages}$$

Hematology

First, convert the percent values to decimal fractions. Then multiply 6,000 by each decimal fraction. The cell counts are reported in numbers of microliter volumes.

```
Total white blood cells                      6,000 per microliter
Segmented neutrophils   0.56 × 6,000 =  3,360  per microliter
Banded neutrophils      0.03 × 6,000 =    180  per microliter
Lymphocytes             0.28 × 6,000 =  1,680  per microliter
Monocytes               0.07 × 6,000 =    420  per microliter
Eosiniphils             0.04 × 6,000 =    240  per microliter
Basophils               0.02 × 6,000 =    120  per microliter
                                        6,000
```

Reporting Confidence

The number with the least significant units is the measurement of the liquid handler, which has three significant figures. The confidence of three significant figures must be applied to the final result. The number reported will be 25.0 units.

Chemistry

$$(Na^+ \text{ concentration} + K^+ \text{ concentration}) - (Cl^- \text{ concentration} + HCO_3^- \text{ concentration})$$
$$(138 + 4.0) - (101 + 23) = 142 - 124 = 18$$

This anion gap (18) is within the normal 10 to 20 range. Some laboratories do not include potassium (K^+) in the measurement of the anion gap. In this case, the reference range is eight to 16, and the foregoing profile excluding K^+ would have an anion gap of 14.

An anion gap outside of the normal range can result from changes in unmeasured anions and cations in blood as a result of conditions such as diabetes or renal disease.

CHAPTER 2

PRACTICE PROBLEM ANSWERS

Equations

Which of the following pairs of values would comprise two sides of the same equation?

1. $2 + 4, 3 + 3$ $6 = 6$, Yes

2. $5 \times 6, \frac{300}{10}$ $30 = 30$, Yes

3. $\frac{3}{9}, \frac{1}{6}$ $\frac{1}{3} \neq \frac{1}{6}$, No

4. $2 \times 0.5, 2.5$ $1.0 \neq 2.5$, No

5. $0.2, \frac{100}{200}$ $0.2 \neq \frac{1}{2}$, No

6. $(\frac{1}{5}) \times 4, \frac{80}{100}$ $\frac{4}{5} = \frac{4}{5}$ or $0.8 = 0.8$, Yes

7. $3x, 6x - 3x$ $3x = 3x$, Yes

8. $x, [(\frac{250 - 240}{10})]x$ $x = 1x$, Yes

9. $0.2x, \frac{x}{2}$ $0.2x \neq \frac{x}{2}$, No

10. $3x + 3y, (5x + 2y) - (2x - y)$ $(3x + 3y) = (3x + 3y)$, Yes

Solving for the Unknown Variable

Solve the following equations for x.

11. $3x + 3 = 9$
$3x = 6$
$x = 2$

12. $5x + 1 = 400 - 394$
$5x = 6 - 1$
$5x = 5$
$x = 1$

13. $\frac{x}{2} = 0.25$
$x = 2 \times 0.25$
$x = 0.5$

14. $(\frac{5x}{3}) = \frac{90}{9}$
$5x = \frac{270}{9}$
$5x = 30$
$x = 6$

15. $(x - 27) = 1,000$

   $x = 1,027$

Use the method of substitution to solve for x and y.

16. $x - 2y = 8; x + y = 11$

   $x = 11 - y$

   $(11 - y) - 2y = 8$

   $11 - 3y = 8$

   $11 - 8 = 3y$

   $3 = 3y$

   $y = 1$

   $x + y = 11$

   $x + 1 = 11$

   $x = 10$

   $x = 10; y = 1$

17. $0.5\,x - y = 25; x = y - 22$

   $0.5\ (y - 22) + y = 25$

   $0.5\ y - 11 + y = 25$

   $1.5\ y = 36$

   $y = 24$

   $x - 24 = -22$

   $x = 2$

   $x = 2; y = 24$

18. $2x + 2y = 36; 3x = 5y + 30$

   $2x = 36 - 2y$

   $x = 18 - y$

   $3x = 5y + 30$

   $3\ (18 - y) = 5y + 30$

   $54 - 3y = 5y + 30$

   $24 = 8y$

   $y = 3$

   $2x + 6 = 36$

   $2x = 30$

   $x = 15$

   $x = 15, yx = 3$

19. $4x + 8y = 17; \dfrac{(32 + 2y)}{2} = 6$

$4x = 17 - 8y$

$x = (\frac{17}{4}) - 2y$

$\dfrac{(32x + 2y)}{2} = 6$

$16x + y = 6$

$16 [(\frac{17}{4}) - 2y] + y = 6$

$68 - 32y + y = 6$

$62 = 31y$

$y = 2$

$4x + 8(2) = 17$

$4x = 1$

$x = 0.25$

$x = 0.25, \ y = 2$

20. $\dfrac{(3x + 3y)}{3} = 11; x + y = 11$

$x = 11 - y$

$(\frac{3x}{4}) = 2y$

$[3(\frac{11 - y}{4})] = 2y$

$(\frac{33 - 3y}{4}) = 2y$

$33 - 3y = 8y$

$33 = 11y$

$y = 3$

$x + y = 11$

$x + 3 = 11$

$x = 8$

$x = 8; \ y = 3$

Use the method of comparison to solve for x and y.

21. $2x - 3y = 12; x + y = 11$

$\begin{array}{r} 2x - 3y = 12 \\ - \ (2x + 2y = 22) \\ \hline - 5y = -10 \end{array}$

$y = 2$

$\begin{array}{r} 2x - 3y = 12 \\ + \ (3x + 3y = 33) \\ \hline 5x = 45 \end{array}$

$x = 9$

$x = 9; \ y = 2$

22. $(x + y) \times 0.2 = 0.6$; $3x + y = 23$

$0.2x + 0.2y = 0.6$

$(x + y) = 3.0$

$$
\begin{array}{r}
3x + y = 23 \\
- \ (x + y = 3) \\
\hline
2x = 20
\end{array}
$$

$x = 10$

$3 (x + y) = 3 (3) = 9$

$3x + 3y = 9$

$$
\begin{array}{r}
3x + y = 23 \\
- \ (3x + 3y = 9) \\
\hline
- 2y = 14
\end{array}
$$

$y = -7$

$x = 10; \ y = -7$

23. $\dfrac{x}{2} + 10 = y - 85$; $y = 5x + 50$

$\dfrac{x}{2} - y = -95$

$0.5x - y = -95$

$y = 5x + 50$

$- 5x + y = 50$

$$
\begin{array}{r}
0.5x - y = -95 \\
+ \ (- 5.0x + y = 50) \\
\hline
- 4.5x = -45
\end{array}
$$

$x = 10$

$- 5x + y = 50$

$- 0.5x + 0.1y = 5.0$

$$
\begin{array}{r}
0.5x - y = -95 \\
+ (- 0.5x + 0.1y = 5.0) \\
\hline
- 0.9y = -90
\end{array}
$$

$y = 100$

$x = 10; \ y = 100$

24. $2x - 3y = 33$; $2x + y = 21$

$$
\begin{array}{r}
-(2x + y = 21) \\
\hline
-4y = 12
\end{array}
$$

$y = -3$

$2x + y = 21$

$6x + 3y = 63$

$$
\begin{array}{r}
2x - 3y = 33 \\
+ \ (6x + 3y = 63) \\
\hline
8x = 96
\end{array}
$$

$x = 12$

$x = 12, \ y = -3$

25. $1,000x + 2y = 1,900; x + y = -48$

$$500x + y = 950$$

$$
\begin{array}{r}
x + y = -48 \\
- (500x + y = 950) \\
\hline
-499x = -998
\end{array}
$$

$$x = 2$$

$$x + y = -48$$
$$1,000x + 1,000y = -48,000$$

$$
\begin{array}{r}
1,000x + 2y = 1,900 \\
- (1,000x + 1,000y = -48,000) \\
\hline
- 998y = 49,900
\end{array}
$$

$$y = -50$$
$$x = 2, \ y = -50$$

Exponents

Convert the following exponential terms to real numbers.

26. $3^1 = 3$

27. $10^1 = 10$

28. $a^0 = 1$

29. $50^{-1} = \dfrac{1}{50} = 0.02$

30. $100^{-2} = \dfrac{1}{10,000} = 0.0001$

31. $10^{-4} = \dfrac{1}{10,000} = 0.0001$

Express the following numbers in exponential form.

32. 25 (base 5) 5^2

33. 64 (base 2) 2^6

34. 100,000 (base 10) 10^5

35. 0.001 (base 10) 10^{-3}

36. 1 (any base a) a^0

Perform the following calculations.

37. $3^2 \times 3^3 = 3^5$

38. $8^2 \times 8^{10} = 8^{12}$

39. $3^2 \times 2^3 = 9 \times 8 = 72$

40. $3^2 + 3^3 = 9 + 27 = 36$

41. $5^2 - 3^2 = 25 - 9 = 16$

42. $\dfrac{(10^2)}{(10^3)} = 10^{-1}$

43. $\frac{(7^9)}{(7^3)} = 7^6$

44. $\frac{(10^{-2})}{(10^3)} = 10^{-5}$

45. $\frac{(10^2)}{(10^{-3})} = 10^5$

46. $\frac{(10^{-1})}{(10^2)} = 10^{-3}$

47. $\frac{(10^2 \times 10^{-2})}{(10^3)} = 10^{-3}$

Express the following numbers in scientific notation.

48. $237 = 2.37 \times 10^2$

49. $415,000 = 4.15 \times 10^5$

50. $60,000,000 = 6.00 \times 10^7$

51. $0,175 = 1.75 \times 10^{-1}$

52. $0.000327 = 3.27 \times 10^{-4}$

Convert the following ratios (A to B) to proportion (A in total/B in total).

53. 1:2 $\frac{1}{3}$ A, $\frac{2}{3}$ B

54. 5:20 $\frac{5}{25}$ or $\frac{1}{5}$ A, $\frac{20}{25}$ or $\frac{4}{5}$ B

55. 9:1 $\frac{9}{10}$ A, $\frac{1}{10}$ B

APPLICATION ANSWERS

Laboratory Automation

1. The ratios of A:B:C are:

3:2:5

The total reagent mix is:

```
3 parts A + 2 parts B + 5 parts C = 10 parts total
```

The proportions of each part in the solution are:

```
3.0 parts A/10 total parts, or 3/10
2.0 parts B/10 total parts, or 1/5
5.0 parts C/10 total parts, or 1/2
```

2. The reagent mix can still be prepared, as long as the proportions are kept the same. Use ratio and proportion in an equation to determine how much of each reagent to use to make 5.0 parts total:

```
3 parts A/10 parts total = x parts A/5 parts total
x = (3/10) × 5 = 1.5 parts A
2 parts B/10 parts total = x parts B/5 parts total
x = (2/10) × 5 = 1.0 part B
5 parts C/10 parts total = x parts A/5 parts total
x = (5/10) x 5 = 2.5 parts C
```

The ratios of A:B:C are:

1.5:1.0:2.5

The total reagent mix is:

```
1.5 parts A + 1.0 parts B + 2.5 parts C = 5 parts total
```

The proportions of each part in the solution are the same as the original procedure.

```
1.5 parts A/5 total parts, or 1.5/5 = 3/10
1.0 parts B/5 total parts, or 1/5 = 2/10
2.5 parts C/5 total parts, or 1/2 = 5/10
```

Because only 1 part B is required to prepare the 5 part mix, there are sufficient reagents to make the mixture.

Computer Maintenance

1. A megabyte is 1,000,000 or 1×10^6 bytes, which in computer memory is supplied as 1,024,000 bytes or 1.024×10^6 bytes; 512 kilobytes is 512,000 bytes or 5.12×10^5 bytes. The upgrade requires addition of:

```
(1.024 x 10⁶) − (5.12 x 10⁵) bytes
or (10.243 × 10⁵) − (5.12 x 10⁵) bytes
= 5.12 × 10⁵ bytes
or, 1,024,000 − 512,000 = 512,000 bytes
```

2. One 512-kilobyte chip will supply sufficient RAM.

CHAPTER 3

PRACTICE PROBLEM ANSWERS

Types of Measurement

Indicate whether the following results are quantitative or qualitative.

1. The presence or absence of a color   qualitative
2. White cells per μL blood   quantitative
3. Glucose blood levels   quantitative
4. Colony morphology   qualitative
5. Blood alcohol content   quantitative

Types of Properties

Indicate whether the following properties are physical or chemical.

6. Mass   physical
7. Odor   physical
8. Solubility   chemical
9. Length   physical
10. Ionization potential   chemical
11. Oxidation state   chemical
12. Freezing point   physical
13. Density   physical
14. Temperature   physical
15. Electronegativity   chemical

Systems of Measure

16. List the three primary units of the metric system for mass, length, and volume. What unit symbol is used with each unit? gram (g), meter (m), liter (L)

For the following SI units:

    a. Indicate whether the unit is basic or derived.
    b. Give the unit and unit symbol for each of the units.

17. Volume   derived   liter (L)
18. Mass   basic   kilogram (kg)
19. Time   basic   second (s)
20. Density   derived   kilograms/liter (kg/L)
21. Current   basic   ampere (A)
22. Concentration   derived   moles per liter; molarity (mol/L)
23. Luminous intensity   basic   candela (cd)

24. Pressure   derived   pascal (Pa; Pa/m²)
25. Temperature   basic   Kelvin (K)

Prefixes

Name the prefix, symbol, and power of 10 for the following orders of magnitude.

26. 0.000001   micro, μ, 10^{-6}
27. 1,000,000   mega, M, 10^6
28. 1,000,000,000   giga, G, 10^9
29. 0.1   deci, d, 10^{-1}
30. 0.001   milli, m, 10^{-3}
31. 1,000   kilo, k, 10^3
32. 0.000000001   nano, n, 10^{-9}
33. 0.000000000001   pico, p, 10^{-12}
34. 1,000,000,000,000   tera, T, 10^{12}
35. 10   deca, da, 10^1
36. 1   no prefix or symbol, 10^0
37. 1 Å = 10^{-10} meter   0.1 nano, n, 0.1×10^{-9}
38. A millimeter is how many meters?   0.001 meter
39. A microliter is how many liters?   0.000001 liter
40. A kilogram is how many grams?   1,000 grams

Heat

41. Temperature is what type of substance characteristic (physical or chemical)?
    physical
42. Motion of particles in matter is thermal energy.
43. True or False? Heat will always move from the cooler to the warmer object.
    False. Give the basis for zero degrees for each of the temperature scales.
44. Fahrenheit freezing temperature of a water-salt mixture
45. Celsius freezing point of pure water
46. Kelvin Absolute zero, temperature at which matter has no more thermal energy to lose

Temperature Scales

47. Which of the three temperature degrees are equal in scale? Celsius and Kelvin
48. 0°C is what temperature on the Fahrenheit scale? 32°F
49. 0°F is what temperature on the Celsius scale? −17.8°C
50. 0 K is what temperature on the Celsius scale? −273°C
51. 0°C is what temperature on the Kelvin scale? 273 K

Temperature Conversions

Convert to Celsius.

52. 100°F   37.8°C

53. 25.0°F   −3.9°C

54. 150°F   65.6°C

55. −25.0°F   −31.7°C

56. 212°F   100°C

57. 50.0 K   −223°C

58. 500 K   227°C

59. 75.0 K   −198°C

60. 100 K   −173°C

Convert to Kelvin.

61. 150°C   423 K

62. −100°C   173 K

63. 25.0°C   298 K

64. 500°C   773 K

65. 22.0°F   267 K

66. 212°F   373 K

67. −10.0°F   250 K

68. 100°F   311 K

69. 0°F   255 K

70. −55.0°F   225 K

Convert to Fahrenheit.

71. 23.0°C   73.4°F

72. −50.0°C   −58.0°F

73. 37.0°C   98.6°F

74. 3.56°C   38.4°F

75. −29.0°C   −20.2°F

76. 20.0 K   −423°F

77. 250 K   −9.40°F

78. 100 K   −279°F

79. 350 K   171°F

80. 0 K   −459°F

81. The laboratory room temperature reads 32.0°C. Is this too warm, too cool, or correct for room temperature (72°F–75°F)?

89.6°F, too warm for room temperature

82. A hot plate is set to 100ᵒF. Will this boil water?

No. 100°F = 44°C. Water boils at 212°F (100°C).

83. Cultures of yeast (optimal growth temperature, 30°C) are placed in an incubator set at 303 K. Is this correct?

Yes. °C = 303 − 273 = 30°C

84. Water-ice mixtures freeze at b: 0°C

85. Will heat-loving (thermophilic) bacteria grow optimally at 300 K?

No. 300K − 273 = 27°C (80.6°F)

86. A body thermometer reads 37°C. Is this normal?

Yes. 37°C = 98.6°F

87. The freezer is set to 20°C. If water freezes at 32°F, is this correct?

No. 20°C = 63°F

88. A water bath in the laboratory is set at 50°F. The protocol calls for a water bath set at 50°C. Should the bath temperature be adjusted up or down?

Up. 50°F = 10°C

89. The freezer alarm has sounded. The freezer was set at –80°C. The temperature inside the freezer must have risen above:

a: 193 K

90. Infectious bacteria grow at human body temperature (98.6°F). Will human cell cultures grow at 310 K?

Yes. 310K = 37°C = 98.6°F

APPLICATION ANSWERS

Hematology

1. Hct is approximately three times the Hb:

   $3 \times 15.5 = 46.5$ (approximately)

2. Hb is approximately $\frac{1}{3}$ the Hct %:

   $41 \div 3 = 14$ (approximately)

3. The RBC count is 5,000,000 RBC/μL = $5 \times 10^6/\mu$L = 5×10^{12}/L

   The MCH is determined using the formula:

   $$MCH = \frac{(Hb\ g/dL) \times 10}{RBC\ count/L}$$

   $$MCH = \frac{(15.0\ g/dL \times 10)}{5.00 \times 10^{12}/L}$$

   $$MCH = \frac{150\ g/\cancel{L}}{5.00 \times 10^{12}/\cancel{L}}$$

   $$MCH = 30 \times 10^{-12}\ g = 30\ pg$$

All these values are within the normal range for an adult RBC index.

Enzymology

$$1\ enzyme\ unit = \frac{1\ \mu mole}{(1\ hour/mL)}$$

$$1\ IU = \frac{1\ \mu mole}{min/mL}$$

The enzyme unit differs from the IU in terms of time. Divide the hour term by 60 to convert the expression to IU.

$$1\ IU = \frac{1\ \mu mole}{(1\cancel{hour}/mL) \times 60\ min/\cancel{hour}}$$

$$1\ IU = 1/60\ enzyme\ units$$

The number of IU in 1,500 enzyme units is:

$$(1/60) \times 1,500 = 25\ IU$$

CHAPTER 4

PRACTICE PROBLEM ANSWERS

Dilutions and Ratios

1. What is the total number of parts in a 1 part in 10 part dilution?

   10 parts

2. What is the total number of parts in a 1 part to 10 part ratio?

   11 parts

3. When substance A is diluted 2/5, how many parts of substance A are in 10 parts total?

   4 parts; 2/5 = 4/10

4. When the substance A: water <u>ratio</u> is 2:5, how many parts of substance A are in 10 parts total?

   2:5 = 2 parts in 7 total parts

   2/7 = x/10

   x = 2.8 parts

5. When the substance A: water <u>ratio</u> is 2:5, how many parts of substance A are in 14 parts total?

   2:5 = 2 parts in 7 total parts

   2/7 = x/14

   x = 4 parts

6. A 1/10 dilution of serum in saline has a ratio of how many parts saline to serum?

   9 parts saline, 1 part serum

7. A 1/10 dilution of serum in saline has a ratio of how many parts serum to saline?

   1 part serum: 9 parts saline

8. A 1:10 ratio of serum to saline has how many parts saline to serum?

   10 parts saline:1 part serum

9. A 1:2 ratio of serum to saline has how many parts serum in 3 parts total?

   1 part: 2 parts = 3 total parts

   1/3 = x/3

   1 part

10. A 1:2 ratio of serum to saline has how many parts serum in 2 parts total?

    1 part:2 parts = 3 total parts

    1/3 = x/2

    0.67 part

Amount of Substance in a Dilution

11. Calculate how many mL of substance A are in 100 mL of the following dilutions of substance A in diluent.

    a. 1/20   5 mL
    b. 1/3   33 mL
    c. 1/30   3.3 mL
    d. 1/1,000   0.1 mL
    e. 9/10   90 mL

12. What is the total volume of a solution in the following dilutions in milliliters?

    a. 1 mL/10 mL   10 mL
    b. 1 mL:4 mL   1 mL + 4 mL = 5 mL
    c. 1 mL/20 mL   20 mL
    d. 1 mL:9 mL   1 mL + 9 mL = 10 mL
    e. 5 mL/10 mL   10 mL

13. Prepare 50 mL of 1/5 substance A in water.

    1/5 = x/50

    x = 10

    Bring 10 mL substance A to 50 mL with water.

14. Prepare 1 L of 70/100 ethanol in water.

    70/100 = x/1,000

    x = 700

    Bring 700 mL ethanol to 1 L with water.

15. What volume of saline is required to make 0.10 mL of a 1/10 serum in saline dilution?

    1/10 = x/0.10

    x = 0.01

    0.10 - 0.01 = 0.09 mL

16. What volume of undiluted reagent is required to make 100 mL of a 1/25 dilution in water?

    1/25 = x/100

    x = 4.0

    4 mL

17. How much plasma is required to make 1.0 mL of a 1/50 dilution of plasma in saline?

    1/50 = x/1.0

    x = 0.02

    0.02 mL

18. The linear range of an instrument requires a 1/100 dilution of normal serum for accurate readings of a test analyte. How much serum is required for each test if the test takes 10 mL total diluted serum?

```
1/100 = x/10
x = 0.1
0.1 mL
```

19. How much diluent is in 100 mL of a 1/200 dilution?

```
1/200 = x/100
x = 0.5
100 - 0.5 = 99.5 mL
```

20. What is the volume of water in 500 mL of a 250 mL/L dilution in water?

```
250/1,000 = x/500
x = 125
500 - 125 = 375 mL
```

21. What is the final dilution if 1 mL of a 1/10 dilution is brought to 10 mL?

```
1/10 x 1/10 = 1/100
```

22. What is the final dilution if 2 mL of a 1/5 dilution is brought to 20 mL?

```
1/5 x 2/20 = 2/100 = 1/50
```

23. What series of three dilutions would make a 1/1,000 dilution? (Note: There are multiple answers; provide one.)

```
1/10, 1/10, 1/10
1/5, 1/10, 1/20
1/100, 1/5, 1/2
and others
```

24. What series of three dilutions would make a 1/5,000 dilution? (Note: There are multiple answers.)

```
1/50, 1/10, 1/10
1/50, 1/20, 1/5
1/20, 1/100, 2/5
and others
```

25. What series of four dilutions would make a 1/20,000 dilution? (Note: There are multiple answers.)

```
1/10, 1/10, 1/10, 1/20
1/50, 1/20, 1/10, 1/2
1/20, 1/100, 1/5, 1/2
and others
```

Dilution Factors

26. What is the dilution factor if 2 mL substance is brought to 10 mL total volume?

```
2/10 = 1/5; dilution factor = 5
```

27. What is the dilution factor if 0.5 mL substance is brought to 1.0 mL total volume?

0.5/1.0 = 1/2; dilution factor = 2

28. What is the dilution factor if 5 mL substance is brought to 15 mL total volume?

5/15 = 1/3; dilution factor = 3

29. What is the dilution factor if 10 mL substance is brought to 20 mL total volume?

10/20 = 1/2; dilution factor = 2

30. What is the dilution factor if 0.01 mL substance is brought to 2.00 mL total volume?

0.01/2.00 = 1/200; dilution factor = 200

Dilution Series

For the following set of dilutions, list:

   a. The tube dilution made in each flask or tube
   b. The resulting sample dilution in each flask or tube
   c. The substance concentration in each flask or tube
   d. The dilution factor for each flask or tube

31. Five milliliters of a 1,000 mg/dL glucose solution is brought to 50 mL with water in flask A, 2 mL of the 1,000 mg/dL glucose solution is brought to 50 mL with water in flask B, and 1 mL of the 1,000 mg/dL glucose solution is brought to 50 mL with water in flask C.

   a. A, 1/10; B, 1/25; C, 1/50
   b. A, 1/10; B, 1/25; C, 1/50
   c. A, 1,000 mg/dL × 1/10 =1,00 mg/dL; B, 1,000 mg/dL × 1/25 = 40 mg/dL; C, 1,000 mg/dL × 1/50 = 20 mg/dL
   d. A, 10; B, 25; C, 50

32. Three milliliters of 10 μg/mL calcium chloride is brought to 30 mL with water in flask A, 2 mL of 10 μg/mL calcium chloride is brought to 60 mL with water in flask B, and 1 mL of 10 μg/mL calcium chloride is brought to 100 mL with water in flask C.

   a. A, 1/10; B, 1/30; C, 1/100
   b. A, 1/10; B, 1/30; C, 1/100
   c. A, 10 μg/mL × 1/10 = 1.0 μg/mL; B, 10 μg/mL × 1/30 = 0.33 μg/mL; C, 10 μg/mL × 1/100 = 0.1 μg/mL
   d. A, 10; B, 30; C, 100

33. Four milliliters of 50 ng/mL dye solution is brought to 5 mL with saline in tube A, 2 mL of the 50 ng/mL dye solution is brought to 5 mL with saline in tube B, 1 mL of the 50 ng/mL dye solution is brought to 5 mL with saline in tube C, and 0.5 mL of the 50 ng/mL dye solution is brought to 5 mL with saline in tube D.

   a. A, 4/5; B, 2/5; C, 1/5; D, 1/10
   b. A, 4/5; B, 2/5; C, 1/5; D, 1/10
   c. A, 50 ng/mL × 4/5 = 40 ng/mL; B, 50 ng/mL × 2/5 = 20 ng/mL; C, 50 ng/mL × 1/5 = 10 ng/mL; D, 50 ng/mL × 1/10 = 5 ng/mL
   d. A, 5/4; B, 5/2; C, 5; D, 10

Serial Dilutions

For the following set of dilutions, list:

    a. The tube dilution made in each flask or tube
    b. The resulting sample dilution in each flask or tube
    c. The substance concentration in each flask or tube
    d. Total volume in each flask or tube after transfer

34. Consider the following dilution series of a 100 µg/mL solution: 1 mL of the solution is brought to 2 mL in tube A, 1 mL of diluted solution in tube A is brought to 10 mL in tube B, and 5 mL of diluted solution in tube B is brought to 10 mL in tube C.

    a. A, 1/2; B, 1/10; C, 1/2
    b. A, 1/2; B, 1/20; C, 1/40
    c. A, 100 µg/mL × 1/2 = 50 µg/mL; B, 100 µg/mL × 1/20 = 5.0 µg/mL; C, 100 µg/mL × 1/40 = 2.5 µg/mL
    d. A, 2 mL − 1 mL = 1 mL; B, 10 mL − 5 mL = 5 mL; C, (10 mL, no transfer)

35. A 5,000 mg/L solution is diluted in the following series: 0.1 mL is brought to 1 mL in tube A, 0.5 mL of the diluted solution in tube A is brought to 10 mL in tube B, and 5 mL of diluted solution in tube B is brought to 50 mL in flask C.

    a. A, 1/10; B, 1/20; C, 1/10
    b. A, 1/10; B, 1/200; C, 1/2,000
    c. A, 5,000 mg/L × 1/10 = 500 mg/L; B, 5,000 mg/L × 1/200 = 25 mg/L; C, 5,000 mg/L × 1/2,000 = 2.5 mg/L
    d. A, 1 mL − 0.5 mL = 0.5 mL; B, 10 mL − 5 mL = 5 mL; C, (50 mL, no transfer)

36. Fifty microliters of 100 µg/mL magnesium chloride solution are brought to 5 mL with water in tube A, 1 mL of the dilution in tube A is brought to 10 mL with water in tube B, and 5 mL of dilution in tube B is brought to 10 mL with water in tube C.

    a. A, 1/100; B, 1/10; C, 1/2
    b. A, 1/100; B, 1/1,000; C, 1/2,000
    c. A, 100 µg/mL × 1/10 = 100 µg/mL; B, 100 µg/mL × 1/1,000 = 0.1 µg/mL; C, 100 µg/mL × 1/2,000 = 0.05 µg/mL
    d. A, 5 mL − 1 mL = 4 mL; B, 10 mL − 5 mL = 5 mL; C, (10 mL, no transfer)

37. One hundred microliters of 580 mg/dL are brought to 10 mL with water in tube A, 1 mL of the dilution in tube A is brought to 100 mL with water in flask B, and 50 mL of dilution in tube B is brought to 200 mL with water in flask C.

    a. A, 1/100; B, 1/100; C, 1/4
    b. A, 1/100; B, 1/10,000; C, 1/40,000
    c. A, 580 mg/dL × 1/100 = 5.80 mg/dL; B, 580 mg/dL × 1/10,000 = 0.058 mg/dL; C, 580 mg/dL × 1/40,000 = 0.014 mg/dL
    d. A, 10 mL − 1 mL = 9 mL; B, 100 mL − 50 mL = 50 mL; C, (200 mL, no transfer)

38. Fifty microliters of 10,000 μg/mL are brought to 50 mL with water in tube A, 2 mL of the dilution in tube A is brought to 10 mL with water in tube B, 5 mL of dilution in tube B is brought to 10 mL with water in tube C, and 2 mL of the dilution in tube C is brought to 10 mL with water in tube D.

a. A, 1/1,000; B, 1/5; C, 1/2; D, 1/5
b. A, 1/1,000; B, 1/5,000; C, 1/10,000; D, 50,000
c. A, 10,000 μg/mL × 1/1,000 = 10 μg/mL; B, 10,000 μg/mL × 1/5,000 = 2.0 μg/mL;
   C, 10,000 μg/mL × 1/10,000 = 1.0μg/mL; D, 10,000 μg/mL × 1/50,000 = 0.2 μg/mL
d. A, 50 mL - 2 mL = 48 mL; B, 10 mL - 5 mL = 5mL; C, 10 mL - 2 mL = 8 mL; D,
   (10 mL, no transfer)

Design of a Dilutions Series

39. A method for preparing an antibody solution requires 10 mL of a 1/10,000 dilution, made with tube dilutions of 1/20, 1/50, and 1/10 in buffer. Only 0.5 mL of antibody solution is available. How can the method be adjusted to achieve the proper dilution?

There are multiple answers. All should result in 10 mL of a final solution dilution of
1/10,000. Example:

Make the first dilution 0.5 in 10, rather than 1/20

Make the second dilution 1/50

Make the third dilution 1/10

40. With 20 mL buffer and 1 mL plasma, how would you prepare 1 mL of a 1/10,000 dilution of plasma in buffer?

There are multiple answers. All should result in 1 mL of a 1/10,000 dilution without
using more than 20 mL buffer. One example is given.
Prepare four 10-fold dilutions in buffer. Bring:

0.5 mL serum to 5 mL in buffer (A)

0.5 mL A to 5 mL (B)

0.5 mL B to 5 mL (C)

0.1 mL C to 1 mL

Fold Dilutions

41. What is the tube dilution in the fifth tube of a fivefold serial dilution?

1/5 (all tube dilutions will be 1/5)

42. What is the tube dilution in the 10th tube of a twofold serial dilution?

1/2 (all tube dilutions will be 1/2)

43. What is the solution dilution in the fifth tube of a 10-fold serial dilution?

1/10 × 1/10 × 1/10 × 1/10 × 1/10 = 1/100,000

44. What is the solution dilution in the 10th tube of a twofold serial dilution?

1/2 × 1/2 × 1/2 × 1/2 × 1/2 × 1/2 × 1/2 × 1/2 × 1/2 × 1/2 = 1/1,024

45. Starting with 1 mL pure substance and making 1-mL transfers, what is the substance volume in the fourth tube of a fivefold serial dilution?

$1/5 \times 1/5 \times 1/5 \times 1/5 = 1/625$

$1/625 \times 1 \text{ mL} = 0.0016 \text{ mL}$

46. Starting with 0.5 mL of a 40 g/L solution in 10 mL (first tube), what is the concentration in the second tube of a 20-fold serial dilution?

$1 \times 0.5/10 = 1/20$ (solution dilution in the first tube)

$1/20 \times 1/20 = 1/400$ (solution dilution in the second tube)

$1/400 \times 40 \text{ g/L} = 0.1 \text{ g/L}$

47. What is the substance concentration in percent in the fourth tube of a 1/5 serial dilution?

$1/5 \times 1/5 \times 1/5 \times 1/5 = 1/625$ (solution dilution in the fourth tube)

$1/625 \times 100\% = 0.16\%$

Corrections for Dilutions

48. A 1/10 dilution of a substance is determined to have a concentration of 10 mg/dL. What is the concentration of the undiluted substance?

$10 \text{ mg/dL} \times 1/(1/10) = 100 \text{ mg/dL}$

49. A 1/100 dilution of nucleic acid is determined to have a concentration of 55 μg/mL. What is the concentration of the undiluted substance?

$55 \text{ μg/mL} \times 1/(1/100) = 5,500 \text{ μg/mL} = 5.5 \text{ mg/mL}$

50. A procedure requires 5 mL volume for concentration reading. Accidentally, 2 mL of the solution is spilled. The remaining 3 mL are brought back to 5 mL with diluent to have adequate volume for the detection device. The reading is 17.0 mg/dL. What is the concentration of the undiluted substance?

$17.0 \text{ mg/dL} \times 1/(3/5) = 28.3 \text{ mg/dL}$

51. A method to detect concentration of a serum protein is designed for analysis of 1/10 dilution of serum, so that the final reading is automatically adjusted to account for the dilution. The serum sample is diluted 1/20 by mistake. The reading is 20.5 μg/mL. What is the concentration of the serum?

$(1/10)/(1/20) = 2$

$20.5 \text{ μg/mL} \times 2 = 41.0 \text{ μg/mL}$

52. A procedure calls for 0.5 mL plasma in 1.0 mL saline for determination of concentration of a plasma component. The final reading is automatically adjusted to account for the dilution. Instead of 0.5 mL, 1.0 mL of undiluted plasma is used. The reading is 3.6 μg/mL. What is the concentration in the plasma?

$3.6 \text{ μg/mL} \times 1/(1.0/0.5) = 1.8 \text{ μg/mL}$

Standards

53. Four 10-fold dilutions of a 500 mg/dL glucose solution are prepared. What is the concentration of each dilution?

50 mg/dL, 5.0 mg/dL, 0.5 mg/dL, 0.05 mg/dL

54. Three twofold dilutions of a 20.0 mg/dL reference standard are prepared. What is the concentration of each dilution?

10 mg/dL, 5.0 mg/dL, 2.5 mg/dL

Antibiotic Resistance

55. Three 10-fold dilutions of antibiotic are added to bacterial cultures. The bacteria grow in the third dilution, but not the first two. What is the antibiotic titer?

1/100 or 100

56. Five twofold dilutions of antibiotic are added to bacterial cultures. The bacteria grow in all dilutions except the first. What is the antibiotic titer?

1/2 or 2

57. A bacterial strain is spread on an agar plate. Discs imbued with antibiotic diluted at 1/5, 1/25, 1/50, 1/100, and 1/250 are placed on the spread. A clear zone of no growth appears only around the disc with the 1/5 dilution of antibiotic. What is the antibiotic titer?

1/5 or 5

Half-life

58. The half-life of an enzyme (specific activity 1,000 units/mL) is 10 days. What is the effective specific activity after 30 days?

30 days = 3 half-lives

1/2 x 1/2 × 1/2 × 1,000 units/mL = 125 units/mL

59. The half-life of ^{32}P is 2 weeks. What is the effective specific activity of a 100 μCi/mL ^{32}P-labeled probe after 14 weeks?

14 weeks = 7 half-lives

1/2 × 1/2 × 1/2 × 1/2 × 1/2 × 1/2 x 1/2 × 100 μCi/mL = 0.8 μCi/mL

60. The half-life of ^{32}P is 2 weeks. What is the effective specific activity of waste containing a total of 10 mCi of ^{32}P probe after 16 weeks?

16 weeks = 8 half-lives

1/2 × 1/2 × 1/2 × 1/2 × 1/2 × 1/2 × 1/2 × 1/2 × 10 mCi = 0.04 mCi

APPLICATION ANSWERS

Molecular Diagnostics

1.

a. The 100-μM reagent must be diluted (2.5 μM/100) = 1/40 to make the 2.5-μM working stock.

> Starting concentration × dilution = Diluted concentration
>
> 100 μM × 1/x = 2.5 μM;
>
> x = 40,

b. Using the 2.5-μM working stock, 1.0 μL is added to each 50-μL reaction mix, a 1/50 dilution. The concentration of the reagent in the reaction mix is then:

> 2.5 μM × 1/50 = 0.05 μM = 50 nM

c. For the 1 mL (=1,000 μL) master mix, determine the equivalent volume:

> 1 μL /50 μL = x/1,000 μL
>
> x = 20 μL

Add 20 μL of the 2.5-μM working stock to the 1-mL master mix.

For using 2 μl instead of 1 μl reagent, include an additional 1/2 dilution of the reagent:

> 20 μL × 1/2 = 10 μL

2. The original dilution is:

> 5/20 × 1/20 = 5/400 = 1/80

A further 1/2 dilution of the 1/80 dilution would be:

> 1/80 × 1/2 = 1/160

A further 1/5 dilution of the 1/80 dilution would be:

> 1/80 × 1/5 = 1/400

One way to achieve the 1/160 final dilution is to increase the total volume of the dilutent (water) in the 1/80 dilution from 20 to 40 μL. A way to provide the 1/400 final dilution is to increase the total volume of the water dilution from 20 to 100 μL. The 1/20 dilution in formamide remains the same.

> 5/40 × 1/20 μL formamide = 5/800 = 1/160
>
> 5/100 × 1/20 μL formamide = 5/2,000 = 1/400

Another way to achieve the 1/160 final dilution is to decrease the total volume of the sample added from 5 to 2.5 μL. For the 1/400 final dilution, decrease the total volume of the sample added from 5 to 1 μL.

> 2.5/20 × 1/20 μL formamide = 2.5/400 = 1/160
>
> 1/20 × 1/20 μL formamide = 1/400

Hematology

The patient's WBC count, expected to be significantly higher than the normal WBC count, will range from 10,000 to 20,000 WBC/μL. For each 0.1-μL volume on the hemocytometer to contain about 100 cells, the diluted WBC concentration should be approximately 1,000 WBC/μL, which is 100 WBC/0.1 μL.

Find the dilution factor for an upper WBC concentration in the patient's blood (20,000 WBC/μL) that would result in 1,000 WBC/μL:

$$20,000 \times 1/x = 1,000$$

$$x = 20$$

After removing the red blood cells by centrifugation or differential hemolysis, start with a 1/20 dilution of the WBC suspension in saline. Apply the sample to the hemocytometer, and observe the cells under the microscope. (If the number of cells in the hemocytometer chamber is above or below the range of 50 to 100 cells per chamber, adjust the dilution as required.)

After counting the cells, multiply the number of cells counted by the dilution factor. Example:

Cells counted per 0.1 μL volume:

$$68, 56, 77, 56, 82, 79, 70, 63, 65, 73$$

Add the 10 counts to obtain the total number of cells/μL:

$$68 + 56 + 77 + 56 + 82 + 79 + 70 + 63 + 65 + 73 = 689$$

(To obtain a measure of uncertainty, the average and standard deviation of the 10 counts may be calculated.)

Multiply the number of WBC/μL in the diluted solution by the reciprocal of the 1/20 dilution factor to determine the patient's WBC concentration:

$$689 \text{ WBC/μL} \times 20 = 13,780 \text{ WBC/μL}$$

Radiation Safety

Ninety-eight days is 7 half-lives (1 half life = 2 weeks = 14 days; $98 \div 14 = 7$). Each half-life is a twofold serial dilution. If the amount of radioactivity present is expressed as 100%, then the amount present after 7 half-lives will be:

$$(1/2 \times 1/2 \times 1/2 \times 1/2 \times 1/2 \times 1/2 \times 1/2) \times 100\% = 0.78\%$$

The amount of radiation after 98 days will be:

$$(1/2 \times 1/2 \times 1/2 \times 1/2 \times 1/2 \times 1/2 \times 1/2) \times 7,500 = 58.5 \text{ dps}$$

Storage of radioactive waste for 7 to 10 half-lives is recommended for this radioisotope before discard. Institutional radiation safety departments supply specific approved methods for disposal.

Molecular Diagnostics

a. The solution dilution in the sixth tube is

$$1/10 \times 1/10 \times 1/10 \times 1/10 \times 1/10 \times 1/10 = 1/1,000,000$$

b. The lowest detectable concentration is 250 nM × $1/10^6$ dilution:

$$(2.5 \times 10^2) \times (10^{-6}) = 2.5 \times 10^{-4} \text{ nM} = 0.25 \text{ pM}$$

c. The number of molecules can be ascertained using Avogadro's number (6.023×10^{23} molecules per mole):

$$02.5 \text{ pM} = 2.5 \times 10^{-13} \text{ moles/L}$$

$$2.5 \times 10^{-13} \text{ ~~moles~~/L} \times 6.023 \times 10^{23} \text{ molecules/~~mole~~} =$$
$$15.0 \times 10^{10} \text{ molecules/L}$$

The reaction volume of the assay was 20 μL.

$$15.0 \times 10^{10} \text{ molecules/~~L~~} \times 20 \times 10^{-6} \text{ ~~L~~} = 30,000 \text{ molecules}$$

If repeated measurement of a $1/10^6$ dilution reproducibly produces signal, then this level is the lowest level of detection or sensitivity of the assay.

CHAPTER 5

PRACTICE PROBLEM ANSWERS

Solutions and Their Components

1. Sodium chloride crystals are dissolved in water. Which is the solute, and which is the solvent?

Sodium chloride is the solute, and water is the solvent.

2. Which of the following will make a true solution?

b. Glucose and water

3. Gelatin and water in a semisolid state form what type of solution?

a. Colloid

4. If agarose in water forms a gel, what are the diameters of the agarose polymers likely to be?

d. Between 1 and 200 nm

5. A solution that loses solute on change in temperature or pressure is <u>supersaturated</u>.

Concentration Expressions

Express the following parts in ppm and percent.

6. 1 part in 100 parts

$1/100 = x/1,000,000$

$x = 10,000$

10,000 ppm;

$1/100 = 1\%$

7. 10 parts in 10,000,000 parts

$10/10,000,000 = x/1,000,000$

$x = 1$

1 ppm;

$10/10,000,000 = x/100$

$x = 0.0001$

0.0001%

8. 5 parts to 10 parts

$5/15 = x/1,000,000$

$x = 333,333$ ppm;

$5/15 = x/100,$

$x = 33.3$

33.3%

9. 10 parts to 90 parts

   10/100 = x/1,000,000

   x = 100,000

   100,000 ppm;

   10/100 = x/100

   x = 10 or

   10%

10. 1 part in 1,000,000,000 parts

    1/1,000,000,000 = x/1,000,000

    x = 0.001

    0.001 ppm;1 ppb

    1/1,000,000,000 = x/100

    x = 0.0000001

    0.0000001%

Express the following as molar concentration.

11. 40 g NaOH in 1.0 L (NaOH MW = 40.00)

    (40 g/L)/(40 g/mole) = 1 mole/L = 1 molar

12. 10 g NaOH in 0.5 L (NaOH MW = 40.00)

    (20 g/L)/(40 g/mole) = 0.5 mole/L = 0.5 molar

13. 58.5 g NaCl in 2.00 L (NaCl MW = 58.44)

    (29.2 g/L)/(58.5 g/mole) = 0.500 mole/L = 0.5 molar

14. 1.00 g KCl in 10.0 mL (KCl MW = 74.55)

    (100 g/L)/(74.6 g/mole) = 1.34 mole/L = 1.34 molar

15. 10.0 mg adenine in 1.00 mL (adenine MW = 135.13)

    (10.0 g/L)/135 g/mole) = 0.074 mole/L = 0.074 molar

Express the following as molal concentration.

16. 5.0 g NaOH in 1.0 kg (NaOH MW = 40.00)

    (5.0 g/kg)/(40 g/mole) = 0.12 mole/kg = 0.12 molal

17. 20.0 g MgCl$_2$ in 1.0 kg (MgCl$_2$ MW = 95.21)

    (20.0 g/kg)/(95.2 g/mole) = 0.210 mole/kg = 0.210 molal

18. 23.0 g NaCl in 1 L of water (NaCl MW = 58.44)

    1 L of water weighs 1 kg

    (23.0g/1.00 kg)/(58.5 g/mole) = 0.393 mole/kg = 0.393 molal

19. 37.2 mg $CuSO_4$ in 100 mL of water ($CuSO_4$ MW = 159.62)

0.100 L of water weighs 0.100 kg

37.2 mg = 0.0372 g

0.0372 g/0.1 kg = 0.372 g/kg

(0.372 g/kg)/(160 g/mole) = 0.00232 mole/kg = 0.00232 molal

What is the molecular weight of the following hydrates?

20. $CaCl_2 \cdot H_2O$

110.98 g/mole + 18.01 g/mole = 128.99 g/mole

21. $CaCl_2 \cdot 10H_2O$

110.98 g/mole + 180.10 g/mole = 291.08 g/mole

22. $Na_3PO_4 \cdot 12H_2O$

163.94 g/mole + 216.12 g/mole = 380.06 g/mole

Express the following as molar concentration.

23. 10.0 g $CaCl_2$ in 1.00 L of water

(10.0g/L)/(110.98 g/mole) = 0.090 mole/L

24. 10.0 g $CaCl_2 \cdot 5H_2O$ in 1.00 L water

$CaCl_2 \cdot 5H_2O$: 110.98 + 90.05 = 201.03 g/mole

(10.0 g/L)/(201 g/mole) = 0.0498 mole/L = 0.49.8 millimole/L = 49.8 mM

25. 100.0 g $NaH_2PO_4 \cdot 10H_2O$ in 1.0 L water

$NaH_2PO_4 \cdot 10H_2O$: 119.98 g/mole + 180.10 g/mole = 300.08 g/mole

(100.0 g/L)/(300 g/mole) = 0.333 mole/L = 0.333 molar = 333 mM

Use molecular weight to calculate the necessary adjustments.

26. What is the molar concentration of 150 g $CuSO_4 \cdot 10H_2O$ in 0.50 L water? Compare this with the concentration of 150 g anhydrous $CuSO_4$ in 0.50 L water.

159.62 g/mole $CuSO_4$ + 180.10 g/mole $10H_2O$ = 339.72 g/mole hydrate

150 g/0.5 L = 300 g/L

(300 g/L)/340 g/mole = 0.88 mole/L = 0.88 molar

160 g/mole $CuSO_4$ anhydrous

150 g/0.5 L = 300 g/L

(300 g/L)/160 g/mole = 1.88 mole/L = 1.88 molar

27. A procedure calls for a 28.0-mM solution of sodium dihydrogen phosphate prepared by mixing 5.00 g NaH_2PO_4 in 1.50 L water. Only $NaH_2PO_4 \cdot 2H_2O$ is available. How would you prepare the solution?

$NaH_2PO_4 \cdot 2H_2O$: 119.98 + 36.02 = 156.00 g/mole

(x g/L)/(156 g/mole) = 0.0280 mole/L

x = 156 g/mole × 0.0280 mole/L = 4.37 g/L

4.37 g/L × 1.50 L = 6.56 g

28. A method requires a 50.0-mM calcium chloride solution prepared by mixing 14.6 g $CaCl_2 \cdot 10H_2O$ in 1.00 L water. Only $CaCl_2 \cdot 1H_2O$ is available. How would you prepare the solution?

$CaCl_2 \cdot 1H_2O$: 110.98 + 18.01 = 128.99 g/mole

(x g/L)/(129 g/mole) = 0.0500 mole/L

x = 129 g/mole × 0.0500 ~~mole~~/L = 6.45g/L

Or use ratio and proportion:

128.99 g/mole monohydrate/ 291.08 g/mole decahydrate = x/14.6 g

x = 6.45 g

Bring 6.45 g $CaCl_2 \cdot 1H_2O$ to 1.00 L.

29. Which has more $CuSO_4$, a 9.0% $^{w/v}$ solution of $CuSO_4 \cdot 5H_2O$ or a 9.0% solution of $CuSO_4$?

9.0%$^{w/v}$ of $CuSO_4 \cdot 5H_2O$ contains 90 g/L $CuSO_4 \cdot 5H_2O$

9.0%$^{w/v}$ of $CuSO_4$ contains 90g/L $CuSO_4$

90g $CuSO_4$/159.62 g/mole = 0.56 mole $CuSO_4$

90g $CuSO_4 \cdot 5H_2O$/249.67 g/mole = 0.36 mole $CuSO_4$

9.0%$^{w/v}$ of $CuSO_4$ contains more $CuSO_4$ than 9.0% $CuSO_4 \cdot 5H_2O$

30. How many grams of $Co(NO_3)_2 \cdot 5H_2O$ are required to make 100 mL of 0.50% $Co(NO_3)_2$? (MW of $Co(NO_3)_2$ is 182.94.)

$Co(NO_3)_2$: 182.94 g/mole

$Co(NO_3)_2 \cdot 5H_2O$: 182.94 + 90.05 = 272.99 g/mole

(0.50 g)/(183 g/mole) = (x g)/(273 g/mole)

x = 0.74 g

Determine the normality of the following solutions.

31. 10 g NaOH in 1.0 L water

(40.00 g/~~mole~~)/(1.0 Eq/~~mole~~) = 40g/Eq

(10 g/L)/(40.00 g/Eq) = 0.25Eq/L = 0.25 N

32. 1.0 g H_2SO_4 in 0.50 L water

(98.08 g/~~mole~~)/(2.0 Eq/~~mole~~) = 49g/Eq

(2.0 g/L)/(49 g/Eq) = 0.04Eq/L = 0.04 N

33. 30 g H_3PO_4 in 3.0 L water

(98.00 g/~~mole~~)/(3.0 Eq/~~mole~~) = 33 g/Eq

(10 g/L)/(33 g/Eq) = 0.30Eq/L = 0.30 N

34. 3.5 g HCl in 0.75 L water

(36.46 g/~~mole~~)/(1.0 Eq/~~mole~~) = 36 g/Eq

3.5 g/0.75 L = 4.7 g/L

(4.7 g/L)/(36 g/Eq) = 0.13 Eq/L = 0.13 N

35. 0.50 g KOH in 100 mL water

(56.10 g/~~mole~~)/(1.00 Eq/~~mole~~) = 56.1 g/Eq

0.5 g/0.10 L = 5.0 g/L

(5.0 g/L)/(56.1 g/Eq) = 0.089 Eq/L = 0.089 N

36. 250 mg $MgCl_2$ in 1 mL water

(95.21 g/~~mole~~)/(2.00 Eq/~~mole~~) = 47.6 g/Eq

0.25 g/0.0010 L = 250.0 g/L

(250 g/L)/(47.6 g/Eq) = 5.2 Eq/L = 5.2 N

Determine the osmolarity of the following solutions.

37. 10 g NaOH in 1.0 L water

(40.00 g/~~mole~~)/(2.0 osmoles/~~mole~~) = 20 g/osmole

(10 g/L)/(20 g/osmole) = 0.50 osmoles/L = 0.50 OsM

38. 50 g HNO_3 in 3.0 L water

(63.01 g/~~mole~~)/(2.0 osmoles/~~mole~~) = 32 g/osmole

(17 g/L)/(32 g/osmole) = 0.53 osmoles/L = 0.53 OsM

39. 5.0 g H_3PO_4 in 5.0 L water

(98.00 g/~~mole~~)/(4.0 osmoles/~~mole~~) = 24.5 g/osmole

(1.0 g/L)/(24.5 g/osmole) = 0.041 osmoles/L = 0.041 OsM = 41 mOsM

40. A 5.0-mL plasma sample with a freezing point of –0.89 °C

1 OsM/–1.86 °C = x osmole/–0.89 °C

x = –0.89/–1.86 = 0.48 OsM = 480 mOsM

41. A 10.0-mL urine sample with a freezing point of –0.65 °C

1.0 OsM/–1.86ºC = x OsM/–0.65°C

x= –0.65/–1.86 = 0.35 OsM = 350 mOsM

42. 250 mOsm glucose (45 g) dissolved in 1 L of a 125-mOsM NaCl solution

125 mOsm NaCl + 250 mOsm glucose = 375 mOsm/L

43. 360 mOsm of NaOH (7.2 g) dissolved in 100 mL water

360 mOsm/0.1 L = 3,600 mOsm/L = 3.6 OsM

Use the following table to answer questions 44 and 45.

	Specific Gravity	Purity (%)
Formic acid	1.20	90
Hydrochloric acid	1.18	37
Nitric acid	1.42	70
Phosphoric acid	1.70	86
Sulfuric acid	1.84	96
Potassium hydroxide	1.46	45

44. How many grams of potassium hydroxide are in 2.0 mL of commercial product?

```
Specific gravity × Purity = g/mL
1.52 × 0.50 = 0.76 g/mL
0.76 g/mL × 2 mL = 1.5 g
```

45. What percent phosphoric acid is 3.0 mL commercial reagent in 100 mL water?

```
1.70 × 0.85 = 1.44 g/mL
3.0 mL × 1.44 g/mL = 4.3 g
4.3 g/100 mL = 4.3 %
```

How would you prepare the following solutions?

46. 10% potassium hydroxide in 50 mL

```
1.52 g/mL × 0.50 = 0.76 g/mL
10% = 10 g/100 mL = 5.0 g/50 mL
5.0 g/(0.76 g/mL) = 6.6 mL
Bring 6.6 mL commercial potassium hydroxide to 50 mL.
```

47. 0.10 M HCl in 200 mL

```
1.18 g/mL × 0.36 = 0.42 g/mL
0.10 mole/L × 36.46 g/mole = 3.6 g/L = 0.72 g/200 mL
0.72 g/(0.42 g/mL) = 1.7 mL
Bring 1.7 mL commercial hydrochloric acid to 200 mL.
```

48. 0.20 N H_2SO_4 in 100 mL

```
1.84 g/mL × 0.85 = 1.6 g/mL
0.20 Eq/L × 49 g/Eq = 9.8 g/L = 0.98 g/100 mL
0.98 g/(1.6 g/mL) = 0.61 mL
Bring 0.61 mL commercial sulfuric acid to 100 mL.
```

49. 0.010 M formic acid, 0.020 M nitric acid in 500 mL (MW of formic acid = 40.02 g/mole; MW of nitric acid = 63.01 g/mole)

```
1.20 g/mL × 0.90 = 1.08 g/mL formic acid
1.42 g/mL × 0.71 = 1.01 g/mL nitric acid
0.01 mole/L × 40 g/mole = 0.40 g/L = 0.20 g/500 mL formic acid
0.02 mole/L × 63 g/mole = 1.26 g/L = 0.63 g/500 mL nitric acid
0.23 g/(1.08 g/mL) = 0.21 mL formic acid
0.63 g/(1.01 g/mL) = 0.62 mL nitric acid
Bring 0.21 mL commercial formic acid plus 0.62 commercial nitric acid to 500 mL.
```

50. A procedure calls for 10 mL of 1.0% phosphoric acid prepared by bringing 100 mg phosphoric acid to 10 mL. How would you prepare this with commercial phosphoric acid solution?

1.70 g/mL × 0.85 = 1.44 g/mL

100 mg = 0.10 g

0.10 g/(1.44 g/mL) = 0.07 mL

Bring 0.07 mL commercial phosphoric acid to 10 mL.

APPLICATION ANSWERS

Body Fluids: Renal Tests

The result will be expressed in mL/minute, so convert hours to minutes to express the urine output as volume per minute:

$$4 \text{ hours} \times 60 \text{ minutes/hour} = 240 \text{ minutes}$$

Use ratio and proportion to determine urine output per minute:

$$320 \text{ mL/240 minutes} = 1.33 \text{ mL/minute}$$
$$C = (U/P) \times V \times (1.73/A)$$
$$C = (140/1.9) \times 1.33 \times (1.73/1.86)$$
$$C = 91.1 \text{ mL plasma cleared/minute}$$

Note: Glomerular filtration rate calculators are now available (e.g., http://www.kidney.org/professionals/kdoqi/gfr_calculator.cfm).

Molecular Diagnostics

1. The lowest concentration was 25 nM with a $1/10^7$ dilution.

$$2.5 \times 10^{-10} \times 10^{-7} = 2.5 \times 10^{-17} \text{ molar} = 0.025 \text{ fM} = 25 \text{ attoM}$$

2. The number of molecules can be ascertained using Avogadro's number (6.023×10^{23} molecules per mole).

$$2.5 \times 10^{-17} \text{ moles/L} \times 6.023 \times 10^{23} \text{ molecules/mole} =$$
$$1.50 \times 10^7 \text{ molecules/L}$$

The reaction volume of the assay was 25 μL.

$$15.0 \times 10^6 \text{ molecules/L} \times 25 \times 10^{-6} \text{ L} = 375 \text{ molecules}$$

If repeated measurement of a $1/10^7$ dilution (in the proper matrix; i.e., solution environment that would be used for patient sample testing) reproducibly produces signal, then this level is the lowest level of detection or sensitivity of the assay.

CHAPTER **6**

PRACTICE PROBLEM ANSWERS

1. How many micrograms are in 10 grams?

1,000,000 µg/1 g = x µg/10 g

x = 10,000,000 µg = 10^7 µg

Or, using exponents

0 − (−6) = 6

10 × 10^6 µg = 10,000,000 µg = 10^7 µg

2. How many centimeters are in 108 micrometers?

−6 − (−2) = −4

108 × 10^{-4} cm = 1.08 × 10^{-2} cm

3. A manufacturer recommends using 1.5 mL reagent A for every 3.0 mL reagent B. You have only 1.0 mL reagent B. How much reagent A should you use?

1.5 mL A/3.0 mL B = x/1.0 mL

x = 0.50 mL reagent A

4. One milliliter (V_1) of solution A with concentration 0.02 mg/dL (C_1) is equivalent to 10 mL (V_2) of solution B. What is the concentration (C_2) of solution B?

V_1 × C_1 = V_2 × C_2

1.0 mL × 0.02 mg/dL = 10 mL × C_2

C_2 = 0.002 mg/dL

5. A test requires 1.00 L of 0.100%$^{w/v}$ of $CuSO_4$. How do you prepare the proper concentration of $CuSO_4$ using $CuSO_4 \cdot H_2O$?

0.100/100 = x/1,000

x = 1.00 g $CuSO_4$ required for 1.00 L

$CuSO_4 \cdot H_2O$ MW = 177.63 and anhydrous $CuSO_4$ MW = 159.62

1/160 = x/178

x = 1.11 g

Bring 1.11 g of $CuSO_4 \cdot H_2O$ to 1,000 mL.

6. A liquid delivery system requires 500 mL of 1%$^{w/v}$ reagent A. Reagent A is supplied in powder form. How do you prepare the proper concentration of reagent A?

1% = 1 g/100 mL

1/100 = x/500

x = 5 g

Bring 5 g of reagent A to 500 mL with diluent.

7. A procedure calls for 150 mL of 0.20%$^{w/v}$ KCl. How do you prepare the proper concentration of KCl?

    0.20%$^{w/v}$ = 0.2 g/100 mL

    0.20/100 = x/150

    x = 0.30 g

    Bring 0.30 g of KCl to 150 mL.

8. Proteins and nucleic acids are separated by sieving through gels. One type of gel is made by mixing powdered agarose in liquid. How do you prepare a 50-mL volume 3%$^{w/v}$ agarose gel?

    3.0% = 3.0 g/100 mL

    3.0/100 = x/50

    x = 1.5 g

    Bring 1.5 g of agarose to 50 mL.

9. A laboratory method calls for 15.0 g of $CaCl_2$ dissolved in 300 mL water. Only $CaCl_2$ dihydrate is available. How do you prepare the proper concentration of $CaCl_2$?

    $CaCl_2$ anhydrous MW = 110.98; $CaCl_2$ dihydrate MW = 147.00

    15.0/111 = x/147

    x = 19.9 g

    Bring 19.9 g of $CaCl_2$ dihydrate to 300 mL.

10. The result of a test was 10.0 mg analyte in 5.00 mL test solution. How much analyte should be added to 45.0 mL of test solution to obtain the same concentration?

    10.0/5.00 = x/45.0

    x = 90 mg in 45 mL

11. How do you make 50 mL of 0.25 N NaOH from 5.0 N NaOH?

    $V_1 \times C_1 = V_2 \times C_2$

    50 mL × 0.25 N = x × 5.0 N

    x = 12.5/5.0 = 2.5 mL

    Bring 2.5 mL 5 N NaOH to 50 mL.

12. How do you make 5.0 mL of 35 mM NaCl from 2.0 M NaCl?

    Because the units must be identical in this $V_1C_1 = V_2C_2$ problem, first convert mM to M:

    35 mM = 0.035 M

    $V_1 \times C_1 = V_2 \times C_2$

    5.0 mL × 0.035 M = x × 2 M

    x = 0.175/2 = 0.0875 mL

    Bring 0.09 mL 2.0 moles/L NaCl to 5.0 mL.

13. A procedure calls for 20 mL of 0.10 N HCl. How do you prepare this from 1.0 N HCl?

    $V_1 \times C_1 = V_2 \times C_2$

    20 mL × 0.10 N = x × 1.0 N

    x = 2.0/1.0 = 2.0 mL

    Bring 2.0 mL 1.0 N HCl to 20 mL.

14. A reagent for use in an instrument is supplied as a $10X$ concentrate (C_1). What volume of reagent is required to make 250 mL (V_2) of $0.10X$ (C_2) solution?

$V_1 \times C_1 = V_2 \times C_2$

$250 \text{ mL} \times (0.10X) = x \times (10X)$

$x = 25/10 = 2.5 \text{ mL}$

Bring 2.5 mL 10X concentrate to 250 mL.

15. How do you prepare 1,000 mL of 0.05 N H_2SO_4 from a 10%$^{w/v}$ H_2SO_4 solution?

First convert % to normality:

$10 \text{ g}/100 \text{ mL} = 100 \text{ g/L}$

$(100 \text{ g/L})/(49 \text{ g/Eq}) = 2.0 \text{ Eq/L}$

$V_1 \times C_1 = V_2 \times C_2$

$1,000 \text{ mL} \times 0.05 \text{ N} = x \times 2.0 \text{ N}$

$x = 50/2.0 = 25 \text{ mL}$

Bring 25 mL 10%$^{w/v}$ H_2SO_4 to 1,000 mL.

16. How do you prepare 100 mL of 1.0%$^{w/v}$ hydrofluoric acid from a commercial hydrofluoric acid solution? (sp gr =1.167 g/mL; purity = 55%)

$1.0\% = 1 \text{ g}/100 \text{ mL}$

$1.167 \text{ g/mL} \times 0.55 = 0.64 \text{ g/mL}$

$1 \text{ g}/0.64 \text{ g/mL} = 1.56 \text{ mL}$

Bring 1.6 mL commercial solution to 100 mL.

17. How do you prepare 50 mL of 0.05 N H_2SO_4 from a commercial H_2SO_4 solution (85% pure; 1.84 g/mL)?

$1.84 \text{ g/mL} \times 0.96 = 1.77 \text{ g/mL}$

$1.77 \text{ g/mL} = 1,770 \text{ g/L}$

$(1,770 \text{ g/L})/(49.00 \text{ g/Eq}) = 36.1 \text{ Eq/L}$

$50 \times 0.05 = x \times 36.1$

$x = 2.5/36.1 = 0.069 \text{ mL}$

Or: $0.05 \text{ Eq/L} \times 49.04 \text{ g/Eq} = 2.45 \text{ g/L}$

$50 \text{ mL} = 0.05 \text{ L}$

$2.45 \text{ g/L} = xg/0.05 \text{ L}$

$x = 0.122 \text{ g } H_2SO_4$ required for 50 mL

$0.122 \text{ g}/1.56 \text{ g/mL} = 0.078 \text{ mL commercial } H_2SO_4$

Bring 0.078 mL commercial solution to 50 mL.

18. How do you prepare 5.0 mL of 0.20 M H_2SO_4 from a 5.0 N H_2SO_4 solution?

$(5.0\text{Eq/L})/(2.0 \text{ Eq/mole}) = 2.5 \text{ moles/L}$

$V_1 \times C_1 = V_2 \times C_2$

$5.0 \text{ mL} \times 0.20 \text{ molar} = x \times 2.5 \text{ molar}$

$x = 1.0/2.5 = 0.4 \text{ mL}$

Bring 0. 4 mL 5.0 N H_2SO_4 commercial solution to 5.0 mL.

19. How do you prepare 10 mL of 2.0 mM NaOH from a commercial NaOH solution with a specific gravity of 1.54 and a purity of 50%?

1.54 g/mL × 0.50 = 0.77 g/mL

0.77 g/mL = 770 g/L in the commercial solution

(770 g/L)/(40.00 g/mole) = 19 moles/L

2.0 mM = 0.0020 M

$V_1 \times C_1 = V_2 \times C_2$

10 mL × 0.0020 molar = x × 19 molar

x = 0.020/19 = 0.0010 mL

Bring 0.0010 mL (1.0 μL) commercial solution to 10 mL.

20. The recommended concentration of a 50-μL reaction mix is 2.0 mM $MgCl_2$. How much 25 mM $MgCl_2$ is required to make this reaction mix?

$V_1 \times C_1 = V_2 \times C_2$

50 μL × 2 mM = x × 25 mM

x = 100/25 = 4.0 μL

Bring 4.0 μL 25 mM $MgCl_2$ to 50 μL.

21. What is the concentration of a mixture of 200 mL 60% alcohol plus 50 mL 80% alcohol?

$(V_1 \times C_1) + (V_2 \times C_2) = V_T \times C_T$

(200 × 60) + (50 × 80) = 250 × C_T

(12,000 + 4,000)/250 = C_T

C_T = 64%

22. What is the concentration of KCl when 500 mL mixed with 350 mL 10%$^{v/v}$ KCl yields 850 mL of a 25%$^{v/v}$ solution?

$(V_1 \times C_1) + (V_2 \times C_2) = V_T \times C_T$

(500 × C_1) + (350 × 10) = 850 × 25

(500 × C_1) + 3,500 = 21,250

500 × C_1 = 17,750

C_1 = 17,750/500

C_T = 35.5%$^{v/v}$

23. How much 3 osmolar salt must be mixed with 2 osmolar salt to yield 10 mL of a 2.5 osmolar salt solution ?

$V_2 = (10 - V_1)$

$(V_1 \times C_1) + (V_2 \times C_2) = V_T \times C_T$

$(V_1 \times 3) + (10 - V_1) \times 2 = 10 \times 2.5$

$(V_1 \times 3) + (20 - 2V_1) = 25$

$3V_1 - 2V_1 = 5$

$V_1 = 5$ mL

$V_2 = 10 - V_1 = 5$ mL

24. What is the final concentration if 10 mL of 2 mg/mL $CuSO_4$ is mixed with 25 mL of 10 mg/mL $CuSO_4$?

$(V_1 \times C_1) + (V_2 \times C_2) = V_T \times C_T$

$(10 \times 2) + (25 \times 10) = 35 \times C_T$

$(20) + (250) = 35 \times C_T$

$270/35 = C_T$

$C_T = 7.71$ mg/mL

25. What is the concentration of a mixture of 20 mL 5 molar $NaCl_2$ plus 30 mL 10 molar $NaCl_2$?

20 mL $\times$ 5 molar + 30 mL $\times$ 10 molar = 50 mL $\times$ x molar

$100 + 300 = 50x$

$400 = 50x$

$x = 8$ molar

Use formulae to do the following calculations.

26. How many equivalents of NaOH are there in 3 L of 0.6 *N* NaOH?

0.6 Eq/L $\times$ 3L = 1.8 Eq

27. Convert 0.30 molar NaCl to grams per liter.

moles/L $\times$ g/mole = g/L

0.30 ~~moles~~/L $\times$ 58.44 g/~~mole~~ = 17 g/L

28. A procedure calls for 1.0 L of 0.50 *N* HCl. How many grams HCl are required?

Eq/L $\times$ g/Eq = g/L

0.50 ~~Eq~~/L $\times$ 35.45 g/~~Eq~~ = 18 g/L

29. A solution containing 30 g/L $MgCl_2$ is what molarity?

(g/L)/(g/mole) = moles/L

(30 ~~g~~/L)/(95.20 ~~g~~/mole) = 0.32 mole/L

30. What is the percent$^{w/v}$ concentration of 1.0 osmolar $CuSO_4$?

% = (g/L)/10

g/L = osmoles/L $\times$ g/osmole

% = (osmoles/L $\times$ g/osmole)/10

% = (1.0 ~~osmole~~/L $\times$ 160 g/~~osmole~~)/10 = 16%$^{w/v}$

31. Convert 10%$^{w/v}$ $CaCl_2$ to molarity.

% $\times$ 10 = g/L

(g/L)/(g/mole) = moles/L

10% $\times$ 10 = 100 g/L

(100 ~~g~~/L)/110.98 ~~g~~/mole = 0.90 moles/L

32. Convert 1.0%$^{w/v}$ HCl to normality.

% × 10 = g/L
(g/L)/(g/Eq) = Eq/L
1.0% × 10 = 10 g/L
(10 g/L)/35.45 g/Eq = 0.28 Eq/L

33. Convert 1.0%$^{w/v}$ H_2SO_4 to normality.

% × 10 = g/L
(g/L)/(g/Eq) = Eq/L
1.0% × 10 = 10 g/L
(10 g/L)/49.04 g/Eq = 0.20 Eq/L

34. Is 5.0 mM MnCl more, less, or equally as concentrated as a 1.0% solution?

% = (g/L)/10
g/L = (moles/L) × (g/mole)
5.0 mM = 0.0050 miles/L
(0.0050 moles/L) × (125.84 g/mole) = 0.63 g/L
0.63 g/L/10 = 0.063%
0.063% is less concentrated than 1.0%

35. What is the % $CaCl_2$ concentration of 10 mM $CaCl_2 \cdot 10H_2O$?

$CaCl_2$ anhydrous MW = 110.98; $CaCl_2 \cdot 10H_2O$ MW = 291.08
% = (g/L)/10
g/L = (moles/L) × (g/mole)
% = [(moles/L) × (g/mole)]/10
10 mM = 0.01 molar
% = [(0.01 ~~mole~~/L) × (291 g/~~mole~~)]/10 = 0.29%
0.29 % hydrate/291 = x % anhydrous/111
0.29 % hydrate × (111/291) = 0.11% anhydrous

36. What is the normality of 20.0%$^{v/v}$ nitric acid? (HNO_3: sp gr = 1.42; assay 70.0%)

%$^{v/v}$ × 10 = mL/L
20.0 × 10 = 200 mL/L
specific gravity × purity = g/mL
1.42 g/mL × 0.700 = 0.994 g/mL
200 ~~mL~~/L × 0.994 g/~~mL~~ = 199 g/L
(g/L)/(g/Eq) = Eq/L
(199 g/L)/(63.01 g/Eq) = 3.16 Eq/L

37. Convert 5.0 osmolar NaCl to molar concentration.

(5.0 osmoles/L)/(2 osmoles/mole) = 2.5 moles/L

38. Convert 250 mOsmolar glucose to percent$^{w/v}$ concentration

(0.25 osmoles/L)/(1 osmoles/mole) = 0.25 moles/L

Perform the following conversions using exponents.

39. 50 g to mg

g → mg: 10^0 → 10^{-3}

0 − (−3) = +3 or 10^3

50 × 10^3 = 50,000 mg

40. 2,500 mL to L

mL → L: 10^{-3} → 10^0

−3 − (0) = −3 or 10^{-3}

2,500 × 10^{-3} = 2.5 × 10^3 × 10^{-3} = 2.5 L

41. 10 nL to μL

nL → μL: 10^{-9} → 10^{-6}

−9 − (−6) = −3 or 10^{-3}

10 × 10^{-3} = 0.010 μL

42. 5.0 mm to nm

mm → nm: 10^{-3} → 10^{-9}

−3 − (−9) = +6 or 10^6

5.0 × 10^6 = 5,000,000 nm

43. 35 pg to μg

pg → μg: 10^{-12} → 10^{-6}

−12 − (−6) = −6 or 10^{-6}

35 × 10^{-6} = 0.000035 μg

44. 7.2 mg/mL to mg/dL

mg/mL → mg/dL: $(10^{-3}/10^{-3})$ → $(10^{-3}/10^{-1})$

[−3 − (−3)] − [−3 − (−1)] = 0 − (−2) = +2 or 10^2

7.2 × 10^2 = 720 mg/dL

45. 48 pg/nL to g/L

pg/nL → g/L: $(10^{-12}/10^{-9})$ → $(10^0/10^0)$

[−12 − (0)] − [−9 − (0)] = −12 − (−9) = −3 or 10^{-3}

48 × 10^{-3} = 0.048 g/L

46. 595 mg/L to μg/mL

mg/L $\rightarrow$ μg/mL: $(10^{-3}/10^0)$ $\rightarrow$ $(10^{-6}/10^{-3})$

$[-3 - (-6)] - [0 - (-3)] = 3 - (3) = 0$ or 10^0

$595 \times 10^0 = 595$ μg/mL

47. 50% to μg/L

g/dL $\rightarrow$ μg/L: $(10^0/10^{-1})$ $\rightarrow$ $(10^{-6}/10^0)$

$[0 - (-6)] - [-1 - 0] = 6 - (-1) = 7$ or 10^7

50% $= 50 \times 10^7$ μg/L

48. 15 mg/mL to %

mg/mL $\rightarrow$ g/dL: $(10^{-3}/10^{-3})$ $\rightarrow$ $(10^0/10^{-1})$

$[(-3) - (0)] - [(-3) - (-1)] = -3 - (-2) = -1$ or 10^{-1}

15 mg/mL $= 15 \times 10^{-1}$ % $= 1.5$%

49. 8,000 square nm to square μm

nm $\rightarrow$ μm: $(10^{-9})/(10^{-6})$

$(-9) - (-6) = -3$

$-3 \times 2 = -6$

8,000 square nm $= 8,000 \times 10^{-6}$ square μm $= 8.0 \times 10^{-3}$ square μm

50. 115 cubic mm to cubic cm

mm $\rightarrow$ cm: $(10^{-3})/(10^{-2})$

$(-3) - (-2) = -1$

$-1 \times 3 = -3$

115 cubic mm $= 115 \times 10^{-3}$ cubic cm $= 1.15 \times 10^{-1}$ cubic cm

APPLICATION ANSWERS

Molecular Diagnostics

1. $(20 + 1)$ ~~reactions~~ $\times 50\ \mu L/$~~reaction~~ $= 1{,}050\ \mu L$
2. 0.01 units$/$~~μL~~ $\times 1{,}050$ ~~μL~~ $= 10.5$ units

$$10.5\ \text{~~units~~}/5\ \text{~~units~~}/\mu L = 2.1\ \mu L\ \text{enzyme}$$

The calculation may also be performed using $V_1C_1 = V_2C_2$:

$$5\ \text{units}/\mu L \times x\ \mu L = 0.01\ \text{units}/\mu L \times 1{,}050\ \mu L$$
$$x = (0.01 \times 1{,}050)/5 = 2.1\ \mu L\ \text{enzyme}$$

Add 2.1 μL concentrated enzyme to the 1,050-μL reaction mix. To be precise, 2.1 μL enzyme should be added to 1,047.9-μL reaction mix. Because the volume of enzyme added is ⅟₅₀₀ the total volume, for most reactions of this type, no adjustment is necessary for the slight change in the final volume of reaction mix from 1,050 to 1,052.1. Always follow the manufacturer's protocol recommendations for the proper preparation of reaction mixes.

Clinical Chemistry

1. Because 0.10 Eq/L NaOH = 0.1 Eq/L acid, a $V_1C_1 = V_2C_2$ equation can be used to determine the acid concentration (C_2) in Eq/L:

$$V_1 \times C_1 = V_2 \times C_2$$
$$3.2 \times 0.10 = 25 \times C_2$$
$$0.32/25 = C_2$$
$$C_2 = 0.013\ \text{Eq/L acid}$$

This value is the same when expressed as normality (mEq/L) or as degrees of acidity. 25 mL 0.013 N acid titrates 3.2 mL 0.10 N NaOH.

2. Use $V_1C_1 = V_2C_2$ to determine the concentration of the sample:

$$(V_1 \times C_1) + (V_2 \times C_2) = V_T \times C_T$$
$$(1\ \text{mL sample} \times x\ \text{mg/dL}) + (19\ \text{mL pooled serum} \times 50\ \text{mg/dL})$$
$$= (20\ \text{mL} \times 65\ \text{mg/dL})$$
$$(x) + 950 = 1{,}300$$
$$x = 350\ \text{mg/dL}$$

Note that the first test was performed on a 1/20 dilution. The results will be different if a 1 part to 20 part ratio (1/21 dilution) is used.

$$(1\ \text{mL sample} \times x\ \text{mg/dL}) + (20\ \text{mL pooled serum} \times 50\ \text{mg/dL})$$
$$= (21\ \text{mL} \times 65\ \text{mg/dL})$$
$$(x) + 1{,}000 = 1{,}365$$
$$x = 365\ \text{mg/dL}$$

CHAPTER 7

PRACTICE PROBLEM ANSWERS

1. What is the base of an exponential expression?

   The base is the number that is multiplied by itself.

2. What is the exponent of an exponential expression?

   The exponent is the number of times by which the base is multiplied by itself.

3. What is the base of natural (Naperian) logarithms?

   The base is e or approximately 2.7182818284.

4. What is the base of common (Briggsian) logarithms?

   The base is 10.

5. For the number 5^3, what is the base and what is the exponent?

   The base is 5 and the exponent is 3.

6. For the number 10^3, what is the base and what is the exponent?

   The base is 10 and the exponent is 3.

7. In expressing the number 10^3 as a common logarithm, what is the characteristic?

   The characteristic is 3.

8. Without using a calculator, find the characteristics of the following numbers.

25	1
25,000	4
377	2
2.5×10^9	9
0.002	-3
7	0
7.237	0
0.27	-1
1.3×10^{-4}	-4
1.000003	0

9. In expressing the number 10^3 as a common logarithm, what is the mantissa?

   The mantissa is 0.0000.

10. Find the <u>mantissas</u> of the following numbers by using a calculator.

25	0.3979
25,000	0.3979
377	0.5763
2.5×10^9	0.3979
0.002	−0.6990
7	0.8451
7.237	0.8596
0.27	0.5687
1.3×10^{-4}	−0.8860
1.000003	0.0000

11. What are the table logarithms of the following numbers?

25	1.3979
25,000	4.3979
377	2.5763
2.5×10^9	9.3979
0.002	−3.3010
7	0.8451
7.237	0.8596
0.27	−0.4314
1.3×10^{-4}	−4.1139
1.000003	0.0000

12. Find the base 10 exponents of the following numbers by using a calculator (i.e., $10^x = 25$, what is x?).

25	1.3979
25,000	4.3979
377	2.5763
2.5×10^9	9.3979
0.002	−2.6990
7	0.8451
7.237	0.8596
0.27	−0.5686
1.3×10^{-4}	−3.8860
1.000003	0.000001

Finish the following equations for logarithms.

13. $\log(xy) =$ log x + log y

14. $\log 1 =$ 0

15. $\log x - \log y =$ log (x/y)

16. $\log (1/x) =$ −log x

17. $\log x^k =$ k × logx

18. $\log_e x =$ ln x

APPLICATION ANSWERS

Physiology

To accommodate the terms in the formula, convert feet and pounds to centimeters and kilograms, respectively, using conversion factors:

6 ~~ft~~ $\times$ 30.5 cm/~~ft~~ = 183 cm = height (H)

235 ~~lb~~ $\times$ 0.454 kg/~~lb~~ = 107 kg = weight (W)

Use the formula to calculate log A.

log A = (0.425 $\times$ log W) + (0.725 $\times$ log H) - 2.144

log A = (0.425 $\times$ log 107) + (0.725 $\times$ log 183) - 2.144

log A = (0.425 $\times$ 2.03) + (0.725 $\times$ 2.26) - 2.144

log A = (0.863) + (1.64) - 2.144 = 0.359

antilog 0.359 = 2.28

A = 2.28 m^2

(The average body surface area is 1.73 m^2.)

CHAPTER 8

PRACTICE PROBLEM ANSWERS

1. Cations have a <u>positive</u> charge.

2. Anions have a <u>negative</u> charge.

3. Cations have more <u>protons</u> than <u>electrons</u>.

4. Anions have more <u>electrons</u> than <u>protons</u>.

5. Cations are attracted to ions with a net <u>negative</u> charge.

6. Cations and anions form <u>ionic</u> bonds.

7. <u>Acids</u> are substances that release hydrogen ions, whereas <u>bases</u> are substances that release hydroxyl ions.

8. A strong acid <u>will</u> almost completely ionize.

9. Loss of a proton from an acid leaves its <u>conjugate base</u>.

10. What are the conjugate bases of the following acids?

Carbonic acid (H_2CO_3)	HCO_3^-
Hydrofluoric acid (HF)	F^-
Formic acid ($HCHO_2$)	CHO_2^-
Acetic acid ($HC_2H_3O_2$)	$C_2H_3O_2^-$
Oxalic acid ($H_2C_2O_4$)	$HC_2O_4^-$

11. What is the hydrogen ion concentration in moles per liter if the concentration of [H+] is 0.01 g/L?

    MW of [H+] = 1.00; therefore, 1 mole [H+] = 1 g and

    0.01 g/L = 0.01 moles/L

Calculate the hydrogen ion concentration in grams per liter of the following solutions.

12. 0.20 *N* acetic acid, 10% ionized

    0.2 × 0.10 = 0.02 g[H+]/L

13. 0.10 molar acetic acid, 1.0% ionized

    0.1 × 0.01 = 0.001 g[H+]/L

14. 0.25 molar hydrochloric acid, 100% ionized

    0.25 × 1.0 = 0.25 g[H+]/L

15. 0.015 molar boric acid, 0.10% ionized

    0.015 × 0.0010 = 0.000015 g[H+]/L

16. What is the pH or pOH corresponding to the following ion concentrations?

$[H^+] = 1.0 \times 10^{-7}$ moles/L

pH = -(-7) = 7 or

pH = b - log a = 7 - log 1 = 7 - 0 = 7

$[H^+] = 1.0 \times 10^{-10}$ moles/L

pH = -(-10) = 10 or

pH = b - log a = 10 - log 1 = 10 - 0 = 10

$[H^+] = 2.5 \times 10^{-2}$ moles/L

pH = -log 0.025 = log (1/0.025) = log 40 = 1.6 or

pH = b - log a = 2 - log 2.5 = 1.6

$[OH^-] = 5.0 \times 10^{-4}$ moles/L

pOH = -log 0.0005 = log (1/0.0005) = log 2,000 = 3.3 or

pOH = b - log a = 4 - log 5.0 = 3.3

$[OH^-] = 2.0 \times 10^{-8}$ moles/L

pOH = -log 0.00000002 = log (1/0.00000002) = log 50,000,000 = 7.7 or

pOH = b - log a = 8 - log 2.0 = 7.7

17. What is the hydrogen ion concentration of water?

Water pH = 7.0, therefore [H+] of water is 10^{-7} g/L = 10^{-7} moles/L

18. An acid solution has a pH of 2.14. What is its hydrogen ion concentration?

pH = b - log a

2.14 = b - log a

2.14 = 3 - log a

log a = 0.86

a = 7.24

$[H^+] = a \times 10^{-b}$

$[H^+] = 7.24 \times 10^{-3}$

19. An acid solution has a pH of 1.88. What is its hydrogen ion concentration?

pH = b - log a

1.88 = b - log a

1.88 = 2 - log a

log a = 0.12

a = 1.32

$[H^+] = a \times 10^{-b}$

$[H^+] = 1.3 \times 10^{-2}$

20. A basic solution has a pH of 10.2. What is its hydrogen ion concentration?

$$pH = b - \log a$$
$$10.2 = b - \log a$$
$$10.2 = 11 - \log a$$
$$\log a = 0.80$$
$$a = 6.31$$
$$[H^+] = a \times 10^{-b}$$
$$[H^+] = 6.31 \times 10^{-11}$$

21. What is the hydroxyl ion concentration of the solution in question 20?

$$[H^+] \times [OH^-] = 10^{-14}$$
$$[OH^-] = 10^{-14}/[H^+]$$
$$[OH^-] = (1.0 \times 10^{-14})/(6.3 \times 10^{-11})$$
$$= 1.6 \times 10^{-4}$$

Convert the following ion concentrations to pH and pOH.

22. $[H^+] = 1.0 \times 10^{-3}$ moles/L

$$pH = b - \log a$$
$$pH = 3 - \log 1 = 3 - 0 = 3$$
$$pOH = 14 - 3 = 11$$

23. $[H^+] = 5.0 \times 10^{-6}$ moles/L

$$pH = 6 - \log 5$$
$$pH = 6 - 0.6990 = 5.3$$
$$pOH = 14 - 5.3 = 8.7$$

24. $[H^+] = 9.8 \times 10^{-12}$ moles/L

$$pH = 12 - \log 9.8$$
$$pH = 12 - 0.9912 = 11$$
$$pOH = 14 - 11 = 3$$

25. $[H^+] = 6.4 \times 10^{-2}$ moles/L

$$pH = 2 - \log 6.4$$
$$pH = 2 - 0.8062 = 1.2$$
$$pOH = 14 - 1.2 = 12.8$$

26. $[H^+] = 15.8 \times 10^{-9}$ moles/L

$$pH = 9 - \log 15.8$$
$$pH = 9 - 1.1986 = 7.8$$
$$pOH = 14 - 7.8 = 6.2$$

27. $[OH^-] = 1.0 \times 10^{-14}$ moles/L

    pOH = 14 − log 1

    pOH = 14 − 0 = 14

    pH = 14 − 14 = 0

28. $[OH^-] = 5.0 \times 10^{-5}$ moles/L

    pOH = 5 − log 5

    pOH = 5 − 0.6990 = 4.3

    pH = 14 − 4.3 = 9.7

29. $[OH^-] = 3.5 \times 10^{-10}$ moles/L

    pOH = 10 − log 3.5

    pOH = 10 − 0.5441 = 9.4

    pH = 14 − 9.5 = 4.6

30. $[OH^-] = 2.1 \times 10^{-7}$ moles/L

    pOH = 7 − log 2.1

    pOH = 7 − 0.3222 = 6.7

    pH = 14 − 6.7 = 7.3

Convert the following ionic concentrations to nM.

31. $[H^+] = 6.4 \times 10^{-2}$

    Convert 6.4 × 10^{-2} moles/L (10^0) to nanomoles/L (10^{-9})

    (0) − (−9) = 9

    6.4 × 10^{-2} × 10^9 = 6.4 × 10^7 nM

32. $[H^+] = 7.3 \times 10^{-8}$

    Convert 7.3 × 10^{-8} molar (10^0) to nM (10^{-9})

    (0) − (−9) = 9

    7.3 × 10^{-8} × 10^9 = 7.3 × 10^1 nM = 73nM

33. $[H^+] = 3.4 \times 10^{-5}$

    Convert 3.4 × 10^{-5} M (10^0) to nM (10^{-9})

    (0) − (−9) = 9

    3.4 × 10^{-5} × 10^9 = 3.4 × 10^4 nM

34. $[OH^-] = 6.8 \times 10^{-9}$

    $[H^+]$ = 1.0 × 10^{-14} / 6.8 × 10^{-9} = 0.15 × 10^{-5}

    Convert 1.5 × 10^{-6} molar (10^0) to nM (10^{-9})

    (0) − (−9) = 9

    1.5 × 10^{-6} × 10^9 = 1.5 × 10^3 nM

35. $[OH^-] = 1.0 \times 10^{-10}$

$[H^+] = 1.0 \times 10^{-14}/1.0 \times 10^{-10} = 1.0 \times 10^{-4}$

Convert 1.0×10^{-4} molar (10^0) to nM (10^{-9})

$(0) - (-9) = 9$

$1.0 \times 10^{-4} \times 10^9 = 1.0 \times 10^5$ nM

36. $[OH^-] = 7.8 \times 10^{-2}$

$[H^+] = 1.0 \times 10^{-14}/7.8 \times 10^{-2} = 0.13 \times 10^{-12} = 1.3 \times 10^{-13}$

Convert 1.3×10^{-13} molar (10^0) to nM (10^{-9})

$(0) - (-9) = 9$

$1.3 \times 10^{-13} \times 10^9 = 1.3 \times 10^{-4}$ nM

Convert the following pH and pOH to nM.

37. pH = 7.3

pH = b - log a

7.3 = 8.0 - log a

0.7 = log a

a = 5.0

$[H^+] = 5.0 \times 10^{-8}$

Convert 5.0×10^{-8} molar (10^0) to nM (10^{-9})

$(0) - (-9) = 9$

$5.0 \times 10^{-8} \times 10^9 = 5.0 \times 10^1$ nM = 50 nM

38. pH = 3.5

pH = b - log a

3.5 = 4.0 - log a

0.5 = log a

a = 3.2

$[H^+] = 3.2 \times 10^{-4}$

Convert 3.2×10^{-4} molar (10^0) to nM (10^{-9})

$(0) - (-9) = 9$

$3.2 \times 10^{-4} \times 10^9 = 3.2 \times 10^5$ nM

39. pOH = 7.3

pH = 14 - 7.3 = 6.7

pH = b - log a

6.7 = 7.0 - log a

0.3 = log a

a = 2.0

$[H^+]$ = 2.0 × 10^{-7}

Convert 2.0 × 10^{-7} molar (10^0) to nM (10^{-9})

(0) - (-9) = 9

2.0 × 10^{-7} × 10^9 = 2.0 × 10^2 nM = 200 nM

40. pOH = 12

pH = 14 - 12 = 2.0

pH = b - log a

2.0 = 3.0 - log a

1.0 = log a

a = 10

$[H^+]$ = 10 × 10^{-3}

Convert 10 × 10^{-3} molar (10^0) to nM (10^{-9})

(0) - (-9) = 9

10 × 10^{-3} × 10^9 = 10 × 10^6 nM = 10^7 nM

41. pOH = 2.0

pH = 14 - 2 = 12

pH = b - log a

12 = 13 - log a

1.0 = log a

a = 10

$[H^+]$ = 10 × 10^{-13}

Convert 10 × 10^{-13} molar (10^0) to nM (10^{-9})

(0) - (-9) = 9

10 × 10^{-13} × 10^9 = 10 × 10^{-4} nM = 10^{-3} nM

Describe how to prepare solutions with the following pH or pOH.

42. One liter HCl, pH = 2.0

pH = b − log a

2 = 3 − log a

1.0 = log a

a = 10

$[H^+]$ = 10 × 10^{-3} = 10^{-2} mole/L

HCl MW = 36.46 g/mole; sp gr 1.18; 36% pure

10^{-2} mole/L × 36.46 g/mole = 0.365 g

0.365g/(0.42 g/mL) = 0.87 mL HCl

Add 0.87 mL HCl to 1 L water.

43. 500 mL H_2SO_4, pH = 1.5

pH = b − log a

1.5 = 2 − log a

0.5 = log a

a = 3.2

$[H^+]$ = 3.2 × 10^{-2} mole/L

H_2SO_4 MW = 98.08 g/mole; sp gr 1.84; 85% pure

3.2 × 10^{-2} mole/L × 98.08 g/mole = 3.14 g/L

3.14 g/(1.56 g/mL) = 2.0 mL HCl/L

Add 1.0 mL H_2SO_4 to 0.5 L (500 mL) water.

44. 700 mL NaOH, pOH = 4.2

pOH = b − log a

4.2 = 5 − log a

0.8 = log a

a = 6.3

$[OH^-]$ = 6.3 × 10^{-5} mole/L

NaOH MW = 40 g/mole

6.3 × 10^{-5} mole/L × 40 g/mole = 2.52 × 10^{-3} g/L = 2.5 mg/L

2.5 mg/L × 0.7 L = 1.8 mg

Bring 1.8 mg NaOH to 0.7 L (700 mL) with water.

45. 2 L NaOH, pOH = 6.0

$$pOH = b - \log a$$
$$6.0 = 7 - \log a$$
$$1.0 = \log a$$
$$a = 10$$
$$[OH^-] = 10 \times 10^{-7} \text{ mole/L} = 10^{-6} \text{ mole/L}$$
$$NaOH \ MW = 40.00 \text{ g/mole}$$
$$10^{-6} \text{ mole/L} \times 40.00 \text{ g/mole} = 4.0 \times 10^{-5} \text{ g/L} = 40 \ \mu g/L$$
$$40 \ \mu g/L \times 2.0 \text{ L} = 80 \ \mu g$$

Bring 80 μg NaOH to 2 L with water.

Use the Henderson-Hasselbalch equation to determine the base:acid ratio in the following buffers.

46. Acetate buffer, pH = 6.00; pK of acetic acid = 4.76

$$pH = pK + \log \frac{[base]}{[acid]}$$

$$\log \frac{[base]}{[acid]} = pH - pK$$

$$\log \frac{[base]}{[acid]} = 6.00 - 4.76$$

$$\log \frac{[base]}{[acid]} = 1.24$$

$$\frac{[base]}{[acid]} = 17.4$$

47. Phosphoric acid buffer, pH = 4.20; pK of H_3PO_4 = 2.16

$$pH = pK + \log \frac{[base]}{[acid]}$$

$$\log \frac{[base]}{[acid]} = pH - pK$$

$$\log \frac{[base]}{[acid]} = 4.20 - 2.16$$

$$\log \frac{[base]}{[acid]} = 2.04$$

$$\frac{[base]}{[acid]} = 110$$

48. Find the molarity of the acid and base necessary to make a 1-mole/L solution of the buffer in questions 46 and 47.

```
Acetate buffer, pH = 6.00; pK of acetic acid = 4.76; [base]/[acid] = 17.4
[base]/[acid] = 17.4
17.4 parts base: 1 part acid
```

$$\frac{\text{Total moles/L acetate + acetic acid}}{\text{moles/L acetic acid}} = \frac{1 \text{ mole/L}}{x \text{ moles/L acetic acid}}$$

$$\frac{18.4}{1.0} = \frac{1 \text{ mole/L}}{x \text{ mole/L acetic acid}}$$

$$x = \frac{1.0}{18.4} = 0.05 \text{ mole/L acetic acid}$$

```
1 - 0.05 = 0.95 mole/L base
Phosphoric acid buffer, pH = 4.20; pK of H₃PO₄ = 2.16
[base]/[acid] = 112
```

$$\frac{\text{Total M phosphate + phosphoric acid}}{\text{M phosphoric acid}} = \frac{1 \text{ mole/L}}{x \text{ mole/L phosphoric acid}}$$

$$\frac{113}{1.0} = \frac{1 \text{ mole/L}}{x \text{ mole/L phosphoric acid}}$$

$$x = \frac{1.0}{113} = 0.009 \text{ mole/L phosphoric acid}$$

```
1 - 0.009 = 0.991 mole/L base
```

49. Calculate the volume of commercial acetic acid (sp gr 1.045 g/mL, 99.5% pure) necessary to make the 1-mole/L solution of the acetate buffer in question 46.

```
Acetate buffer, pH = 6.00; pK of acetic acid = 4.76; [base]/[acid] = 17.4; 0.06 moles/L
acetic acid
0.06 moles/L × 60.00 g/mole = 3.6 g/L
1.045 g/mL × 0.995 = 1.04 g/mL
(3.6 g)/(1.04 g/mL) = 3.46 mL
```

50. Calculate the volume of commercial phosphoric acid (sp gr 1.7 g/mL, 85% pure) necessary to make the 1-mole/L solution of the phosphate buffer in question 47. Phosphate buffer, pH = 6.00; pK of phosphoric acid = 2.16; [base]/[acid] = 112; 0.009 molar phosphoric acid

```
0.009 m̶o̶l̶e̶s̶/L × 98.00 g/m̶o̶l̶e̶s̶ = 0.88 g/L
1.70 g/mL × 0.85 = 1.44 g/mL
(0.88 g̶)/(1.44 g̶/mL) = 0.61 mL
```

APPLICATION ANSWERS

Clinical Chemistry

The pK of carbonic acid is 6.1.

$$pH = pK + \log \frac{([HCO_3^-]}{[a \times Pco_2])}$$

$$7.60 = 6.1 + \log \frac{([HCO_3^-]}{0.03 \times 39)}$$

$$1.5 = \log \frac{([HCO_3^-]}{1.17)}$$

$$32 = \frac{[HCO_3^-]}{1.17}$$

$$[HCO_3^-] = 1.17 \times 32 = 37$$

The high pH results from the high carbonate level.

The body may compensate for this high carbonate level by retaining or increasing CO_2 levels in the lung. Suppose the pH had been measured at 7.43 (within normal range) with the same carbonate level.

$$7.43 = 6.10 + \log (37\ 0.03 \times Pco_2)$$

$$1.33 = \log (\ 37\ 0.03 \times Pco_2)$$

$$21 = \frac{37}{(0.03 \times Pco_2)}$$

$$21 \times (0.03 \times Pco_2) = 37$$

$$0.63 \times Pco_2 = 37$$

$$Pco_2 = 37/0.63 = 59$$

The high carbonate level was compensated with a high venous CO_2, resulting in the normal pH.

Microbiology

Use the Henderson-Hasselbalch equation to determine the relative concentrations of the dipotassium and monopotassium phosphates:

$$pH = pK + \log \frac{[base]}{[acid]}$$

$$7.5 = 7.2 + \log \frac{[K_2HPO_4]}{[KH_2PO_4]}$$

$$0.3 = \log \frac{[K_2HPO_4]}{[KH_2PO_4]}$$

$$2.0 = \frac{[K_2HPO_4]}{[KH_2PO_4]}$$

The relative concentrations are:

> 2 parts $[K_2HPO_4]$ to 1 part $[KH_2PO_4]$

Use ratio and proportion to determine the number of moles of each component:

$$\frac{2 \text{ parts } K_2HPO_4}{3 \text{ parts total}} = \frac{x \text{ moles } K_2HPO_4}{0.15 \text{ moles total}}$$

$x = 0.3/3 = 0.1$ mole K_2HPO_4

moles $KH_2PO_4 = 0.15$ moles total $- 0.1$ mole $K_2HPO_4 = 0.05$ moles of KH_2PO_4

According to the labels, the molecular weight of K_2HPO_4 is 174.2 g/mole and the molecular weight of KH_2PO_4 is 136.1 g/mole. Use molecular weight to convert moles/L to grams/L to determine how much of each component to add.

(g/~~mole~~) × (~~mole~~/L) = g/L

(174.2 g/~~mole~~) × (0.1 ~~mole~~/L) = 17.4 g/L K_2HPO_4

(136.1g/~~mole~~) × (0.05 ~~mole~~/L) = 6.8 g/L KH_2PO_4

Bring 17.4 g K_2HPO_4 and 6.8 g KH_2PO_4 to 1 L with culture medium.

CHAPTER **9**

PRACTICE PROBLEM ANSWERS

1. Derive Beer's Law from the formula, $I = I_o \times 10^{-abc}$, given $T = I/I_o$ and $A = -\log T$.

$I = I_o \times 10^{-abc}$

$T = I/I_o$

$I/I_o = 10^{-abc}$

$\log T = \log I/I_o$

$\log I/I_o = \log 10^{-abc}$

$\log T = \log 10^{-abc}$

$\log T = -abc$

$A = -\log T$

$A = -(-abc) = abc$

2. Absorbance = 0.280 with a path length of 1.0 cm. The molar absorptivity is 55,000.

$A = a\ b\ c$

$c = A/(b\ a)$

$c = 0.280/1 \times 55,000$

$c = 5.1 \times 10^{-6}$ moles/L $= 5.1$ μM

3. Absorbance = 0.500 with a path length of 1.0 cm. The molar absorptivity is 55,000.

$c = A/(b\ a)$

$c = 0.500/1 \times 55,000$

$c = 9.1 \times 10^{-6}$ moles/L $= 9.1$ μM

4. Absorbance of a $\frac{1}{50}$ dilution = 0.150 with a path length of 1.0 cm. The molar absorptivity is 55,000.

$c = A/(b\ a)$

$c = (0.150 \times 50)/1 \times 55,000$

$c = 1.4 \times 10^{-4}$ moles/L $= 0.14$ mM

5. Absorbance of 0.750 with a path length of 1.50 cm. The molar absorptivity is 125,000.

$c = A/(b\ a)$

$c = 0.750/(1.50 \times 125,000)$

$c = 4.00 \times 10^{-6}$ mole/L $= 4.00$ μM

6. Absorbance of 0.750 with a path length of 1.00 cm. The millimolar absorptivity (E) is 125.

$c = A/(b\ E)$

$c = 0.750/(1.00 \times 125)$

$c = 6.00 \times 10^{-3}$ mM $= 6.00$ μM

7. Absorbance of a $\frac{1}{100}$ dilution = 0.420 with a path length of 1.50 cm. The millimolar absorptivity is 75.

$c = A/(b\ E)$

$c = (0.420 \times 100)/(1.50 \times 75)$

$c = 0.373\ mM = 373\ \mu M$

8. Absorbance = 0.280 with a path length of 1.5 cm. The 100 mg/mL standard reads 0.280 with a path length of 1.0 cm.

$c_u = (c_s\ b_s)/b_u$

$c_u = (100 \times 1.0)/1.5 = 67\ mg/mL$

9. Absorbance = 0.280 with a path length of 0.8 cm. The 100 mg/mL standard reads 0.280 with a path length of 1.00 cm.

$c_u = (c_s\ b_s)/b_u$

$c_u = (100 \times 1.0)/0.8 = 125\ mg/mL$

10. Absorbance = 0.280 with a path length of 1.9 cm. The 100 mg/mL standard reads 0.280 with a path length of 1.00 cm.

$c_u = (c_s\ b_s)/b_u$

$c_u = (100 \times 1.0)/1.9 = 52.6\ mg/mL$

11. Absorbance of a $\frac{1}{20}$ dilution = 0.180 with a path length of 2.00 cm. The 100 mg/mL standard reads 0.180 with a path length of 1.00 cm.

$c_u = (c_s\ b_s)/b_u$

$c_u = (100 \times 1.00)/2.00 = 50.0\ mg/mL$

$50.0\ mg/mL \times 20 = 1,000\ mg/mL = 1.00\ g/mL$

12. Absorbance of a $\frac{1}{10}$ dilution = 0.080 with a path length of 1.5 cm. The 50 mg/mL standard reads 0.080 with a path length of 1.00 cm.

$c_u = (c_s\ b_s)/b_u$

$c_u = (50 \times 1.00)/1.50 = 33.3\ mg/mL$

$33.3\ mg/mL \times 10 = 333\ mg/mL$

13. Absorbance = 0.280 with a path length of 1.00 cm. The 100 mg/mL standard reads 0.250 with a path length of 1.00 cm.

$c_u = (A_u\ c_s)/A_s$

$c_u = (0.280 \times 100)/\ 0.250 = 112\ mg/mL$

14. Absorbance = 0.125 with a path length of 1.00 cm. The 100 mg/mL standard reads 0.250 with a path length of 1.00 cm.

$c_u = (A_u\ c_s)/A_s$

$c_u = (0.125 \times 100)/\ 0.250 = 50\ mg/mL$

15. Absorbance = 0.380 with a path length of 1.00 cm. The 200 μg/mL standard reads 0.500 with a path length of 1.00 cm.

```
c_u = (A_u c_s)/A_s
c_u = (0.380 × 200)/0.500 = 152 μg/mL
```

16. Absorbance of a $\frac{1}{5}$ dilution = 0.290 with a path length of 1.50 cm. The 200 mg/mL standard reads 0.500 with a path length of 1.50 cm.

```
c_u = (A_u c_s)/A_s
c_u = (0.290 × 200)/0.500 = 116 mg/mL
116 mg/mL × 5 = 580 mg/mL
```

17. Absorbance of a $\frac{1}{20}$ = 0.045 with a path length of 1.50 cm. The 100 mg/mL standard reads 0.250 with a path length of 1.50 cm.

```
c_u = (A_u c_s)/A_s
c_u = (0.045 × 100)/0.250 = 18.0 mg/mL
18.0 mg/mL × 20 = 360 mg/mL
```

18. Derive the formula for conversion of transmittance to absorbance from percent transmittance, starting with $A = -\log T$.

```
A = -logT
%T = T × 100
T = %T/100
A = -[log(%T/100)]
  = -(log %T - log 100)
  = -(log %T - 2)
A = -log %T + 2 = 2 - log %T
```

19. 80%

```
A = 2 - log %T
A = 2 - log 80
A = 2 - 1.903
A = 0.097
```

20. 20%

```
A = 2 - log 20
A = 2 - 1.301
A = 0.699
```

21. 50%

```
A = 2 - log 50
A = 2 - 1.699
A = 0.301
```

22. 100%

    $A = 2 - \log 100$

    $A = 2 - 2$

    $A = 0.000$

23. 10%

    $A = 2 - \log 10$

    $A = 2 - 1$

    $A = 1.0$

24. 0.80

    $A = -\log T$

    $0.80 = -\log T$

    $6.31 = 1/T$

    $T = 0.158$

25. 0.15

    $A = -\log T$

    $0.15 = -\log T$

    $1.41 = 1/T$

    $T = 0.709$

26. 0.55

    $A = -\log T$

    $0.55 = -\log T$

    $3.55 = 1/T$

    $T = 0.282$

27. 0.400

    $A = -\log T$

    $0.40 = -\log T$

    $2.51 = 1/T$

    $T = 0.398$

28. 0.60

    $A = -\log T$

    $0.60 = -\log T$

    $3.98 = 1/T$

    $T = 0.251$

29. 0.459

    $0.459 = 2.00 - \log \%T$

    $\log \%T = 2.00 - 0.459$

    $\log \%T = 1.54$

    $\%T = 34.7$

30. 0.255

    $0.255 = 2.00 - \log \%T$

    $\log \%T = 2.00 - 0.255$

    $\log \%T = 1.74$

    $\%T = 55.0$

31. 0.100

    $0.100 = 2.00 - \log \%T$

    $\log \%T = 2.00 - 0.100$

    $\log \%T = 1.90$

    $\%T = 79.4$

32. 0.999

    $0.999 = 2.00 - \log \%T$

    $\log \%T = 2.00 - 0.999$

    $\log \%T = 1.00$

    $\%T = 10.0$

33. 0.080

    $0.080 = 2.00 - \log \%T$

    $\log \%T = 2.00 - 0.080$

    $\log \%T = 1.92$

    $\%T = 83.2$

34. 0.859

    $0.859 = 2.000 - \log \%T$

    $\log \%T = 2.000 - 0.859$

    $\log \%T = 1.141$

    $\%T = 13.8$

35. 0.300

    $0.30 = 2.00 - \log \%T$

    $\log \%T = 2.00 - 0.30$

    $\log \%T = 1.70$

    $\%T = 50.1$

36. 0.057

$$0.057 = 2.000 - \log \%T$$
$$\log \%T = 2.000 - 0.057$$
$$\log \%T = 1.943$$
$$\%T = 87.7$$

37. 0.950

$$0.950 = 2.00 - \log \%T$$
$$\log \%T = 2.00 - 0.95$$
$$\log \%T = 1.05$$
$$\%T = 11.2$$

38. 0.125

$$0.125 = 2.000 - \log \%T$$
$$\log \%T = 2.000 - 0.125$$
$$\log \%T = 1.875$$
$$\%T = 75.0$$

39. A_{330} of a 1.00-μM solution is 0.020 (1.00-cm path length).

$$a = A/(bc)$$
$$= 0.020/(1.00 \times 10^{-6})$$
$$= 2 \times 10^4 = 20,000$$

40. A_{330} of a 1.00-M solution diluted $\frac{1}{10,000}$ is 0.320 (1.00-cm path length).

$$a = A/(bc)$$
$$= 0.320/[1.00 \times (1.00 \times 10^{-4})]$$
$$= 3.2 \times 10^3 = 3,200$$

41. A_{330} of a 1.00-molar solution diluted $\frac{1}{10,000}$ is 0.300 (1.50-cm path length).

$$a = A/(bc)$$
$$= 0.320/[1.50 \times (1.00 \times 10^{-4})]$$
$$= 2.13 \times 10^3 = 2,133$$

42. A_{330} of a 0.50-molar solution diluted $\frac{1}{10,000}$ is 0.100 (1.00 cm path length).

$$a = A/(bc)$$
$$= 0.100/[1.00 \times (1.00 \times 10^{-4})]$$
$$= 1.00 \times 10^3 = 1,000$$

43. A_{330} of a 1.50-molar solution diluted $\frac{1}{1,000}$ is 0.350 (1.90-cm path length).

$$a = A/(bc)$$
$$= 0.350/[1.90 \times (1.5 \times 10^{-3})]$$
$$= 1.23 \times 10^2 = 123$$

44. A_{330} of a 0.200-molar solution diluted $\frac{1}{100}$ is 0.100 (0.80-cm path length).

$a = A/(bc)$

$= 0.100/[0.80 \times (0.20 \times 10^{-2})]$

$= 0.625 \times 10^2 = 62.5$

45. A_{330} of a solution is 0.147; $a_{330} = 55,000$ (1.00-cm path length).

$c = A/(b\ a)$

$= 0.147/[1.00 \times (5.5 \times 10^4)]$

$= 2.67 \times 10^{-6}$ moles/L $= 2.67$ μM

46. A_{310} of a solution is 0.850; $a_{310} = 45,000$ (1.00-cm path length).

$c = A/(b\ a)$

$= 0.850/[1.00 \times (4.5 \times 10^4)]$

$= 1.89 \times 10^{-5}$ moles/L $= 18.9$ μM

47. A_{250} of a solution diluted $\frac{1}{100}$ is 0.351; $a_{250} = 65,000$ (1.00-cm path length).

$c = A/(b\ a)$

$= 0.351/[1.00 \times (6.5 \times 10^4) \times (1/100)]$

$= 5.40 \times 10^{-4}$ M $= 0.54$ mM $= 540$ μM

48. A_{350} of a solution diluted $\frac{1}{1,000}$ is 0.782; $a_{350} = 25,000$ (1.00-cm path length).

$c = A/(b\ a)$

$= 0.782/[1.00 \times (2.5 \times 10^4) \times (1/1,000)]$

$= 3.13 \times 10^{-2}$ moles/L $= 31.3$ mM

49. A_{250} of a solution diluted $\frac{1}{100}$ is 0.282; $a_{250} = 5,000$ (1.50-cm path length).

$c = A/(b\ a)$

$= 0.282/[1.50 \times (5.0 \times 10^3) \times (1/100)]$

$= 3.76 \times 10^{-3}$ moles/L $= 3.76$ mM

50. A_{300} of a solution diluted $\frac{1}{100}$ is 0.282; $E_{300} = 5.00$ (1.50-cm path length).

$c = A/(b\ E)$

$= 0.282/[(1.50 \times 5.00) \times (1/100)]$

$= 3.76$ mM

APPLICATION ANSWERS

Molecular Diagnostics

The oligonucleotide has two adenines, one cytosine, three guanines, and two thymines. The E for this oligonucleotide is:

$$E_{GGTAACGT} = (2 \times 15.1) + (1 \times 7.4) + (3 \times 11.7) + (2 \times 8.7)$$
$$= 30.2 + 7.4 + 35.1 + 17.4 = 90.1$$

The concentration c of the solution is:

$$c = (A_{260})/(b\ E)$$
$$c = 0.286/(1 \times 90.1)$$
$$= 3.17 \times 10^{-3}\ mM = 3.17\ \mu M$$

The concentration of the supplied oligonucleotide is 3.17 μM and will have to be diluted to obtain the desired 2-μM solution. To obtain 100 μL of a 2-μM solution, use ratio and proportion:

$$2.00/3.17 = x/100$$
$$x = 100 \times (2.00/3.17)$$
$$x = 100 \times 0.631 = 63.1\ \mu L$$

Alternatively, $V_1 \times C_1 = V_2 \times C_2$ may be used:

$$x \times 3.17 = 100 \times 2.00$$
$$x = (100 \times 2.00)/3.17$$
$$x = 63.1\ \mu L$$

To make 100 μL of the 2.00-μM solution, bring 63.1 μL of the supplied reagent to 100 μL.

Enzymology

$$IU\ /mL = [(\Delta A \times V_t)/(6.22 \times V_s)]$$
$$0.291 - 0.288 = 0.003 = \Delta A$$
$$c = A/(ab)$$
$$I\ U/mL = [0.003 \times 5/(6.22 \times 1)]$$
$$= 2.41 \times 10^{-3}\ IU/mL$$

CHAPTER 10

PRACTICE PROBLEM ANSWERS

Write the y coordinates for the following relationships.

1. $x = y$, when $x = 0.5$, $x = 2$, $x = 19$

   y = 0.5, y = 2, y = 19, respectively

2. $y = x + 3.0$, when $x = 0.5$, $x = 2$, $x = 19$

   y = 3.5, y = 5, y = 22, respectively

3. $y = x - 3.0$, when $x = 0.5$, $x = 2$, $x = 19$

   y = -2.5, y = -1, y = 16, respectively

4. $2.0y = x$, when $x = 0.5$, $x = 2$, $x = 19$

   y = x/2.0
   y = 0.25, y = 1, y = 9.5, respectively

5. $3.0y + 2.0x = 10$, when $x = 0.5$, $x = 2$, $x = 19$

   3.0y = 10 - 2.0x
   y = (10 - 2.0x)/3.0
   y = 3.0, y = 2.0, y = -9.3, respectively

Plot a curve that describes the following relationships, using x = 0.0, x = 5.0, and x = 10.

6. $y = x + 2.0$

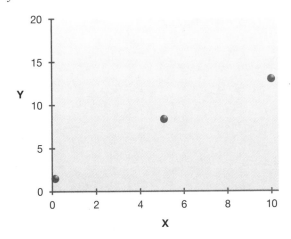

7. $y = x - 2$

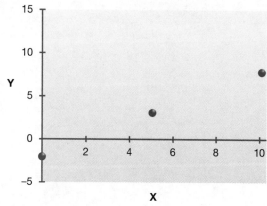

8. $2y = x$

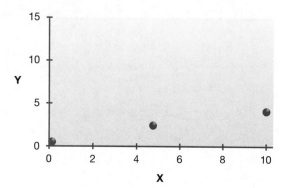

9. $y = -\left(\dfrac{10x}{5}\right)$

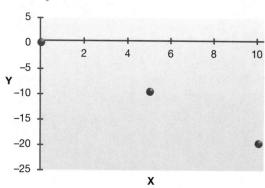

10. $y = -3x + 10$

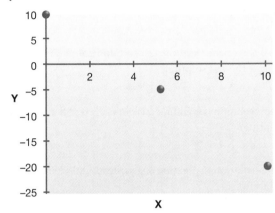

11. Match the following terms.

Abscissa: Independent variable
Origin: (0,0)
y-axis: Perpendicular line
Slope: m = (y - b)x
Ordinate: Dependent variable
Extrapolation: Outside plotted coordinates
y intercept: x = 0

12. How much glucose is required to make 50 mL of a stock standard of 10 mg/mL?

10 mg/mL × 50 mL = 500 mg

13. Calculate how to make a working standard of 2 mg/mL from a 40 mg/mL stock standard.

(40 mg/mL)/(2 mg/mL) = 20 (dilution factor)

Dilute the stock standard 1/20 (1 part stock + 19 parts diluent)

14. Calculate how to make a working standard of 25 mg/mL from a 50 g/L stock standard.

50 g/L = 50 mg/mL

(50 mg/mL)/(25 mg/mL) = 2 (dilution factor)

Dilute the stock standard 1/2 (1 part stock + 1 part diluent)

15. How much of the 10 mg/mL stock standard is required to make 100 mL of a working standard of 50 μg/mL?

50 μg/mL × 100 mL = 10,000 μg/mL × x mL

x = 5,000/10,000 = 0.5 mL

16. Which type of blank (reagent or specialized) is used for an analyte in a diluent such as water that does not absorb light at the test wavelength?

Reagent blank

17. Which type of blank (reagent or specialized) is used for an analyte diluted in a buffer mix that contains a component that absorbs light at the same wavelength as the analyte?

Specialized blank

18. If a specialized blank reads 0.010 absorbance and the test solution containing analyte reads 0.325 absorbance, what is the corrected absorbance reading of the test solution?

`0.325 - 0.010 = 0.315`

19. If a reagent blank is used to set the 0 concentration at 0 absorbance and the test solution containing analyte reads 0.325 absorbance, what is the absorbance reading of the test solution?

`0.325`

20. If a specialized blank reads 0.050 absorbance and the test solution containing analyte reads 0.158 absorbance, what is the corrected absorbance reading of the test solution?

`0.158 - 0.050 = 0.108`

21. If a specialized blank reads 0.000 absorbance and the test solution containing analyte reads 0.097 absorbance, what is the corrected absorbance reading of the test solution?

`0.097 - 0.000 = 0.097`

22. If a specialized blank reads 90.0% transmittance and the test solution containing analyte reads 35.8% transmittance, what is the corrected absorbance reading of the test solution?

`A = -log T`

`A = -log 0.900 = 0.046 for the blank`

`A = -log 0.358 = 0.446 for the test solution with analyte`

`0.446 - 0.046 = 0.400`

23. Use the graph in Figure 10-9 to estimate concentrations with the following readings:

0.055	`360 mg/dL`
0.150	`120 mg/dL`
0.200	`160 mg/dL`
0.700	`450 mg/dL`
0.900	`(cannot extrapolate)`

24. Consider the following equation for absorbance (y) versus concentration in milliliters per deciliter (x):

`y = 0.0015x`

Find the concentrations of the following unknowns with the following absorbances.

0.088	`58.7 mg/dL`
0.500	`333 mg/dL`
0.345	`230 mg/dL`
0.125	`83.3 mg/dL`
0.199	`133 mg/dL`

25. Consider the following equation for absorbance (y) versus concentration in milligrams per deciliter (x):

`y = 0.0015x`

Find the concentrations of the following unknowns with the following % transmittances.

`70% = 0.155 absorbance`	`103 mg/dL`
`45% = 0.347 absorbance`	`231 mg/dL`
`60% = 0.222 absorbance`	`148 mg/dL`
`25% = 0.602 absorbance`	`401 mg/dL`
`15% = 0.824 absorbance`	`549 mg/dL`

APPLICATION ANSWERS

Pharmacology

1. The drug concentrations are:

Time (hours)	High-Dose Concentration (μg/mL)	Medium-Dose Concentration (μg/mL)	Low-Dose Concentration (μg/mL)
2	30	20	12
3	15	10	6.0
4	7.5	5.0	3.0

2. Because the drug concentration decreases by one half within each hour of time, the half-life of the drug is 1 hour. This half-life is independent of the dosage amount as shown in the previous table. This is an example of a drug obeying first-order kinetics. Not all drugs have this property.

Molecular Diagnostics

1. The lowest concentration was 25 nM with a $1/10^7$ dilution factor.

$$1.6 \times 10^{-8} \text{ mole/L} \times 10^{-7} = 2.5 \times 10^{-15} \text{ mole/L} = 2.5 \text{ fM}$$

2. The number of molecules can be ascertained using Avogadro's number (6.02×10^{23} molecules per mole).

$$(2.5 \times 10^{-15} \text{ ~~moles~~/L}) \times (6.02 \times 10^{23} \text{ molecules/~~mole~~}) =$$

$$15.0 \times 10^8 \text{ molecules/L}$$

The reaction volume of the assay was 25 μL.

$$(1.5 \times 10^9 \text{ molecules/L}) \times (25 \times 10^{-6} \text{ L}) = 37,500 \text{ molecules}$$

If repeated measurement of a $1/10^7$ dilution (in the proper matrix, that is, the solution environment that would be used for patient sample testing), reproducibly produces signal, then this level is the lowest level of detection or sensitivity of the assay.

General Laboratory

1. Draw a graph of both readings (y-axis) compared with c_s (x-axis).

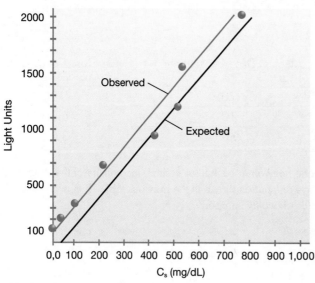

2. Which is the independent variable?

   c_s

3. Using the expected readings and the formula $y = mx + b$, what is the slope of the curve if $b = 0$?

   In the equation, $y = mx + b$, m is the slope. Because the graph yields a straight line, any point on the graph may be used to determine the slope; b is given as 0.

   $y = mx + 0$

   $125 = m \times 50$

   $m = 2.5$

4. Is the relationship between c_s and light units linear?

   Yes. The line is straight within the point tested.

5. How should the instrument be adjusted?

   b. Adjust concentrations downward.

Molecular Diagnostics

1. A fragment that travels faster will travel farther than one that travels slower. The fragment traveling 9 cm is smaller than the fragment traveling 3 cm.

2. Using the graph, 6 cm corresponds to approximately 250 bp. Capillary gel electrophoresis is often used instead of gel electrophoresis. The DNA fragments appear as peaks of fluorescence, rather than as bands on the gel. Similar to the gel, the short fragments travel through the capillary faster than the long fragments. Capillary instruments automatically determine fragment size by using a molecular weight ladder run simultaneously with the sample. In this case, the fragment sizes are determined in the instrument software and are displayed under each peak.

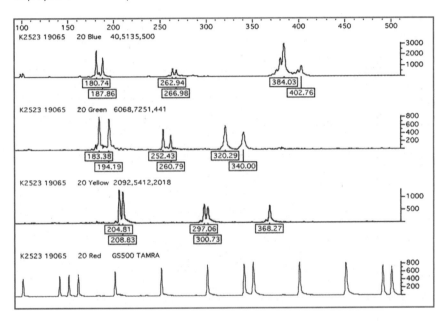

CHAPTER **11**

PRACTICE PROBLEM ANSWERS

1. Find the mean, median, and mode of the following data:
26, 52, 37, 22, 24, 45, 58, 28, 39, 60, 25, 47, 23, 56, 28

Mean: **38**

Median: **37**

Mode: **28**

2. Do the data in question 1 demonstrate central tendency (normal distribution)?

No. The mean, median, and mode are not the same.

3. Find the mean, median, and mode of the following data:
126, 125, 130, 122, 124, 125, 125, 128, 129, 130, 125, 124, 123, 126, 125

Mean: **125.8**

Median: **125**

Mode: **125**

4. Do the data in question 3 demonstrate central tendency (normal distribution)?

Yes. The mean, median, and mode are approximately equal.

5. Find the mean, median, and mode of the following data:
0.38, 0.52, 0.55, 0.32, 0.37, 0.38, 0.38, 0.35, 0.29, 0.38, 0.28, 0.39, 0.40, 0.38, 0.38, 0.38

Mean: **0.38**

Median: **0.38**

Mode: **0.38**

6. Do the data in question 5 demonstrate central tendency (normal distribution)?

Yes. The mean, median, and mode are the same.

7. What is *n* for the number sets in questions 1, 3, and 5?

1. n = 15

3. n = 15

5. n = 16

8. If the standard deviation of is 8.90 and the mean is 127, what is the coefficient of variation (%CV)?

%CV = (8.90/127) × 100 = 0.07 × 100 = 7.0

9. Given the following standard deviations, what is the %CV for the data in questions 1, 3, and 5?

1. s = 14.0; %CV = (14.0/38.0) × 100 = 36.8%

3. s = 2.43; %CV = (2.43/125.8) × 100 = 1.93%

5. s = 0.07; %CV = (0.07/0.38) × 100 = 18.4%

10. What are the values for the mean −2s and mean +2s for question 1?

38.0 ± 2(14.0) = 10.0 − 66.0

11. What are the values for the mean +1s and mean −1s for question 3?

    123.4 − 128.2

12. What are the values for the mean +3s and mean −3s for question 5?

    0.17 − 0.59

13. Find the mean, median, and mode of the following data:
    0.76, 1.89, 0.88, 1.12, 0.07, 1.62, 0.11, 0.02, 0.13, 0.01

    Mean: 0.66

    Median: 0.44

    Mode: (No mode)

14. Do the data in question 13 demonstrate central tendency (normal distribution)?

    No. The mean and median are different, and there is no mode.

15. Find the mean, median, and mode of the following data:
    9, 8, 9, 10, 9, 9, 10, 8, 9, 8, 10, 9

    Mean: 9

    Median: 9

    Mode: 9

16. Do the data in question 15 demonstrate central tendency (normal distribution)?

    Yes. The mean, median, and mode are the same.

17. If the standard deviation of the values in question 13 is 0.70, what is the variance?

    Variance = s^2 = 0.70^2 = 0.49

18. If the standard deviation of the values in question 15 is 0.74, what is the variance?

    Variance = s^2 = 0.74^2 = 0.55

19. What is the %CV for the data in question 13?

    %CV = (0.70/0.66) × 100 = 106%

20. What is the %CV for the data in question 15?

    %CV = (0.74/9) × 100 = 8.2%

21. Compare the %CV in questions 19 and 20. Which data set has the highest variability?

    The %CV of the data described in question 19 is 106%, which is significantly more than 8.2%, which is the %CV of the data described in question 20.

22. Which would describe data with the greatest precision?

    b. Low standard deviation, large mean

    Precision increases as the standard deviation decreases. In the %CV, the standard deviation relative to the mean value of the data is normalized to allow comparison of data measured and expressed in different units.

Hematocrit is a measure of the percent (%) of blood volume that consists of red blood cells.

23. What are the mean % values for males and females?

    Males 43.9; females 38.2

24. What are the median % values for males and females?

Males 43.5; females 38

25. What are the mode values for males and females?

Males 41, 45; females 38

26. If the standard deviations are 4.6 for males and 2.3 for females, what would be the range that would include 95.4% of values based on the numbers given?

Males 34.7 to 53.1; females 33.6 to 42.8

27. What is the %CV for the test for males and females?

Males 10.5%; females 6.0%

28. If s = 2.5 and the mean is 20, what is the mean ±2s?

20 − (2 × 2.5) = 15 and 20 + (2 × 2.5) = 25
15 − 25

29. If s = 3.0 and the mean is 20, what is the mean ±1s?

20 − (3.0) = 17 and 20 + (3.0) = 23
17 − 23

30. If s = 17 and the mean is 298, what is the mean ±3s?

298 − (3 × 17) = 247 and 298 + (3 × 17) = 349
247 − 349

31. If ±1s is the control limit, what does the plot show?

c. There is a systemic error.

32. Which of the following rules is violated?

d. 2_{1s}

33. Compare the cusum plot with the Levey-Jennings plot. What characteristic of the cusum plot suggests error in values for runs 1 to 5?

The positive slope of the cusum plot: Even though most of the values are within the control limits in the Levey-Jennings plot, they are all above the mean, and this affects the slope of the cusum plot. The slope may alert the technologist of a systemic error.

34. What does the cusum plot suggest for runs 6 to 10?

The negative slope shows systemic error below the mean.

35. Which of the following rules is violated over the course of 15 runs?

a. 3_{2s}
c. R_{4s}

36. What does the cusum plot suggest for runs 4 to 7?

The slope of the line suggests a systemic error for these runs. Because the error is cumulative, the slope will increase with added error. When the results move to the other side of the mean, the slope decreases.

37. Which rule is violated over the course of 15 runs?

    b. Five consecutive run control results have fallen above the mean.
       Because this is a cusum plot, the actual control values are not available. The cumulative sum of the differences between the control values and the mean are plotted. If the difference between consecutive run control values and the mean is repeatedly negative, a negative slope will result on the cusum plot.

38. Which type of error is apparent?

    d. Systemic error
       Random error with control values above and below the mean does not produce the slope shown in the cusum plot. Systemic error causes a repeated error to one side of the mean.

39. Which rule(s) is/are violated over the course of 20 runs?

    c. R_{4s}
       There are not 4 consecutive values that appear to be outside of the 3s control limits. No values are outside 4s. R_{4s}, however, is violated between runs 5 and 6.

40. Which type of error is apparent?

    a. Acceptable random error
       Control values fall to either side of the mean, but not outside of the 3s limits.

Observe the following plot:

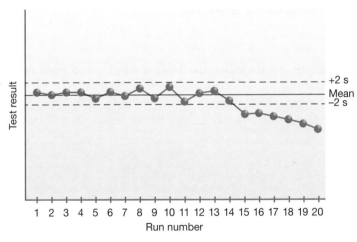

41. Which rule(s) is/are violated over the course of 20 runs?

    a. 2_{2s}
    b. 5_T
    c. 3_{2s}

42. Which type of error is apparent?

    d. Unacceptable systemic error

43. If each of two technologists performed every other run, what could be the cause of the observed results?

    b. Reagent preparation
    d. Instrument failure
    More likely, a reagent is not prepared or diluted properly, or a new lot number of reagent was installed. An instrument failure is likely to result in loss of signal or low results, but this is not always the case, such as if a power surge caused a false increase in sensitivity by increasing light intensity.

44. Which rule(s) is/are violated over the course of 15 runs?

    a. 2_{2s}
    c. 3_{2s}
    d. R_{2s}

45. Which type of error is apparent?

    d. Unacceptable systemic error

46. Based on the information given, which of the following could be the cause of the observed results?

    b. The new reagent lot

47. What does the cusum plot indicate for runs 1 to 12?

    There is acceptable random error in runs 1 to 12.

48. Which type of error is apparent from a cusum plot for runs 13 to 15?

    d. Unacceptable systemic error

49. Which of the following changed in runs 13 to 15 with the new reagent lot?

    a. Accuracy of control results
    d. Unacceptable systemic error

50. What would be the predicted error in the measurement of the patient specimens in runs 13 to 15, based on the effect of the new reagent lot on the controls?

    c. Results will be inaccurate and high.

APPLICATION ANSWERS

1. The 15 test results are within 2s of the mean. The method is within control limits in this regard, if results from all shifts are taken together. For each shift separately, however, the method is showing systemic error.
2. Results obtained on the first shift are consistently higher than the mean, whereas results from the second and third shifts are all less than the mean. If the shift values were taken separately, a systemic error would be apparent. That is, five consecutive measurements are on the same side of the mean.

This observation has various explanations. Reagents may be prepared on the first shift and used on later shifts. The freshly prepared solutions would have maximum activity on first shift with some loss of activity over the course of the day. Alternatively, the test may be subject to the technologists' skill and speed of work. If so, differences would be shift-specific because different technologists would perform the test on different shifts.

Although this method overall looks to be in control if results from all three shifts are monitored sequentially, the repetitive pattern in the Levey-Jennings and cusum plots suggests that offsetting systemic errors are occurring. Draw Levey-Jennings charts and cusum plots for each shift separately. Compare the slope of the cusum plots with the plots pictured for all three shifts.

SYMBOLS

Symbol	Meaning	Symbol	Meaning
+	Plus, add to	Σ	The sum of
−	Minus, subtract from	Δ	Change
±	Plus or minus	()	Parentheses
=	Equals	[]	Brackets
≠	Is/are not equal to	{}	Braces
≈	Approximately equal to	σ	Standard deviation
≅	Similar to	X	Multiply, times
∴	Therefore	*	Multiply (in spreadsheets)
∞	Infinity, unending	÷, /	Divide
%	Percent	||	Absolute value
::	Is proportional to	#	Number, pound
:	Ratio, is to; also designates range in spreadsheets	√	Square root

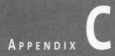
GREEK ALPHABET

Letter	Symbol	Meaning
Alpha	A, α	First, primary, false-positive rate
Beta	B, β	Second, secondary, false-negative rate
Gamma	Γ, χ	Third, tertiary, gamma rays, photon
Delta	Δ, δ	Change, density, heat
Epsilon	E, ε	Molar absorptivity, random error
Zeta	Z, ζ	Viscous friction (polymer science)
Eta	H, η	Viscosity, efficiency
Theta	Θ, θ	Plane angle, potential temperature (thermodynamics)
Iota	I, ι	Computer language function
Kappa	K, κ	Thermal conductivity, curvature
Lambda	Λ, γ	Wavelength, microliter (obsolete)
Mu	M, μ	Population mean, micrometer (obsolete)
Nu	N, ν	Frequency (physics)
Xi	Ξ, ξ	Random variable
Omicron	O, o	
Pi	Π, π	Type of covalent bond, circumference to diameter ratio
Rho	P, ρ	Resistivity, termination factor (molecular biology),
Sigma	Σ, σ	Summation, standard deviation
Tau	T, τ	Interval of time; mean lifetime
Upsilon	Y, υ	
Phi	Φ, φ	Phenyl group (chemistry); electric potential
Chi	X, χ	Statistical term (X^2)
Psi	Ψ, ψ	Used in quantum mechanics
Omega	Ω, ω	Electrical resistance (SI units)

ROMAN NUMERALS

Roman	Arabic	Roman	Arabic
I, i	1	X	10
V, v	5	XX	20
X, x	10	XXX	30
L, l	50	XL	40
C, c	100	L	50
D, d	500	LX	60
M, m	1,000	LXX	70
I	1	LXXX	80
II	2	XC	90
III	3	C	100
IV	4		
V	5		
VI	6		
VII	7		
VIII	8		
IX	9		
X	10		

APPENDIX E

CONSTANTS

Symbol	Constant	Value
p	Pi	3.14159...
i	Imaginary number	$\sqrt{-1}$
e	Natural logarithm base	2.71828
Å	Angstrom	1^{-10} m
A	Avogadro's number	6.022×10^{23}
mol	Mole	6.022×10^{23} molecules
amu	Atomic mass unit	1.6605×10^{-27} kg

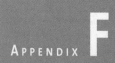
PERIODIC TABLE

IA																	Inert
H 1.01	IIA																He 4.00
Li 6.94	Be 9.01											IIIA	IVA	VA	VIA	VIIA	
Na 22.99	Mg 24.30	IIIB	IVB	VB	VIB	VIIB	VIIIB			IB	IIB	B 10.81	c 12.01	N 14.01	O 16.00	F 19.00	Ne 20.18
K 39.10	Ca 40.08	Sc 44.96	Ti 47.90	V 50.94	Cr 52.00	Mn 54.94	Fe 55.85	Co 58.93	Ni 58.70	Cu 63.55	Zn 65.38	Al 26.98	Si 28.08	P 30.97	S 32.06	Cl 35.45	Ar 39.95
Rb 85.47	Sr 87.62	Y 88.91	Zr 91.22	Nb 92.91	Mo 95.94	Tc (98.0)	Ru 101.07	Rh 102.90	Pd 106.4	Ag 107.87	Cd 112.40	Ga 69.72	Ge 72.59	As 74.92	Se 79.96	Br 79.90	Kr 83.80
Cs 132.90	Ba 137.33		Hf 178.49	Ta 180.95	W 183.85	Re 186.21	Os 190.20	Ir 192.22	Pt 195.09	Au 196.97	Hg 200.59	In 114.82	Sn 118.69	Sb 121.75	Te 127.60	I 126.90	Xe 131.30
Fr (223)	Ra 226.02		Rf (267)	Db (268)	Sg (271)	Bh (272)	Hs (270)	Mt (276)	Ds (281)	Rg (280)	Cn (285)	Tl 204.37	Pb 207.20	Bi 208.98	Po (209.0)	At (210)	Rn (222)
												Fl (289)			Lv (293)		

	La 138.90	Ce 140.12	Pr 140.91	Nd 144.24	Pm (145)	Sm 150.36	Eu 151.96	Gd 157.25	Tb 158.92	Dy 162.50	Ho 164.93	Er 167.26	Tm 168.93	Yb 173.04	Lu 174.97
	Ac (227)	Th 232.04	Pa 231.04	U 238.03	Np 237.05	Pu (244)	Am (243)	Cm (247)	Bk (247)	Cf (251)	Es (254)	Fm (257)	Md (258)	No (259)	Lr (260)

Atomic weights are shown beneath the element symbols.

Elements are arranged according to molecular mass and valence groups (IA–VIIIB).

International Union of Pure and Applied Chemistry, 2012.

HALF-LIFE OF NUCLIDES USED IN MEDICINE

Radionuclide	Half-Life	Radionuclide	Half-Life
^{3}H	4,500 days	^{90}Y	64.1 hours
^{14}C	1.830 hours	^{76}Br	16.0 hours
^{18}F	59.41 days	^{109}Cd	463.26 days
^{32}P	14.26 days	^{111}In	2.805 days
^{33}P	25.34 days	^{123}I	13.224 days
^{35}S	87.51 days	^{124}I	100.2 hours
^{60}Co	1,925 days	^{125}I	59.41 days
^{64}Cu	12.7 hours	^{131}I	8.0197 days
^{67}Cu	2.6 days	^{133}Ba	3,853.6 days
^{67}Ga	3.261 days	^{186}Re	89.25 hours
^{88}Y	106.63 days	^{188}Re	17.02 hours

SYSTEMS OF
MEASUREMENT
CONVERSIONS

Multiply the original units by the factors given to obtain the converted units.

Original Unit	Converted Unit	Factor
Angstroms	Centimeters	1×10^{-8}
	Inches	3.937×10^{-9}
Centimeters	Inches	0.3937
Cubic centimeters	Liters	0.001
	Ounces (U.S. fluid)	0.0338
Cubic inches	Cubic centimeters	28,317
	Gallons (U.S. liquid)	0.004329
	Liters	0.016387
Cubic millimeters	Cubic centimeters	1×10^{6}
	Cubic inches	6.10237×10^{-5}
Drams (avoirdupois)	Grams	1.7718
	Ounces (avoirdupois)	0.0625
Drams (U.S. fluid)	Cubic centimeters	3.6967
	Milliliters	3.6966
	Ounces	0.125
Feet	Centimeters	30.48
	Inches	12
	Yards	0.3333

Original Unit	Converted Unit	Factor
Gallons (U.S. liquid)	Cubic centimeters	3,785.4
	Liters	3.7854
	Ounces	128
	Quarts (U.S. liquid)	4
	Pints (U.S. liquid)	8
Grains	Grams	0.064799
	Carats (metric)	0.32399
	Drams (avoirdupois)	0.0365714
	Ounces (avoirdupois)	0.0022857
Grams	Kilograms	0.001
	Carats (metric)	5
	Tons (metric)	1×10^{-6}
	Drams (avoirdupois)	0.56438
	Ounces (avoirdupois)	0.035273962
	Pounds (avoirdupois)	0.0022046
Hands	Centimeters	10.16
	Inches	4
Inches	Angstroms	2.54×10^{8}
	Centimeters	2.54
	Feet	0.08333
	Meters	0.0254
Kilograms	Tons (metric)	0.001
	Grains	15,432.4
	Ounces (avoirdupois)	35.2734
	Pounds (avoirdupois)	2.205
Kilometers	Centimeters	100,000
	Feet	3,280.84
	Meters	1,000
	Miles (statute)	0.62137
	Yards	1,093.613
Liters	Cubic centimeters	1,000
	Cubic inches	61.0237
	Drams (U.S. fluid)	270.512
	Gallons (U.S. liquid)	0.264172
	Ounces (U.S. fluid)	33.814
	Pints (U.S. liquid)	2.1134
	Quarts (U.S. liquid)	1.0567

Continued

Original Unit	Converted Unit	Factor
Meters	Angstrom units	1×10^{10}
	Centimeters	100
	Feet	3.2808
	Inches	39.3701
	Miles (statute)	0.0006214
	Yards	1.0936
Microns (micrometers)	Angstrom units	10,000
	Meters	1×10^{-6}
	Feet	3.2808×10^{-6}
	Inches	3.9370×10^{-5}
Miles (statute)	Centimeters	160,934
	Meters	1,609.3
	Feet	5,280
	Yards	1,750
Millimeters of Hg (0°)	Grams/square centimeter	1.3595
	Pounds/sq ft	2.7845
	Pounds/sq in	0.01933
Minutes (mean solar)	Days (mean solar)	0.0006944
	Hours (mean solar)	0.0167
Ounces (avoirdupois)	Grams	28.3495
	Ounces (apothecary or troy)	0.9114
	Pounds (avoirdupois)	0.0625
Parts per million	Milligrams/liter	1
Pints (U.S. liquid)	Cubic centimeters	473.176
	Gallons (U.S. liquid)	0.125
	Liters	0.4732
	Quarts	0.5
Pounds (avoirdupois)	Grams	453.59
	Ounces (avoirdupois)	16
	Pounds (apothecary or troy)	1.2153
	Tons (metric)	0.0004536
Quart (U.S. liquid)	Cubic centimeters	946.353
	Liters	0.9463
	Gallons (U.S. liquid)	0.2909
	Pints (U.S. liquid)	2

Original Unit	Converted Unit	Factor
Square feet	Square centimeters	929.0304
	Square meters	0.9290
	Square inches	144
	Square yards	0.1111
Square inches	Square centimeters	6.4516
	Square meters	0.00064516
	Square feet	0.006944
Square kilometers	Square meters	1×10^6
	Square feet	1.07639×10^7
	Square yards	1.19599×10^{-6}
Square meters	Square centimeters	10,000
	Square kilometers	1×10^{-6}
	Square feet	10.7639
	Square yards	1.19599
Square yards	Square centimeters	8,361.274
	Square meters	0.8361
	Square feet	9
	Square inches	1,296
Tons (metric)	Kilograms	1,000
	Pounds (avoirdupois)	2,204.623
Yards	Centimeters	91.44
	Meters	0.9144
	Feet	3
	Inches	36
Years (calendar)	Days (mean solar)	365
	Hours (mean solar)	8,670
	Months (lunar)	12
	Weeks (mean calendar)	52.1428

FORMULAE

TEMPERATURE

$$°F = [(9/5) \times °C] + 32°$$
$$°C = (°F - 32°) \times 5/9$$
$$9 \times °C = 5 \times °F - 160°$$
$$°C = K - 273$$

DILUTIONS

$$\frac{\text{Amount of substance}}{\text{Total volume of dilution}} \times \text{Specified volume of dilution} = \text{Volume of substance}$$

$$\frac{\text{Starting concentration}}{\text{Dilution factor}} = \text{Dilution concentration}$$

$$\text{Diluted concentration} \times \text{Dilution factor} = \text{Starting concentration}$$

CONCENTRATION

$$\frac{\text{g/mole (molecular weight)}}{\text{Eq/mole}} = \text{g/Eq (normal weight)}$$

$$\frac{\text{g/mole (molecular weight)}}{\text{Particles/mole}} = \text{g/osmole (osmolar weight)}$$

$$\frac{1 \text{ osmole}}{-1.86°C} = \frac{x \text{ osmole}}{\text{Freezing point}}$$

Specific gravity $\times$ Purity (decimal) $=$ g/mL

$V_1 \times C_1 = V_2 \times C_2$

g/mole $\times$ moles/L $=$ g/L

g/Eq $\times$ Eq/L $=$ g/L

$$\text{moles/L} = \frac{\text{g/L}}{\text{g/mole}}$$

$$\text{g/mole} = \frac{\text{g/Eq}}{\text{Eq/mole}}$$

$$\text{g/L} = \frac{\text{moles/L}}{\text{g/mole}}$$

% $\times$ 10 (dL/L) $=$ g/L

METRIC CONVERSIONS

Exponent of converted units $=$ Exponent of original units $-$ Exponent of the desired units

$$\text{Converted units} = \text{Original units} \times \frac{\text{Exponent to convert the top unit}}{\text{Exponent to convert the bottom unit}}$$

EXPONENTS AND LOGS

$x^a \times x^b = x^{(a + b)}$

$x^a \div x^b = x^{(a - b)}$

$(x^a)^b = x^{(ab)}$

$x^0 = 1$

$x^1 = x$

$\log(xy) = \log x + \log y$

$\log(x/y) = \log x - \log y$

$\log(1/x) = -(\log x)$

$\log x^n = n \times \log x$

$\log 1 = 0$

IONIC SOLUTIONS

Dissociation constants:

$$K_a = \frac{[H^+] \times [A^-]}{[HA]}$$

$$K_b = \frac{[B^+] \times [OH^-]}{[BOH]}$$

Hydrogen/hydroxyl ion concentration:

$pH = \log 1/[H^+] = -\log[H^+]$

$pOH = \log 1/[OH^-] = -\log[OH^-]$

$pH = b - \log a$

$cH = [H+] \times 10^9$

Henderson-Hasselbalch:

$$pH = pK + \frac{[base]}{[acid]}$$

$$pH = pK + \log \frac{([HCO_3^-])}{\left[a \times P_{CO_2} \right]}$$

SPECTROPHOTOMETRY

Beer's Law:

$$T = 10^{-abc}$$
$$A = -\log T$$
$$A = abc$$

Direct colorimetry:

$$c_u = (A_u / A_s) \times c_s$$

Absorbance-transmittance:

$$A = 2 - \log \%T$$

Molar absorptivity:

$$c = A/(ab)$$

Millimolar absorptivity:

$$c = A/(\mathcal{E}b)$$

GRAPHING

Slope:

$$m = \frac{\Delta x}{\Delta y}$$

Straight line equation:

$$y = mx + b$$

STATISTICS AND QUALITY CONTROL

Mean:

$$\bar{x} = \Sigma x_i / n$$

Standard deviation:

$$s = \sqrt{\frac{\sum (x_i - \bar{x})^2}{n - 1}}$$

Variance:

$$s^2 = \sqrt{\frac{\sum\left(x_i - \bar{x}^2\right)}{n}}$$

Coefficient of variation:

$$\%CV = s/\bar{x} \times 100$$

Quality control:

$$\text{Sensitivity} = [TP/(TP + FN)] \times 100$$
$$\text{Specificity} = [TN/(TN + FP)] \times 100$$
$$\text{Accuracy} = [(TN + TP)/(TN + TP + FN + FP)] \times 100$$

JULIAN DAY
CALENDARS

REGULAR YEARS

	Jan	Feb	Mar	Apr	May	Jun	Jul	Aug	Sep	Oct	Nov	Dec
1	1	32	60	91	121	152	182	213	244	274	305	335
2	2	33	61	92	122	153	183	214	245	275	306	336
3	3	34	62	93	123	154	184	215	246	276	307	337
4	4	35	63	94	124	155	185	216	247	277	308	338
5	5	36	64	95	125	156	186	217	248	278	309	339
6	6	37	65	96	126	157	187	218	249	279	310	340
7	7	38	66	97	127	158	188	219	250	280	311	341
8	8	39	67	98	128	159	189	220	251	281	312	342
9	9	40	68	99	129	160	190	221	252	282	313	343
10	10	41	69	100	130	161	191	222	253	283	314	344
11	11	42	70	101	131	162	192	223	254	284	315	345
12	12	43	71	102	132	163	193	224	255	285	316	346
13	13	44	72	103	133	164	194	225	256	286	317	347
14	14	45	73	104	134	165	195	226	257	287	318	348
15	15	46	74	105	135	166	196	227	258	288	319	349
16	16	47	75	106	136	167	197	228	259	289	320	350
17	17	48	76	107	137	168	198	229	260	290	321	351
18	18	49	77	108	138	169	199	230	261	291	322	352
19	19	50	78	109	139	170	200	231	262	292	323	353
20	20	51	79	110	140	171	201	232	263	293	324	354
21	21	52	80	111	141	172	202	233	264	294	325	355
22	22	53	81	112	142	173	203	234	265	295	326	356
23	23	54	82	113	143	174	204	235	266	296	327	357
24	24	55	83	114	144	175	205	236	267	297	328	358
25	25	56	84	115	145	176	206	237	268	298	329	359
26	26	57	85	116	146	177	207	238	269	299	330	360
27	27	58	86	117	147	178	208	239	270	300	331	361
28	28	59	87	118	148	179	209	240	271	301	332	362
29	29		88	119	149	180	210	241	272	302	333	363
30	30		89	120	150	181	211	242	273	303	334	364
31	31		90		151		212	243		304		365

LEAP YEARS (2012, 2016, 2020, 2024, ...)

	Jan	Feb	Mar	Apr	May	Jun	Jul	Aug	Sep	Oct	Nov	Dec
1	1	32	61	92	122	153	183	214	245	275	306	336
2	2	33	62	93	123	154	184	215	246	276	307	337
3	3	34	63	94	124	155	185	216	247	277	308	338
4	4	35	64	95	125	156	186	217	248	278	309	339
5	5	36	65	96	126	157	187	218	249	279	310	340
6	6	37	66	97	127	158	188	219	250	280	311	341
7	7	38	67	98	128	159	189	220	251	281	312	342
8	8	39	68	99	129	160	190	221	252	282	313	343
9	9	40	69	100	130	161	191	222	253	283	314	344
10	10	41	70	101	131	162	192	223	254	284	315	345
11	11	42	71	102	132	163	193	224	255	285	316	346
12	12	43	72	103	133	164	194	225	256	286	317	347
13	13	44	73	104	134	165	195	226	257	287	318	348
14	14	45	74	105	135	166	196	227	258	288	319	349
15	15	46	75	106	136	167	197	228	259	289	320	350
16	16	47	76	107	137	168	198	229	260	290	321	351
17	17	48	77	108	138	169	199	230	261	291	322	352
18	18	49	78	109	139	170	200	231	262	292	323	353
19	19	50	79	110	140	171	201	232	263	293	324	354
20	20	51	80	111	141	172	202	233	264	294	325	355
21	21	52	81	112	142	173	203	234	265	295	326	356
22	22	53	82	113	143	174	204	235	266	296	327	357
23	23	54	83	114	144	175	205	236	267	297	328	358
24	24	55	84	115	145	176	206	237	268	298	329	359
25	25	56	85	116	146	177	207	238	269	299	330	360
26	26	57	86	117	147	178	208	239	270	300	331	361
27	27	58	87	118	148	179	209	240	271	301	332	362
28	28	59	88	119	149	180	210	241	272	302	333	363
29	29	60	89	120	150	181	211	242	273	303	334	364
30	30		90	121	151	182	212	243	274	304	335	365
31	31		91		152		213	244		305		366

INDEX

Note: Illustrations are indicated by *(f)*; tables by *(t)*; boxes by *(b)*.